Work and Social Inequalities in Health in Europe

P.I.E. Peter Lang

Bruxelles · Bern · Berlin · Frankfurt am Main · New York · Oxford · Wien

SALTSA

A Joint Programme for Working Life Research in Europe

SALTSA is a programme of partnership in European working life research run by the Swedish Confederations of Trade Unions (LO), Professional Employees (TCO) and Professional Associations (SACO). SALTSA was a cooperation venture of these three confederations and Swedish National Institute for Working Life until the Swedish government closed NIWL in 2006. The SALTSA programme continues in new forms.

The aim of SALTSA is to generate applicable research results of a high academic standard and relevance. Research is largely project-based.

Research is carried out in three areas:
* the labour market
* work organisation
* the work environment

The Work Environment and Health Programme

Research on work environment and health focuses instruments and methods for healthier working conditions, the effects of certain risks in current working life as well as the conditions of selected groups of workers. Projects are designed with the ambition to contribute to the political debate and decision-making, applied occupational health and work environment management as well as participatory processes involving social partners in European working life.

Chairman of the SALTSA Programme is Professor Lars Magnusson and programme secretary for this area is Charlotta Krafft.

Ingvar LUNDBERG, Tomas HEMMINGSSON
& Christer HOGSTEDT (eds.)

Work and Social Inequalities in Health in Europe

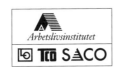

Arbetslivsinstitutet

SALTSA — JOINT PROGRAMME
FOR WORKING LIFE RESEARCH IN EUROPE
The National Institute for Working Life and The Swedish Trade Unions in Co-operation

"Work & Society"
No.58

The work was financially supported by SALTSA.

© P.I.E. PETER LANG S.A.
Éditions scientifiques internationales
Brussels, 2007
1 avenue Maurice, 1050 Brussels, Belgium
info@peterlang.com; www.peterlang.com

ISSN 1376-0955
ISBN 978-90-5201-372-5
D/2007/5678/52

Printed in Germany

Bibliographic information published by "Die Deutsche Bibliothek"

"Die Deutsche Bibliothek" lists this publication in the "Deutsche Nationalbibliografie"; detailed bibliographic data is available on the Internet at <http://dnb.ddb.de>.

CIP available from the British Library, GB and the Library of Congress, USA.

Contents

PART II
SPECIAL THEMES

PART III
SUMMARY AND CONCLUSIONS

Preface

For those working within, or interested in, occupational health, the question of work-related conditions as causes of social inequalities in health is often considered a non-issue or an issue of limited interest. The reason is that there has been abundant occupational health research which has been successful in identifying risk factors and has also implied preventive efforts that have largely benefited manual workers and thus led to reductions in social class differences in health, other things being equal. Could it not be that occupational health research is sufficient? Why bother with social class differences? We think there are at least two arguments in favour of the social class approach.

- Social classes are discernible groups in society, regardless of whether they are based on occupation, education, income, or ownership of/ control over different types of assets. The effects of different changes in society are commonly described for such groups. For most people, the large differences in health between social classes are not acceptable. This is also a starting point for occupational health research.

- While occupational health research has been extremely successful in identifying and reducing chemical risk factors in the work environment in Europe there has been no comparable success in the prevention of psychosocial risk factors. This could be partly due to the fact that the identification of such risk factors is more complicated than for chemical hazards. However, another reason is probably that the psychosocial work environment contains elements that are directly linked to the class structure itself. Hence, preventive efforts without problem conceptualisation that is also based in social class research may become shallow and less fruitful.

The purpose of this project was to try to link occupational health research to research on social class inequalities in health. We have done so by compiling data on labour market and working conditions in relation to social class and health outcomes from a number of European countries. Selection of the countries (Denmark, France, Germany, Netherlands, Norway, Spain, Sweden, UK) was based on country size, geographical location, and on the existence of previous research into these matters. Researchers from these countries and from Massachusetts in the USA were invited to an initial meeting in Stockholm in September 2002. At that meeting we discussed the purpose of the project and what information could be compiled from the different countries. We were particularly interested in data that were nationally or regionally representative, in order to see whether work-related social inequalities differed between countries. A second seminar was held in October 2003 to discuss preliminary versions of the chapters from different countries and to provide further guidelines for the final versions of these chapters. Moreover, the intended content of two chapters – on the importance of globalisation for work-related social inequalities in health and on the interactions between social class and gender for work-related social inequalities – was discussed. After this meeting, new versions of the different chapters have been reviewed by reviewers from the different countries as well as by the editors. Finally, all chapters have been linguistically edited.

The project has been supported financially by SALTSA (www.saltsa.se), which was an organisation for cooperation between major Swedish trade unions and the Swedish National Institute for Working Life regarding work-life issues of common interest between European countries.

The book starts with an introductory chapter, where literature relevant to the associations between work and labour market conditions, social class and health is reviewed. The chapters on the situation in the different countries are presented in the next section, followed by the two topical chapters mentioned above. The summary chapter at the end of the book provides a discussion of themes in the different chapters that are of common interest.

Stockholm, February 2006

Ingvar Lundberg   Tomas Hemmingsson   Christer Hogstedt

Introductory Review and Background

Ingvar LUNDBERG, Tomas HEMMINGSSON
& Christer HOGSTEDT

Introduction

Social inequalities in health have probably existed throughout most of the history of man and have been described by many authors during more recent centuries. During the 1970s it was widely believed that socio-economic differences in health had disappeared, or become minor, due to the fact that severe poverty had almost disappeared from the welfare societies. It is suggested that health inequalities reached their narrowest around 1950 (Pamuk 1985, Davey Smith and Lynch 2004). However, the importance of social class for health was 'rediscovered' with the Black report in 1980 (Townsend and Davidson 1982, Smith *et al.* 1990). Since then, interest in social inequalities in health has increased tremendously and this has led to a large number of papers and books that aim to explain these differences.

In recent decades a widening of the relative differences in death rates between higher and lower socio-economic groups has been reported from several European countries. During the same period of time there has been an increase in life expectancy in most of those countries. Data from the UK show that the increase in life expectancy has been more pronounced in upper social positions since the mid-1950s, resulting in a larger gap between those in upper and lower socio-economic positions (Davey Smith and Lynch 2004). The association between social position and coronary heart disease and mortality is well documented in several industrialised countries. During the past few decades the incidence of coronary heart disease has decreased in Western countries, while social differences seem to have increased. The background to the social inequalities in health within and between countries has been discussed extensively but the full explanation is as yet unknown. A number of potential explanatory factors have been proposed. Such factors include differences in work environment, social environment, access to health care, and health behaviours. The focus of this volume is the possible impact of working life circumstances on social differences in health.

This introductory chapter will initially review topical data on social class differences in health in Europe. In the subsequent sections we will discuss the relations between previous health status, accumulation of risk factors before labour market entry and social class, as well as the importance of health and risk factors for ill-health for varying possibilities to remain on the labour market in different social classes. We will review the literature on work, social class and health.

1. Socio-economic Position, Mortality, Heart Disease, and Self-reported Health in Europe

A series of studies from the group around Kunst and Mackenbach have shown that manual workers have a higher rate of all-cause mortality, cardiovascular mortality and poor self-rated health compared with non-manual employees in Western European countries (Mackenbach *et al.* 1997, Kunst *et al.* 1998a, Kunst *et al.* 1998b, Mackenbach *et al.* 1999, Mackenbach *et al.* 2000, Mackenbach *et al.* 2003, Mackenbach *et al.* 2004, Kunst *et al.* 2005). The following countries were included in those studies for one or more health outcomes: Austria, Denmark, England, Finland, France, Germany, Italy, Ireland, Netherlands, Norway, Portugal, Spain, Sweden, and Switzerland. Socio-economic differences in mortality have also been investigated for different periods during recent decades, and in relative terms it seems as if inequalities have increased. The studies showed that the health differences in Scandinavian welfare states were greater than in many other countries, although the interpretations concerning these findings are a subject of controversy (Vagero and Erikson 1997).

Most European collaborative studies have compared only manual and non-manual workers. However, several other studies have shown that inequalities are seen not only between broad groups of manual and non-manual workers. Rather, a dominant feature of the health situation in Western countries is the social gradient in mortality and morbidity: the higher you climb on the social ladder, the better is your health (Erikson 2002, Kitigawa and Hauser 1973). In the British Whitehall studies based on a sample of white-collar workers in London, a social gradient based on seven levels was evident (Marmot *et al.* 1991).

Different measures of social position have been in use. The most common measures are based on occupation, education, or income. Although the different measures characterise the same underlying social structure and have similar associations with health outcomes, they are also different in some respects (Erikson 2002). A measure of social position based on occupation is an indicator of employment status, employment relations, working conditions. However, when using this measure, only those who are employed can be classified into a social class. Education might be a better indicator of the social and cultural standing of the parental home and cultural interests in adulthood. Income is an indicator of material conditions.

2. Linking Work to Social Class and Health

It is self-evident that most health-related working conditions will be socially distributed in such a way that lower social strata are disadvantaged. Therefore, in an editorial in *Journal of Epidemiology and Community Health*, Moncada pointed out that the contribution of work to social class inequalities in health "could be central" (Moncada 1999). However, as will be shown in this chapter, work and working conditions have attracted surprisingly little interest when trying to understand the roots of social inequalities in health.

The Italian physician Bernardino Ramazzini wrote in the preface to his book *Diseases of Workers*, which first appeared in 1700, "… for we must admit that the workers in certain arts and crafts sometimes derive from them grave injuries, so that where they hoped for a subsistence that would prolong their lives and feed their families, they are too often repaid with the most dangerous diseases and finally, uttering curses on the profession to which they had devoted themselves, they desert their post among the living" (Ramazzini 1964).

A large majority of those exposed to dangerous chemicals were, and are, male blue-collar workers; and chemical exposures such as silica or asbestos have contributed to social class differences in silicosis, and lung cancer and mesothelioma, a malignant pleural tumour with very long induction-latency time after first exposure, and a very low incidence in the absence of asbestos exposure. The use of asbestos increased rapidly in industrialised countries after the Second World War; however, the health hazards were gradually discovered and regulations were gradually imposed. In Sweden there was an almost universal ban on asbestos in 1975 and regulations limiting asbestos exposure were imposed in most countries in the following decades. The incidence of mesothelioma has been increasing continuously for many decades. There are, however, signs that the incidence of mesothelioma has reached its peak in Sweden at around 120 cases per year but there are as yet no signs of a decline (Burdorf *et al.* 2004). In Britain the peak is calculated to occur around 2011-2015, when 1950-2450 mesothelioma deaths are estimated per year. Between 1968 and 2050 there will be around 90,000 mesothelioma deaths in Great Britain (Hodgson *et al.* 2005). The number of lung cancers caused by asbestos by far outnumbers the number of mesothelioma cases. Hence, the asbestos bans are major achievements in disease prevention and have mainly benefited male blue-collar workers.

Fatal accidents at work have to a very large extent occurred among manual workers. In the EU states, such accidents have become less and less common, which can be seen mainly as an indication of structural changes in working life, with a diminishing number of hazardous jobs. This is also a case where the development should have resulted in lower social class differences in health. In figure 1 we have compiled data on the incidence of fatal accidents (standardised for age and branch sizes) in recent years in a number of EU countries. The figure shows that incidences of fatal accidents are higher in southern than in northern European countries. It also shows that there is a tendency for the number of fatal accidents to diminish rapidly in most countries.

The number of workers exposed to high levels of dangerous chemicals is rapidly decreasing in Western Europe due to the reduced need for workers in industry and due to the movement of remaining workers further away from the production process (Lundberg *et al.* 2005). Other things being equal, this development will also reduce socio-economic differences in diseases caused by industrial chemicals.

Figure 1. Number of fatal occupational accidents/10,000 workers 1994-2002 in different European countries

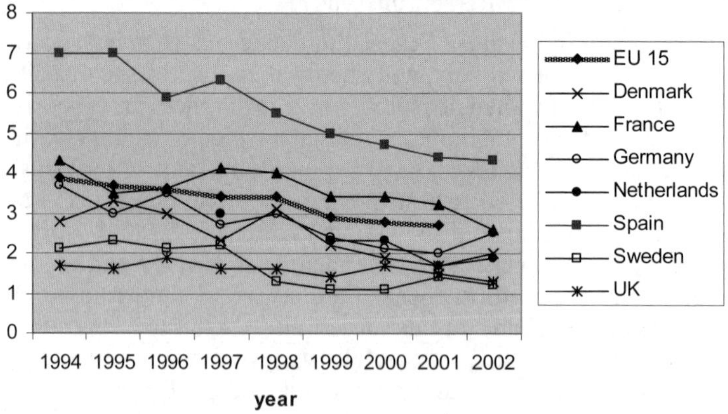

Source: http://epp.eurostat.cec.eu.int/

Factors directly related to manual labour, such as carrying heavy loads and work with repetitive movements or in bent or twisted positions, are also much more common in lower than in higher social strata. Hence, musculoskeletal disorders will be more common in lower than in higher strata; the extent to which they produce inequalities is dependent on their importance as risk factors.

During recent decades there has been an increasing interest in how stressful events, or psychosocial factors, in the work environment may contribute to, or cause, disease (Marmot *et al.* 2002). The association between psychosocial stress at work and coronary heart disease has been particularly in focus (Marmot *et al.* 2002, Belkic *et al.* 2004). Psychosocial, or stress-generating, factors are more difficult to observe and detect compared with chemical agents in the work environment or factors related to heavy physical workload or monotonous work. Rather, theoretical concepts are needed to analyse the nature of work in order to identify particular stressful job characteristics (Marmot *et al.* 2002). The empirical expressions of these concepts should be possible to identify in a wide range of occupations. Information concerning psychosocial factors is most often collected through questionnaires, although observation and structured interviews are also used. The research field must still be regarded as a theoretical and methodological challenge (Marmot *et al.* 2002, Siegrist and Marmot 2004).

In table 1 we have compiled some working conditions in relation to certain occupational categories in EU countries in the year 2000. These occupational categories are not always possible to translate to social class, but social classes are still discernible.

**Table 1: Prevalence of certain working conditions (%)
in occupational groups in the EU countries in the year 2000**

Occupational group	Occupational exposure				
	Noise	Vapours, dust etc.	Painful positions	Monotonous tasks	Learning new things
Legislators and managers	20	13	29	36	78
Professionals	17	11	32	25	92
Technicians	18	15	38	28	85
Clerks	7	5	30	43	76
Service workers and sales workers	17	15	49	39	63
Agricultural workers	39	34	75	45	59
Craft-related trades workers	60	47	65	44	72
Plant and machine operators	59	42	60	57	56
Elementary occupations	33	28	58	57	38
Armed forces	37	20	44	39	91

Source: Paoli and Merllié 2000.

Most studies of work as an explanation of social class differences in health have focused on the impact of psychosocial work environment conditions. The definition of the psychosocial concept is somewhat unclear. Here it will be used to define and identify working conditions that are thought to exert their effects on health through psychological mechanisms. There are currently two widely used theoretical models for psychosocial working conditions that are believed to induce different forms of ill health. The first, and most studied, is the demand-control model of Karasek and Theorell (Karasek and Theorell 1990, Karasek *et al.* 1981). This model suggests that work demands such as time pressure or level of complexity, and control in terms of decision authority about different aspects of work, as well as the opportunity to learn and use skills and acquire new knowledge at work, are conditions that will affect health. The combination of low control and high demands has some-times been regarded as particularly hazardous.

The effort-reward model claims that if efforts put into work are not reciprocally rewarded this will affect health negatively (Siegrist 1996). Included in the model are rewards in terms of wages, esteem, career opportunities and job security, as well as a coping pattern of over-commitment to work. The links between the psychosocial work envi-ronment and social inequalities in health constituted the subject of a recent review by Siegrist and Marmot (Siegrist and Marmot 2004). Both models could be hypothesised to exert their effects either as direct effects on body functions or as effects on behaviour, e.g. propensity to smoke or to give up smoking (Marmot and Theorell 1988). There is evidence linking both models to an increased relative risk of coronary heart disease, depression, and alcohol problems. It is obvious that psychosocial risk factors such as job control must be strongly linked to social class. In fact, decision authority and skill discretion at work may often be an integrated part of a definition of social class. For psycho-logical demands and social support at work the class relations are not self-evident.

3. Health-related Selection

Social class differences in health, and also health differences be-tween occupations, have most commonly been viewed as a result of either social causation or social selection. The causation issue is most often discussed in relation to adult life experiences, e.g. working life circumstances. The issue of causation-selection has been central to the determination of the roots of socio-economic differences in psychiatric disorders for many decades (Illsley 1955, Dohrenwend *et al.* 1992). The question to be answered is whether ill health is caused by the (generally adult) environment under study, or by health-related characteristics among those recruited to and remaining in the same environment.

The social-selection model for explaining social class differences in health is concerned with recruitment into social classes (West 1991). Studies of social selection often investigate the effects on social differences in health of health-related social mobility. The model postulates that inequalities in health between social classes remain because individuals with poor health move from higher to lower social positions, whereas those with good health move in the opposite direction. Intra-generational mobility occurs when social position changes during adult life. Inter-generational social mobility occurs between generations and is most frequent at the time of transition from adolescent to adult life, i.e. at ages 16-25 (West 1991).

There has been little doubt that illness can result in downward social mobility and that people in good health are relatively more likely to be upwardly mobile (Illsley 1955, West 1991, Power *et al.* 2002a). To contribute to social-class inequalities in health, direct health-related selection must involve a process where ill compared with healthy people more often end up as manual workers (Lundberg 1991b). A relationship has been reported between psychiatric illness (Dohrenwend *et al.* 1992) and severe illness during childhood (Wadsworth and Kuh 1997) on the one hand, and inter-generational downward mobility on the other. During adult life, illness is much more likely to result in exclusion from the labour market than in downward (intra-generational) mobility (Dahl 1994, Lundberg 1991b). Based on data from the British 1958 birth cohort, Power & Peckman (1990) concluded that although poor health does have an adverse effect on people's life chances and social mobility, it does not make a very large contribution to the observed class differences in mortality.

In the occupational health field, the 'healthy worker' effect is a concept used to express the idea that people who hold a job within the regular labour market, and are able to stay there, are – on average – healthier than those who are outside the labour market (McMichael 1976, Ostlin 1989). Specifically, the healthy worker effect refers to a bias in mortality studies, where occupational groups are compared with the entire population. In such studies it is generally shown that the mortality among unskilled workers is lower than in the entire population because of the strong influence on mortality rates from people who are not inside the labour market. There are several roots of the healthy worker effect, i.e. that people whose health is poor have difficulties in finding jobs, or that people will be excluded from the labour market because of ill health, which could also be due to work environment problems. Moreover, it is highly likely that people with poor health in occupations within lower social classes will often have greater difficulties in adjusting their work situation to their health than people with a similar health status in higher social classes (Johansson and Lundberg 2004). This means that the healthy worker effect would generally act to conceal social class differences in comparison with a situation where individuals are classified according to, for example, their last occupation.

4. Risk-factor-associated Selection

In risk-factor-associated selection (also referred to as indirect selection), mobility is not associated with illness but rather with factors that might later cause illness, sometimes called health potential (Lundberg 1991b, West 1991). Such factors influence both health and social position. Several studies have shown that unfavourable lifestyle factors established in adolescence, such as smoking, alcohol consumption and low physical activity, are related to low future social position, Hemmingsson *et al.* 1999). Such studies suggest that to some extent the socio-economic distribution of behavioural factors is already established at the time of labour market entry. A similar pattern is seen for some, but not all, known risk factors for e.g. coronary heart disease (Batty and Leon 2002). Hemmingsson & Lundberg (2005) showed that risk factors measured in childhood and late adolescence had a strong effect on socio-economic differences in coronary heart disease and cardiovascular mortality 30 to 40 years later. There is, however, evidence that behavioural factors at one point in time can be regarded as outcomes of previous circumstances. Childhood adversities are strongly related to negative social, behavioural and health outcomes in adult life (Felitti *et al.* 1998). Therefore negative behavioural factors in adolescence (such as smoking, overweight and heavy alcohol consumption) may be regarded partly as outcomes of previous childhood circumstances. Smoking in adulthood relates to childhood experiences such as emotional, physical and sexual abuse, parental divorce, and parental substance abuse (Anda *et al.* 1999). In Swedish males the number of cigarettes smoked at age 18-20 was strongly related to the prevalence of low mental health (psychiatric diagnosis, low emotional control and self-reported use of drugs for nervous problems), other substance abuse (alcohol and drugs), as well as parental divorce (Hemmingsson and Kriebel 2003). Other studies have shown a relationship between factors of psychological distress in childhood, and adult mortality and morbidity (Felitti *et al.* 1998, Poulton *et al.* 2002).

5. Life-course Approaches

In recent years, what have been called life-course perspectives on adult health have attracted considerable attention (Marmot *et al.* 2001, Kuh and Ben Shlomo 1997, 2004, Davey Smith and Lynch 2004). It has been suggested that social class differences in health may partly have their roots in differential exposure to health-damaging factors over the entire life course (Davey Smith and Lynch 2004), starting in foetal life (Barker 1991).

Three models for how circumstances in early life might be related to adult health inequalities have been identified (Kuh and Ben Shlomo 2004). The 'accumulation of risk' model assumes that risk factors can occur both in childhood and in adulthood, and that they accumulate during the life course and result in an increased risk of ill health. The pathway model is a special version of the accumulation model. Unfavourable conditions in childhood may be a link in a chain where less favourable circumstances accumulate. Some of those circumstances might be unfavourable just because they increase the likelihood of future exposure to risk factors. For example, an advantageous situation in childhood and adolescence may be linked to better school results, and a more privileged social position in adult life may imply less exposure to health-damaging environments. In this model, childhood circumstances by themselves are not necessarily a major source of poor health in adulthood (Marmot *et al.* 2001).

In the 'critical period' model ('latency model', 'biological programming'), a discrete event early in life, even before birth, is seen as possibly having a strong independent effect on a person's health situation later in life. Several such links have been proposed, i.e. by Barker *et al.* (Barker 1991).

Several studies show a link between indicators of adverse social circumstances in childhood, and coronary heart disease and mortality in adulthood (Galobardes *et al.* 2004). Behavioural risk factors such as smoking, poor diet, and low physical activity are often established in childhood and adolescence, and are important in shaping socio-economic differences in coronary heart disease risk (Blane *et al.* 1996). Conventional CHD risk factors, such as blood pressure, obesity and blood cholesterol measured in adolescents and young adults, predict CHD risk many decades later (Davey Smith and Lynch 2004).

So far there is limited evidence that early life exposures have contributed in explaining socio-economic health differences. However, a study on Swedish middle-aged men suggested that a main part of the socio-economic differences in coronary heart disease and CVD mortality could be attributed to indictors of poor childhood circumstances and

19

negative behaviour established in adolescence (Hemmingsson and Lundberg 2005).

A topical debate has discussed the relative importance of 'psychosocial' and 'material' factors for the explanations of social inequalities in health. The increased relative risk of e.g. CHD is not elevated only among the poor, but demonstrates a finely graded association with social position (Erikson 2002). This is apparent in the British Whitehall studies including civil servants who are not expected to be poor, but where position in the hierarchy showed a strong correlation with mortality risk (Marmot 2003). It has been concluded that this association cannot be explained by differences in material goods and that psychosocial factors probably play a central role (Marmot 2003). In one study, the grade differences in CHD could be explained to a great extent by differences between the grades concerning exposure to psychosocial factors, i.e. level of job control (Marmot *et al.* 1997). The interpretation of this finding has raised some criticism. Some have argued that the strong association between job control and CHD may be explained by residual confounding, primarily from negative childhood circumstances (Davey Smith *et al.* 2002). However, this hypothesis has rarely been tested. Recent studies have investigated the extent to which the association between psychosocial factors at work and CVD mortality could be attenuated by adjustment for indicators of early life disadvantage with divergent results (Brunner *et al.* 2004, Hemmingsson and Lundberg 2006).

6. Working Life, Social Class and Health

Marmot *et al.* have pointed to four important benefits of work and occupation for individuals in advanced industrialised societies (Marmot *et al.* 2002). The first is that work provides income, which in turn determines a wide range of life chances. Second, training for a job and achievement of occupational status are the most important goals of socialisation and give a core social identity outside the family. Moreover, occupation is a most important criterion of social stratification and determines esteem and social approval in interpersonal relations. Self-direction at work will also influence behavioural patterns in other areas such as family life and political activity (Kohn and Schooler 1973). Finally, work absorbs the largest amount of active time during adult life. Work is obviously a most important part of mid-life. But how does work affect health? We have already pointed to several working conditions such as chemical exposures and physical load that affected health in lower social classes. When considering the influence of work on health in modern societies, the importance of such conditions must have diminished, since fewer people are exposed. This may not, however, be the case for psychosocial conditions, as defined mainly by the demand-control and effort-reward models.

The demand-control model was introduced in 1979 (Karasek 1979). There is abundant evidence that this model, also when it is expanded to contain social support at work, is related to a number of health outcomes such as coronary heart disease, musculoskeletal disorders and psychological distress and psychiatric disorders (Hemingway and Marmot 1999, Stansfeld *et al*. 1999, Punnett and Wegman 2004). The effort-reward model introduced around 1990 has mainly been related to heart disease and risk factors for heart disease, but psychiatric symptoms and self-reported health have also been investigated (Kuper *et al*. 2002, Marmot *et al*. 2002). The results show an association between this model and the health outcomes investigated. However, in recent years there has been a debate concerning the extent to which the effects found may really be attributed to psychosocial working conditions. Other researchers claim that living conditions, particularly in childhood and adolescence, may determine psychosocial working conditions. Work control is for obvious reasons strongly related to social class. Several authors also consider low social class to be practically inseparable from work control (Lynch and Kaplan 2000, Davey Smith and Lynch 2004). Accordingly, these authors argue that the effects attributed to work control may in fact have been due to residual confounding from other conditions (Davey Smith and Lynch 2004).

7. Studies Examining the Effects of Working Conditions on Social Class Differences in Health

Today there is a vast amount of literature on social inequalities in health. However, it is obvious that the notion of work as an explanation for this has only been examined to a limited extent. Working conditions will explain social class differences in health if they are true risk factors for the illness concerned and this is more common in lower than in higher social classes. The studies reviewed in this chapter are all, at least implicitly, based on this conception.

A. Studies of Self-reported Health

Self-reported health (SRH) is intended as a global health measure and low SRH is usually the response "fair", "poor" or "very poor" to the question: "How do you regard your health at present?". The studies performed have found quite considerable effects of working conditions on SRH. This is true for studies from Sweden (Lundberg 1991a), Denmark (Borg and Kristensen 2000), the Netherlands (Schrijvers *et al*. 1998) and Spain (Borrell *et al*. 2004). When some measure of muscular load was studied separately this explained more of the social class differences than other working conditions (Lundberg 1991a, Schrijvers *et al.* 1998, Borg and Kristensen 2000). In the Whitehall study, financial insecurity, but not job insecurity, explained 15-30% of the social class differences in SRH. Power *et al.* studied the contribution of different factors for social class differences in SRH in the British birth cohort. Many factors contributed to the explanation of social class differences, but job strain (a combination of three questions on job control and one question on job demands) belonged to the most influential factors, together with adolescent socio-emotional adjustment, class at birth and educational qualifications (Power *et al.* 1998).

A cross-sectional study from Finland showed that low job control as well as high psychological demands at work were related to poor SRH, as well as limiting long-standing illness (LLSI) among both men and women. The relationship between social class and SRH and LLSI was considerably attenuated in both sexes when job control was controlled for. However, controlling for job demands strengthened the same relationship in both sexes. When job control and job demands were controlled for simultaneously, the relationship between social class and SRH was somewhat attenuated in both sexes, while the relationship between social class and LLSI was attenuated among women and strengthened among men. These effects reflect the social class distributions of job control and job demands. High control as well as high demands are more common, the higher the social class (Rahkonen *et al.* 2006).

Except for the studies from Denmark (Borg and Kristensen 2000) and the UK (Power *et al.* 1998), these studies were cross-sectional. In cross-sectional studies it is not possible to determine the extent to which working conditions and health-related mobility are the actual determinants of the social class differences in SRH. However, as mentioned above, the studies performed show that downward intra-generational mobility due to bad health is uncommon (Lundberg 1991b).

B. Studies of Coronary Heart Disease

In studies of almost 3000 Danish men, no relation was found between decision authority, psychological demands or social support at work and myocardial infarction, and these psychosocial conditions consequently did not explain anything of the social class gradient in myocardial infarction (Suadicani *et al.* 1993, Suadicani *et al.* 1995, 1997). Adjustment for exposure to soldering fumes and organic solvents changed the relative risk associated with lower social class from 1.4 to 1.2 which was no longer significant, indicating an effect of these exposures on ischaemic heart disease. However, neither soldering fumes nor organic solvents are recognised risk factors for ischaemic heart disease.

Marmot *et al.* showed that low job control accounted for most of the increased odds ratio of 1.5 for coronary heart disease incidence in the Whitehall study (Marmot *et al.* 1997). In a case-control study among Czech men, Bobak *et al.* showed that educational level and low job decision latitude were significantly related to myocardial infarction risk (Bobak *et al.* 1998). Decision latitude at work explained a substantial part of the association between educational level and myocardial infraction.

In a recent Danish study, Andersen *et al.* showed that the prevalence of decision authority as well as skill discretion, determined through a job-exposure matrix, diminished with decreasing socio-economic group and was related to increased risk of myocardial infarction (Andersen *et al.* 2004). However, only skill discretion, and not decision authority, seemed to mediate the effects of socio-economic group on myocardial infarction.

In a cross-sectional study, Ferrie *et al.* showed that job insecurity and financial insecurity were unimportant for the employment grade gradient in blood pressure, serum cholesterol and BMI (Ferrie *et al.* 2003).

So far the evidence for an effect of working conditions on social inequalities in coronary heart disease rests on the studies by Marmot *et al.* (Marmot *et al.* 1997), Bobak *et al.* (Bobak *et al.* 1998) and Andersen *et al.* (Andersen *et al.* 2004), where the only working condition contributing to explain such differences was job control. However, job control is part of the characteristics of social class and may therefore be difficult to separate from social class. Residual unmeasured confounding from previous or present living conditions is possible.

C. Studies of Psychological Distress

There are three studies on this issue, which provide separate estimates for the contribution of working conditions to social class differences in depression, available from the Whitehall study and three studies from the British 1958 birth cohort. No studies exist from other countries. Three of the Whitehall studies concerned mainly psychosocial working conditions as explanations. In the first cross-sectional study from Whitehall phase I, skill discretion and decision authority explained the entire social class difference in psychological well-being in both sexes, and the entire social class difference in depression among men (Stansfeld *et al.* 1998). In a longitudinal study based on data from Whitehall III and V, explanations of differences in anxiety and depression in phase V were examined based on exposure data and data on depression and anxiety from phase III (Griffin *et al.* 2002). Decision latitude explained 50-70% of the grade difference in depression, as well as anxiety in both sexes, when other factors were taken into account.

In a longitudinal analysis over around 10 years in the Whitehall study, phase I and phase V, Stansfeld *et al.* (2003) found that the grade gradient in depressive symptoms at time II was entirely explained by work characteristics (job-strain and effort-reward imbalance), material disadvantage, social support and health behaviours at phase I, in both women and men (Stansfeld *et al.* 2003).

The importance of job insecurity and financial security for the grade gradient in depression was studied cross-sectionally in Whitehall phase V (Ferrie *et al.* 2003). Job insecurity explained 10-20% of the social class gradient in both sexes, and financial insecurity around 15% of the gradient among women and 50% among men. Since the study is cross-sectional, job and financial insecurity may be caused by and may also cause depression.

The first of the studies from the British 1958 birth cohort found in both sexes that 30% of the social class gradient in psychological distress at age 33 was explained by psychological distress at age 23. Psychosocial work conditions explained about 50% of the remaining gradient among men and about 10% of the remaining gradient among women (Matthews *et al.* 2001). In the second study on the same material, Matthews and Power examined the effects of work and home factors on social class differences in psychological distress among women. Odds ratios for low compared with high social class were attenuated by 33% by accounting for psychological distress at age 23, and with a further 15% by accounting for psychosocial work factors. Home factors were comparatively unimportant for class differences (Matthews and Power 2002).

In the third study from the British birth cohort, Power *et al.* found that psychological status was related to subsequent social mobility among 16-year-olds but that this had no effect on adult social class differences in psychological distress. The authors then examined the effects of conditions at different stages of life on psychological distress at age 33. Previous unemployment and job strain at age 33 were important in explaining the social class differences among men, while job insecurity at age 33 was the only important work factor among women (Power *et al.* 2002b).

D. Studies of Other Outcomes

Martikainen *et al.* (1999) examined decline in mental and physical functioning in social classes between phases III and V in the Whitehall study. Among men there was an obvious social class gradient in decline in both types of functioning, while for women there was a gradient only for physical functioning. Health behaviours were the most important determinants for social class differences in decline of physical functioning among men, followed by decision latitude and material problems. For social class differences in decline of mental functioning among men, material problems and job decision latitude were the most important determinants. Among women, none of the factors examined had any importance for social class differences in terms of decline in physical functioning (Martikainen *et al.* 1999).

In a study mentioned above based on risk factors from Whitehall II phase I and employment grade in phase V, Stansfeld *et al.* (2003) found that work characteristics only explained a minor part of the grade gradient in physical functioning at phase V (Stansfeld *et al.* 2003).

In their study of sickness absence, Vahtera *et al.* pointed to the possibility that different 'cultures' may exist at different workplaces, which may be important determinants of social class differences in sickness absence (Vahtera *et al.* 1999).

E. Studies of Interactions between Social Class and Working Conditions in the Causation of Disease

When the combination of some working condition and low social class exerts a joint effect on an outcome variable that is higher than the combination of the separate effects of the working condition and social class, considering all confounding factors, there is an interaction between social class and the working conditions. Interactions are mainly a statistical concept and it is largely unknown how they relate to biological or social mechanisms, apart from the fact that they indicate increased susceptibility in certain groups. However, they are interesting from a preventive point of view. If there is an interaction, the effects of a similar improvement in the working condition would benefit lower classes more than higher classes, i.e. would diminish social class differences in health.

A limited number of papers have considered such interactions. In a study based on the Swedish Surveys of Living Conditions, Johnson and Hall (1988) used cross-sectional data to show that prevalence ratios associated with the combination of high work demands and low work control, or the combination of high job demands, low work control, and low work social support were much higher among blue-collar than white-collar males. Among women there were no such differences (Johnson and Hall 1988). In the Swedish SHEEP study, Hallqvist *et al.*, examining incident male cases of myocardial infarction and controls, found an interaction between psychological work demands and job decision latitude, i.e. job strain, among manual but not non-manual workers. There also seemed to be an interaction, although not significant, between low socio-economic group and job strain in the causation of myocardial infarction (Hallqvist *et al.* 1998). However, in an 11-year follow-up study based on the Whitehall II material, no interaction was found between low socio-economic status and job strain, job demands or job decision latitude, to increase the incidence of coronary heart disease (Kuper and Marmot 2003). In another study from Whitehall II, Kuper *et al.* made the same analysis but now with the effort-reward imbalance model as the exposure under study (Kuper *et al.* 2002). High effort in comparison with reward was associated with an increased incidence of coronary heart disease. There was a tendency for low socio-economic status to interact with effort-reward imbalance to increase the incidence of coronary heart disease, but not of low physical or mental functioning.

Interactions might result from a higher correlation of risk factors in lower classes than in higher classes. If so, every new risk factor associated with social class will interact with lower social class because of its association with other, unknown, risk factors. Such correlations in lower social classes may appear for example if unfavourable psychosocial working conditions lead to higher alcohol consumption and more smoking in lower than in higher social classes (Marmot and Theorell 1988, Marmot *et al.* 2002, Kouvonen *et al.* 2005), while these factors remain unmeasured.

References

ANDA, R. F., J. B. CROFT, V. J. FELITTI, D. NORDENBERG, W. H. GILES, D. F. WILLIAMSON, and G. A. GIOVINO. 1999. "Adverse childhood experiences and smoking during adolescence and adulthood", *Jama* 282: 1652-8.

ANDERSEN, I., H. BURR, T. S. KRISTENSEN, M. GAMBORG, M. OSLER, E. PRESCOTT, and F. DIDERICHSEN. 2004. "Do factors in the psychosocial work environment mediate the effect of socioeconomic position on the risk of myocardial infarction? Study from the Copenhagen Centre for Prospective Population Studies", *Occup Environ Med* 61: 886-92.

BARKER, D. J. 1991. "The foetal and infant origins of inequalities in health in Britain", *J Public Health Med* 13: 64-8.

BATTY, G. D. and D. A. LEON. 2002. "Socio-economic position and coronary heart disease risk factors in children and young people. Evidence from UK epidemiological studies", *Eur J Public Health* 12: 263-72.

BELKIC, K. L., P. A. LANDSBERGIS, P. L. SCHNALL, and D. BAKER. 2004. "Is job strain a major source of cardiovascular disease risk?", S*cand J Work Environ Health* 30: 85-128.

BLANE, D., C. L. HART, G. D. SMITH, C. R. GILLIS, D. J. HOLE, and V. M. HAWTHORNE. 1996. "Association of cardiovascular disease risk factors with socioeconomic position during childhood and during adulthood", *BMJ* 313: 1434-8.

BOBAK, M., C. HERTZMAN, Z. SKODOVA, and M. MARMOT. 1998. "Association between psychosocial factors at work and nonfatal myocardial infarction in a population-based case-control study in Czech men", *Epidemiology* 9: 43-7.

BORG, V. and T. S. KRISTENSEN. 2000. "Social class and self-rated health: can the gradient be explained by differences in life style or work environment?", *Soc Sci Med* 51: 1019-30.

BORRELL, C., C. MUNTANER, J. BENACH, and L. ARTAZCOZ. 2004. S"ocial class and self-reported health status among men and women: what is the role of work organisation, household material standards and household labour?", *Soc Sci Med* 58: 1869-87.

BRUNNER, E. J., M. KIVIMAKI, J. SIEGRIST, T. THEORELL, R. LUUKKONEN, H. RIIHIMAKI, J. VAHTERA, J. KIRJONEN, and P. LEINO-ARJAS. 2004. "Is the effect of work stress on cardiovascular mortality confounded by socioeconomic factors in the Valmet study?", *J Epidemiol Community Health* 58: 1019-20.

BURDORF, A., B. JARVHOLM, and A. ENGLUND. 2004. "Explaining differences in incidence rates of pleural mesothelioma between Sweden and the Netherlands", *Int J Cancer* 113: 298-301.

DAVEY SMITH, G. and J. LYNCH. 2004. Life course approaches to socioeconomic differentials in health, pp. 77-115. *In* D. Kuh and Y. Ben-Shlomo [eds.], *A life course approach to chronic disease epidemiology*. Oxford University Press, New York.

DAVEY SMITH, G., Y. BEN SHLOMO, and J. LYNCH. 2002. "Life course approaches to inequalities in coronary heart disease risk", in M. S. STANSFELD and M. MARMOT (eds.), *Stress and the heart. Psychosocial pathways to coronary heart disease*. BMJ Books, London, pp. 20-49.

DOHRENWEND, B. P., I. LEVAV, P. E. SHROUT, S. SCHWARTZ, G. NAVEH, B. G. LINK, A. E. SKODOL, and A. STUEVE. 1992. "Socioeconomic status and psychiatric disorders: the causation-selection issue", *Science* 255: 946-52.

ERIKSON, R. 2002. "Why do graduates live longer? Education, occupation, family and mortality during the 1990s", in J. O. JONSSON and C. MILLS (eds.), *Cradle to grave. Life-course change in modern Sweden*. Sociologypress, Durham, pp. 211-227.

FELITTI, V. J., R. F. ANDA, D. NORDENBERG, D. F. WILLIAMSON, A. M. SPITZ, V. EDWARDS, M. P. KOSS, and J. S. MARKS. 1998. "Relationship of childhood abuse and household dysfunction to many of the leading causes of death in adults. The Adverse Childhood Experiences (ACE) Study", *Am J Prev Med* 14: 245-58.

FERRIE, J. E., M. J. SHIPLEY, S. A. STANSFELD, G. D. SMITH, and M. MARMOT. 2003. "Future uncertainty and socioeconomic inequalities in health: the Whitehall II study", *Soc Sci Med* 57: 637-46.

GALOBARDES, B., J. W. LYNCH, and G. DAVEY SMITH. 2004. "Childhood socioeconomic circumstances and cause-specific mortality in adulthood: systematic review and interpretation", *Epidemiol Rev* 26: 7-21.

GRIFFIN, J. M., R. FUHRER, S. A. STANSFELD, and M. MARMOT. 2002. "The importance of low control at work and home on depression and anxiety: do these effects vary by gender and social class?", *Soc Sci Med* 54: 783-98.

HALLQVIST, J., F. DIDERICHSEN, T. THEORELL, C. REUTERWALL, and A. AHLBOM. 1998. "Is the effect of job strain on myocardial infarction risk due to interaction between high psychological demands and low decision latitude? Results from Stockholm Heart Epidemiology Program (SHEEP)", *Soc Sci Med* 46: 1405-15.

HEMINGWAY, H. and M. MARMOT. 1999. "Evidence based cardiology: psychosocial factors in the aetiology and prognosis of coronary heart disease. Systematic review of prospective cohort studies", *BMJ* 318: 1460-7.

HEMMINGSSON, T. and D. KRIEBEL. 2003. "Smoking at age 18-20 and suicide during 26 years of follow-up: how can the association be explained?", *Int J Epidemiol* 32: 1000-4.

HEMMINGSSON, T. and I. LUNDBERG. 2005. "How far are socioeconomic differences in coronary heart disease hospitalization, all-cause mortality and cardiovascular mortality among adult Swedish males attributable to negative childhood circumstances and behaviour in adolescence?", *Int J Epidemiol* 34: 260-7.

HEMMINGSSON, T. and I. LUNDBERG. 2006. "Is the association between low job control and coronary heart disease confounded by risk factors measured in childhood and adolescence among Swedish males 40-53 years of age?", *Int J Epidemiol*.

HEMMINGSSON, T., I. LUNDBERG, and F. DIDERICHSEN. 1999. "The roles of social class of origin, achieved social class and intergenerational social mobility in explaining social-class inequalities in alcoholism among young men", *Soc Sci Med* 49: 1051-9.

HODGSON, J., D. MCELVENNY, A. DARNTON, M. PRICE, and J. PETO. 2005. "The expected burden of mesothelioma mortality in Great Britain from 2002 to 2050", *Br J Cancer* 92: 587-593.

ILLSLEY, R. 1955. "Social class selection and class differences in relation to stillbirths and infant deaths", *Br Med J*: 1520-4.

JOHANSSON, G. and I. LUNDBERG. 2004. "Adjustment latitude and attendance requirements as determinants of sickness absence or attendance. Empirical tests of the illness flexibility model", *Soc Sci Med* 58: 1857-68.

JOHNSON, J. V. and E. M. HALL. 1988. "Job strain, work place social support, and cardiovascular disease: a cross-sectional study of a random sample of the Swedish working population", *Am J Public Health* 78: 1336-42.

KARASEK, R. 1979. "Job demands, job decision latitude, and mental strain: An implication for job redesign", *Adm Sci Q* 24: 285-307.

KARASEK, R. and T. THEORELL. 1990. *Healthy work. Stress, productivity, and the reconstruction of working life*. Basic Books, New York.

KARASEK, R., D. BAKER, F. MARXER, A. AHLBOM, and T. THEORELL. 1981. "Job decision latitude, job demands, and cardiovascular disease: a prospective study of Swedish men", *Am J Public Health* 71: 694-705.

KITIGAWA, E. M. and P. M. HAUSER. 1973. *Differential mortality in the United States: A study in socio-economic epidemiology*. Harvard University Press, Cambridge.

KOHN, M. S. and C. SCHOOLER. 1973. "Occupational experience and psychological functioning: An assessment of reciprocal effects", *American Sociological Review* 38: 97-118.

KOIVUSILTA, L., A. RIMPELA, and M. RIMPELA. 1998. "Health related lifestyle in adolescence predicts adult educational level: a longitudinal study from Finland", *J Epidemiol Community Health* 52: 794-801.

KOUVONEN, A., M. KIVIMAKI, M. VIRTANEN, J. PENTTI, and J. VAHTERA. 2005. "Work stress, smoking status, and smoking intensity: an observational study of 46,190 employees", *J Epidemiol Community Health* 59: 63-9.

KUH, D. and Y. BEN SHLOMO (eds.). 1997. *A life course approach to chronic disease epidemiology*. Oxford University Press, Oxford.

KUH, D. and Y. BEN SHLOMO (eds.). 2004. *A life course approach to chronic disease epidemiology*. Oxford University Press, Oxford.

KUNST, A. E., F. GROENHOF, and J. P. MACKENBACH. 1998a. "Mortality by occupational class among men 30-64 years in 11 European countries. EU Working Group on Socioeconomic Inequalities in Health", *Soc Sci Med* 46: 1459-76.

KUNST, A. E., F. GROENHOF, J. P. MACKENBACH, and E. W. HEALTH. 1998b. "Occupational class and cause specific mortality in middle aged men in 11 European countries: comparison of population based studies. EU Working Group on Socioeconomic Inequalities in Health", *BMJ* 316: 1636-42.

KUNST, A. E., V. BOS, E. LAHELMA, M. BARTLEY, I. LISSAU, E. REGIDOR, A. MIELCK, M. CARDANO, J. A. DALSTRA, J. J. GEURTS, U. HELMERT, C. LENNARTSSON, J. RAMM, T. SPADEA, W. J. STRONEGGER, and J. P. MACKENBACH. 2005. "Trends in socioeconomic inequalities in self-assessed health in 10 European countries", *Int J Epidemiol* 34: 295-305.

KUPER, H. and M. MARMOT. 2003. "Job strain, job demands, decision latitude, and risk of coronary heart disease within the Whitehall II study", *J Epidemiol Community Health* 57: 147-53.

KUPER, H., A. SINGH-MANOUX, J. SIEGRIST, and M. MARMOT. 2002. "When reciprocity fails: effort-reward imbalance in relation to coronary heart disease and health functioning within the Whitehall II study", *Occup Environ Med* 59: 777-84.

LUNDBERG, I., C. HOGSTEDT, C. LIDÉN, and G. NISE. 2005. "Organic solvents and related compounds", in L. ROSENSTOCK, M. CULLEN, C. BRODKIN and C. REDLICH (eds.), *Textbook of Clinical Occupational and Environmental Medicine*. Elsevier, Saunders, Philadelphia, pp. 9991-1010.

LUNDBERG, O. 1991a. "Causal explanations for class inequality in health – an empirical analysis", *Soc Sci Med* 32: 385-93.

LUNDBERG, O. 1991b. "Childhood living conditions, health status, and social mobility: A contribution to the health selection debate", *European Sociological Review* 7: 149-162.

LYNCH, J. and G. A. KAPLAN. 2000. "Socioeconomic position", in L. BERKMAN and I. KAWACHI (eds.), *Social epidemiology*. Oxford University Press, New York, pp. 13-35

MACKENBACH, J. P., A. E. CAVELAARS, A. E. KUNST, and F. GROENHOF. 2000. "Socioeconomic inequalities in cardiovascular disease mortality; an international study", *Eur Heart J* 21: 1141-51.

MACKENBACH, J. P., A. E. KUNST, A. E. CAVELAARS, F. GROENHOF, and J. J. GEURTS. 1997. "Socioeconomic inequalities in morbidity and mortality in western Europe. The EU Working Group on Socioeconomic Inequalities in Health", *Lancet* 349: 1655-9.

MACKENBACH, J. P., V. BOS, O. ANDERSEN, M. CARDANO, G. COSTA, S. HARDING, A. REID, O. HEMSTROM, T. VALKONEN, and A. E. KUNST. 2003. "Widening socioeconomic inequalities in mortality in six Western European countries", *Int J Epidemiol* 32: 830-7.

MACKENBACH, J. P., A. E. KUNST, F. GROENHOF, J. K. BORGAN, G. COSTA, F. FAGGIANO, P. JOZAN, M. LEINSALU, P. MARTIKAINEN, J. RYCHTARIKOVA, and T. VALKONEN. 1999. "Socioeconomic inequalities in mortality among women and among men: an international study", *Am J Public Health* 89: 1800-6.

MACKENBACH, J. P., M. HUISMAN, O. ANDERSEN, M. BOPP, J. K. BORGAN, C. BORRELL, G. COSTA, P. DEBOOSERE, A. DONKIN, S. GADEYNE, C. MINDER, E. REGIDOR, T. SPADEA, T. VALKONEN, and A. E. KUNST. 2004. "Inequalities in lung cancer mortality by the educational level in 10 European populations", *Eur J Cancer* 40: 126-35.

MARMOT, M. and T. THEORELL. 1988. "Social class and cardiovascular disease: the contribution of work", *Int J Health Serv* 18: 659-74.

MARMOT, M., T. THEORELL, and J. SIEGRIST. 2002. "Work and coronary heart disease", in M. S. STANSFELD and M. MARMOT (eds.), *Stress and the heart. Psychosocial pathways to coronary heart disease*. BMJ Books, London, pp. 50-71

MARMOT, M., M. SHIPLEY, E. BRUNNER, and H. HEMINGWAY. 2001. "Relative contribution of early life and adult socioeconomic factors to adult morbidity in the Whitehall II study", *J Epidemiol Community Health* 55: 301-7.

MARMOT, M. G. 2003. "Understanding social inequalities in health", *Perspect Biol Med* 46: S9-23.

MARMOT, M. G., H. BOSMA, H. HEMINGWAY, E. BRUNNER, and S. STANSFELD. 1997. "Contribution of job control and other risk factors to social variations in coronary heart disease incidence", *Lancet* 350: 235-9.

MARMOT, M. G., G. D. SMITH, S. STANSFELD, C. PATEL, F. NORTH, J. HEAD, I. WHITE, E. BRUNNER, and A. FEENEY. 1991. "Health inequalities among British civil servants: the Whitehall II study", *Lancet* 337: 1387-93.

MARTIKAINEN, P., S. STANSFELD, H. HEMINGWAY, and M. MARMOT. 1999. "Determinants of socioeconomic differences in change in physical and mental functioning", *Soc Sci Med* 49: 499-507.

MATTHEWS, S. and C. POWER. 2002. "Socio-economic gradients in psychological distress: a focus on women, social roles and work-home characteristics", *Soc Sci Med* 54: 799-810.

MATTHEWS, S., C. POWER, and S. A. STANSFELD. 2001. "Psychological distress and work and home roles: a focus on socio-economic differences in distress", *Psychol Med* 31: 725-36.

MCMICHAEL AJ. 1976. "Standardized mortality ratios and the 'healthy worker effect': Scratching beneath the surface", *J Occup Med* 18: 165-8.

MONCADA, S. 1999. "Working conditions and social inequalities in health", *J Epidemiol Community Health* 53: 390-1.

OSTLIN, P. 1989. "The 'health-related selection effect' on occupational morbidity rates", *Scand J Soc Med* 17: 265-70.

PAMUK, E. 1985. "Social class inequality in mortality from 1921 to 1972 in England and Wales", *Population studies* 39: 17-31.

PAOLI, P. and D. MERLLIÉ. Third European Survey on Working Conditions 2000. European Foundation for the Improvement of Working and Living Conditions 2000. www.Eurofound.eu.int.

POULTON, R., A. CASPI, B. J. MILNE, W. M. THOMSON, A. TAYLOR, M. R. SEARS, and T. E. MOFFITT. 2002. "Association between children's experience of socioeconomic disadvantage and adult health: a life-course study", *Lancet* 360: 1640-5.

POWER, C. and C. PECKHAM. 1990. "Childhood morbidity and adulthood ill health", *J Epidemiol Community Health* 44: 69-74.

POWER, C., S. MATTHEWS, and O. MANOR. 1998. "Inequalities in self-rated health: explanations from different stages of life", *Lancet* 351: 1009-14.

POWER, C., O. MANOR, and L. LI. 2002a. "Are inequalities in height underestimated by adult social position? Effects of changing social structure and height selection in a cohort study", BMJ 325: 131-4.

POWER, C., S. A. STANSFELD, S. MATTHEWS, O. MANOR, and S. HOPE. 2002b. "Childhood and adulthood risk factors for socio-economic differentials in psychological distress: evidence from the 1958 British birth cohort", *Soc Sci Med* 55: 1989-2004.

PUNNETT, L. and D. H. WEGMAN. 2004. "Work-related musculoskeletal disorders: the epidemiologic evidence and the debate", *J Electromyogr Kinesiol* 14: 13-23.

RAHKONEN, O., M. LAAKSONEN, P. MARTIKAINEN, E. ROOS, and E. LAHELMA. 2006."Job control, job demands, or social class? The impact of working conditions on the relation between social class and health", *J Epidemiol Community Health* 60: 50-4.

RAMAZZINI, B. 1964. *Diseases of the worker. Translated from the Latin text De Morbis Artificum of 1713.* Hafner Publishing Company, New York, London.

SCHRIJVERS, C. T., H. D. VAN DE MHEEN, K. STRONKS, and J. P. MACKENBACH. 1998. "Socioeconomic inequalities in health in the working population: the contribution of working conditions", *Int J Epidemiol* 27: 1011-8.

SIEGRIST, J. 1996. "Adverse health effects of high-effort/low-reward conditions", *J Occup Health Psychol 1*: 27-41.

SIEGRIST, J. and M. MARMOT. 2004. "Health inequalities and the psychosocial environment – two scientific challenges", *Soc Sci Med* 58: 1463-73.

SMITH, G. D., M. BARTLEY, and D. BLANE. 1990. "The Black report on socioeconomic inequalities in health 10 years on", *BMJ* 301: 373-7.

STANSFELD, S. A., J. HEAD, and M. G. MARMOT. 1998. "Explaining social class differences in depression and well-being", *Soc Psychiatry Psychiatr Epidemiol* 33: 1-9.

STANSFELD, S. A., R. FUHRER, M. J. SHIPLEY, and M. G. MARMOT. 1999. "Work characteristics predict psychiatric disorder: prospective results from the Whitehall II Study", *Occup Environ Med* 56: 302-7.

STANSFELD, S. A., J. HEAD, R. FUHRER, J. WARDLE, and V. CATTELL. 2003. "Social inequalities in depressive symptoms and physical functioning in the Whitehall II study: exploring a common cause explanation", *J Epidemiol Community Health* 57: 361-7.

SUADICANI, P., H. O. HEIN, and F. GYNTELBERG. 1993. "Are social inequalities as associated with the risk of ischaemic heart disease a result of psychosocial working conditions?", *Atherosclerosis* 101: 165-75.

SUADICANI, P., H. O. HEIN, and F. GYNTELBERG. 1995. "Do physical and chemical working conditions explain the association of social class with ischaemic heart disease?", *Atherosclerosis* 113: 63-9.

SUADICANI, P., H. O. HEIN, and F. GYNTELBERG. 1997. "Strong mediators of social inequalities in risk of ischaemic heart disease: a six-year follow-up in the Copenhagen Male Study", *Int J Epidemiol* 26: 516-22.

TOWNSEND, P. and N. DAVIDSON. 1982. *Inequalities in health: The Black report.* Penguin, Harmondsworth.

WADSWORTH, M. E. 1997. "Health inequalities in the life course perspective", *Soc Sci Med* 44: 859-69.

WADSWORTH, M. E. and D. J. KUH. 1997. "Childhood influences on adult health: a review of recent work from the British 1946 national birth cohort study, the MRC National Survey of Health and Development, *Paediatr Perinat Epidemiol* 11: 2-20.

VAGERO, D. and R. ERIKSON. 1997. "Socioeconomic inequalities in morbidity and mortality in western Europe", *Lancet* 350: 516; author reply 517-8.

VAHTERA, J., P. VIRTANEN, M. KIVIMAKI, and J. PENTTI. 1999. "Workplace as an origin of health inequalities", *J Epidemiol Community Health* 53: 399-407.

WEST, P. 1991. "Rethinking the health selection explanation for health inequalities", *Soc Sci Med* 32: 373-84.

PART I

COUNTRY CHAPTERS

Introduction

The studies on working conditions as determinants of social class differences in health that are reviewed in the introductory chapter came from a few countries, about half of them from the UK and a number from Denmark. Four countries provided one or a few papers each, but we were unable to find any papers from large EU-15 countries such as France, Germany, Italy and Belgium. Hence it is obvious that the issue of understanding working conditions as determinants of social class differences in health has been of major interest mainly in one country. This calls for studies also in other countries to explore whether explanations of social class differences are similar to those in the Whitehall and British birth cohort studies.

The purpose of the project reported in this volume was to compile data on the social distribution of working conditions that are presumed to be risk factors for ill health, in a number of European countries. We also wished to provide some estimates of the potential of these working conditions to explain social class differences in health. Changes in the occurrence of such conditions in social classes over recent decades were compiled. In addition, information was collected regarding conditions such as unemployment rates that may affect these relations in the participating countries. The specific request for information from the different countries is reproduced in Appendix 1.

Denmark

Eva STØTTRUP HANSEN

Introduction

Significant social inequalities are a disgrace to any society and the presence of such inequalities clashes with our ideas of humanity, democracy, and justice. Unfortunately, marked social inequalities are present within the Danish population, and the demonstration of inequalities in health has stained the image of the Danish welfare state.

Work is intimately associated with social status and because the working conditions of many people may constitute a hazard to their health, inequality in working conditions is likely to contribute to social inequality in health. It is the purpose of the present paper to review some aspects of this complex of problems.

The paper covers more or less the last three decades of the 20th century providing a rough outline of the Danish labour market, the labour force, the working conditions, the social structure, and the social security system. Further, the paper presents social group data on the health-related parameters covered by the "Winner-project", including data on mortality, self-rated health, self-reported long-standing illness, and notification data on occupational injuries. The discussion focuses on the complex interrelatedness of work, occupational hazards, socio-economic status, and registered health status, the conclusion being that – because of a strong health-based selection of the labour force – the main burden of work-related disease is likely not to be found among occupationally active people, but among those who are no longer occupationally active. Finally, an attempt is made to depict a realistic future scenario based on the prevailing political and economic trends. The manuscript was finished in December 2003.

The paper is based on literature studies, as the funding allowed for no new studies or data analyses. The main data sources employed in the paper include:

National data on socio-economic indicators, from Statistics Denmark (Johansen and Jacobsen 2001, Statistics Denmark 2003a, Statistics Denmark 2003b, Statistics Denmark 2003c).

National follow-up data on mortality 1970-1980, 1981-5, 1986-90, and 1991-5 in relation to job-title at baseline, from Statistics Denmark (Andersen 1985, Ingerslev *et al.* 1994, Andersen *et al.* 2001).

National data on notified work-related diseases, from the National Working Environment Authority (National Working Environment Authority 2002).

National data on notified occupational accidents with injury, from the National Working Environment Authority (National Working Environment Authority 2002).

National follow-up data on somatic hospitalisations in relation to job-title at baseline, from the National Institute of Occupational Health (Tüchsen *et al.* 1992, Bach *et al.* 2002, National Institute of Occupational Health 2003a).

National follow-up data on cancer incidence 1970-9, 1970-80, 1970-87, and 1970-97 in relation to job-title at baseline, from the Danish Cancer Registry and the National Working Environment Authority (Olsen and Jensen 1987, Lynge and Thygesen 1990, Engholm *et al.* 1996, Andersen *et al.* 1999, Hansen and Meerson 2003).

Follow-up data on morbidity and mortality of population samples (Parving *et al.* 1983, Ostri and Parving 1991, Hein *et al.* 1992a, Hein *et al.* 1992b, Suadicani *et al.* 1995, Suadicani *et al.* 1997, Borg and Kristensen 2000, Suadicani *et al.* 2001).

Surveys and panel studies on self-reported health and working conditions of population samples, from the National Institute of Public Health, The National Institute of Occupational Health, and the National Institute of Social Research (Rasmussen *et al.* 1988, Kjøller *et al.* 1995, Borg and Burr 1997, Bonke 1997, Burr *et al.* 2000, Kjøller and Rasmussen 2002, National Institute of Occupational Health 2003b).

1. The Danish Labour Market

A. Economic Structure

Within the last few decades, the economic structure of Danish society has changed from being dominated by agriculture and industry to being dominated by service trades. This profound transformation, which has significant implications for the living conditions of most people, has taken place primarily through a generational change.

Around the beginning of the third millennium, the service sector constitutes approximately 3/4 of the labour market, while industry and construction account for 1/5, and agriculture and fishing 1/20 (table 1).

**Table 1: The Danish labour force 2002, by trade and gender:
Percentages with absolute numbers (thousands) in brackets**

Trade	Males	Females	Total
Agriculture, fishing, and mining	5 (79)	2 (23)	4 (102)
Industry	21 (308)	11 (146)	16 (454)
Construction	11 (156)	1 (17)	6 (173)
Retail trades, hotels, and Restaurants	19 (278)	17 (217)	18 (495)
Transportation, postal and telecommunication services	9 (130)	4 (49)	6 (179)
Finance and management	14 (205)	13 (171)	13 (376)
Teaching and care (incl. nursing and looking after children)	21 (309)	51 (666)	35 (974)
Other or unknown	1 (19)	1 (10)	1 (29)

Source: Statistics Denmark 2003a.

The Service Sector

Private enterprises, which account for about 60% of the jobs in the service sector, provide services within the retail and wholesale trades, shipping, banking and financial services, management, advertising, hotels and restaurants, emergency services, cleaning, care, nursing, looking after children, and transportation of goods and people. The relative size of the private service sector has increased moderately within the last few decades.

The public service sector covers teaching, health care, nursing, looking after children, emergency services, police, courts and prison services, armed forces, religious services, postal and telecommunication services, broadcasting and television, maintenance of roads, highways, and other infrastructure, public transportation, heating, electricity, and water supplies, sewerage and wastewater treatment, refuse disposal, and administration at the national, county, and municipality level. The relative size of the public service sector has increased from covering about 10% of all jobs in 1960 to about 30% in 2002. Within recent years, however, the public service sector has been stagnant/reduced in response to an economic policy involving strict limitations of public expenditure combined with outsourcing of publicly financed services to private entrepreneurs. Public services that have been subject to outsourcing include public transportation (buses, trains, and ferries), cleaning and laundering in public hospitals and nursing homes, telephone and postal services, television and broadcasting, refuse disposal and sewerage services, emergency services, education for adults, kindergartens, home help, and medical services.

Industry and Construction

Within the last decades, major cutbacks have affected the Danish shipyard industry, steel industry, textile industry, and fish manufacturing industry. Overall, the number of jobs in the manufacturing industry has been steadily decreasing, while the number of jobs in the construction sector has been rather stable for several years.

Agriculture and Fishing

Traditionally, agriculture has constituted the dominating economic sector in Denmark, with most people earning their living from farming. Today, however, the number of people working in this sector has decreased to less than 4% of the labour force, a change reflecting an immense structural transition that has taken place within a few decades.

Today, huge-scale mono-production is predominant in Danish agriculture, and about 50% of the arable land is owned by big agricultural enterprises of 100 hectares or more (Johansen and Jacobsen 2001, Statistics Denmark 2003a). In many respects, these huge production units, e.g. pig farms, chicken farms or wheat farms, compare with industrial plants. The previously predominant mixed farming in smaller production units ('family farms') still exists but its importance is rapidly decreasing (Johansen and Jacobsen 2001, Statistics Denmark 2003a).

Previously, Denmark also had a large fishing fleet and a fish manufacturing industry, but within the last decade, the size of the fishing fleet has been reduced by 40%, and today the trade employs less than 1% of the labour force (Johansen and Jacobsen 2001, Statistics Denmark 2003a).

B. Business Cycle and Unemployment

During the first decades following World War II, Denmark experienced rapidly increasing economic activity, and in the 1960s the unemployment rate was extremely low (1-2%). This came to an end with the oil crisis in the early 1970s, after which ten years of recession and increasing unemployment rates (up to 12%) followed. Political measures brought about a temporary stabilisation in 1983-4, but from 1985 on, the unemployment rate grew again and reached 14% in 1994. However, during the last half of the 1990s, the unemployment rate was reduced to 4-5%, a development that was opposite to the general trend in the European Union (EU). At present, the Danish unemployment rate is on the increase again, and for the year 2003, it is expected to reach 6%.

However, comparing unemployment rates over time, one should remember that these figures reflect not only the economic activity but also the effect of (i) various labour market programmes, (ii) alterations in the welfare system, and (iii) demographic changes. For instance, early retirement (from age 60) has been optional since 1979, and in the year 2000, the number of early-retired people exceeded the number of people registered as being unemployed. About one third of those who retire before the age of ordinary retirement, retire from long-term unemployment. Furthermore, many de facto unemployed people are today no longer included in the unemployment figures; having been without employment for a rather long period, people are removed from the list and are transferred from unemployment benefit to social benefit.

Generally speaking, the unemployment rates are slightly higher for women than for men; higher for immigrant workers than for native Danes; higher among people with no education beyond basic school; and higher among people over 55 years of age than among others (Statistics Denmark 2003a).

C. Conclusion

Within a few decades, the Danish labour market has undergone a profound structural transition from being dominated by agriculture and industry to a situation in which 3/4 of the jobs are in the service trades. Recently, a number of tax-financed public services have been transferred from the public to the private service sector. Several industries have been seriously affected by closures, while agricultural production has become more and more industrialised. During the last decade, the unemployment rate has been relatively low (4-5%), but within the most recent years it has increased slightly.

2. The Danish Labour Force

Since the 1960s, the Danish labour force has grown significantly, mainly because of a rapid increase in the occupational activity of women (figure 1, table 2).

Figure 1: Number of people in the Danish labour force, 1970-2002

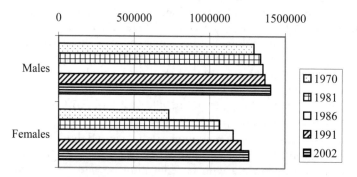

Source: Statistics Denmark 2003a, Andersen 1985, Andersen et al. 2001.

Table 2: Percentage of occupationally active people, by year, gender, and age group (%)

Year	Males		Females	
	25-44 yrs.	45-64 yrs.	25-44 yrs.	45-64 yrs.
1940	98	92	38	29
1950	98	94	–	–
1960	98	95	37	34
1970	96	91	56	43
1979	96	84	83	53
1990	91	82	88	67
1995	90	79	84	66
2002	89	No data	85	No data

Source: Statistics Denmark 2003a, Bonke 1997.

Further, the frequency of part-time employment has decreased from 21% in 1975 to 15% in 2002, solely due to a significant reduction in the percentage of women working part-time, while an opposite trend is seen for males (table 3).

Table 3: Percentage of the labour force in part-time employment, by year and gender (%)

	Males	Females	Total
1975	4	44	21
1980	8	36	20
1990	9	26	17
2002	13	17	15

Source: Statistics Denmark 2003a, Bonke 1997.

Formally, full-time work means 37 hours per week, but the average is higher, and if part-time employees are included, the overall average amounts to 36 hours per week.

The vast majority of the occupationally active women are salaried employees or unskilled manual workers, most of them being employed in service trades and industry (tables 1 and 4). For comparison, the occupationally active males are more uniformly distributed over the various trades and job types (tables 1 and 5). In 2002, immigrant workers constituted 6% of the labour force.

Table 4: The female labour force 1970-1995, by year and socio-economic group: Percentages (%) with absolute numbers (thousands) in brackets

	1970	1980	1990	1995
Self-employed	5(42)	4(45)	4(48)	4(48)
Assisting spouses	11(93)	6(67)	3(36)	2(24)
Salaried employees, upper level	15(127)	15(168)	19(230)	22(265)
Salaried employees, lower level	34(287)	35(392)	37(448)	34(410)
Skilled manual workers	-	1(11)	2(24)	2(24)
Unskilled manual workers	33(279)	26(291)	23 (279)	21(253)
Domestic servants	2(17)	-	-	-
Others/Unspecified	-	12(135)	12(145)	15(181)

Source: Bonke 1997.

Table 5: The male labour force 1970-1995, by year and socio-economic group: Percentages (%) with absolute numbers (thousands) in brackets

	1970	1980	1990	1995
Self-employed in agriculture	9 (132)	7 (100)	5 (72)	4 (58)
Self-employed in other industries	12 (176)	9 (129)	7(101)	8 (115)
Salaried employees, upper level	19 (279)	23 (329)	25 (360)	24 (346)
Salaried employees, lower level	9 (132)	14 (200)	15 (216)	13 (188)
Skilled manual workers	20 (294)	19 (272)	19 (273)	18 (260)
Unskilled manual workers	27 (397)	18 (257)	18 (259)	19 (274)
Workers in agriculture	4 (59)	2 (29)	1 (14)	1 (14)
Others/Unspecified	-	8 (114)	10 (144)	13 (188)

Source: Bonke 1997.

A. Educational Level

A large proportion of the Danish labour force is well educated and trained, and younger generations tend to receive longer education than the previous ones did, a trend that is particularly marked for women. Still, about one third has no education or training beyond basic school (table 6). Labour force participation is associated with educational background (table 7).

Table 6: Educational background of people aged 15-69 years in 2001, by highest completed education and gender (%)

	Men	Women
Basic school (9 years)	33	37
Upper secondary school (12 years)	8	9
Vocational training	38	30
Short- and medium-cycle higher education	13	18
University	6	4
No information	3	3

Source: Statistics Denmark 2003c.

Table 7: Education and occupational activity in 1991 among men and women aged 20-64 years (%)

Education*		Labour force participation in 1991		
		Active	Inactive	Total number
Basic school	Males	80	20	631,289
	Females	70	30	765,986
Vocational training	Males	93	7	627,995
	Females	89	11	455,173
Short-cycle higher education	Males	92	8	74,557
	Females	90	10	99,504
Medium-cycle higher education	Males	90	10	121,346
	Females	88	12	146,187
University	Males	84	16	115,073
	Females	72	28	65,467
Total	Males	87	13	1,570,260
	Females	79	21	1,532,317

* *Completed or completing, i.e. the figures for e.g. "University" include university students, a group that is typically "occupationally inactive".*
Source: Andersen et al. 2001.

B. Flexibility

Unlike many other industrialised countries, Denmark has no tradition of job security, and the labour market is characterised by very high flexibility.

No data are available as regards the prevalence of precarious jobs and short-term employment. It is likely, however, that these contracts are not prevalent because most employers may quickly and easily dismiss people employed on ordinary contracts. Nevertheless, precarious jobs are likely to predominate within the grey and black labour market, but data on this topic are not available.

C. Retirement

The age of ordinary retirement is 67 years (to be reduced to 65 years) for both men and women, but many people retire at an earlier age (optional from the age of 60). This is particularly the case for unskilled manual workers and low-level salaried employees. Occupational activity is rather low among people aged 60-66 years: in 2002, 44% were on early retirement benefit and 26% were receiving a disability pension, while 29% were still active.

D. Political Measures Influencing the Occupational Activity Rate

Depending on the economic and political situation, changing governments have attempted to influence the balance between economic activity and the size, structure, and qualifications of the labour force. Various labour market programmes have involved e.g. subsidised jobs in the public and private sectors, and various types of training. Other remedies have included alterations of the conditions for receiving welfare payments plus changes in the compensation level.

E. Trade Unions

The Danish unionisation rate is almost 80% and the unions, most of which are more or less formally associated with the social democrat party, may influence the political processes. However, most Danish unions are primarily concerned with collective bargaining issues, work environment issues, and international issues, but not very much with social inequality in health.

F. Conclusion

Within the last few decades, the size of the Danish labour force has grown dramatically because the vast majority of women have become occupationally active, mainly in the service sector, and most of them in full-time jobs. On average, the educational level of the labour force is quite high, and it is increasing in subsequent birth cohorts, a trend that is most marked for women. The Danish labour market is extremely flexible because of a very low level of job security.

3. Socio-economic Structure

In this paper, socio-economic status is generally defined in terms of association with the labour market. It might have been preferable to base the socio-economic grouping on a more stable parameter such as e.g. educational background, but being based on a review of the literature, this paper has had to adopt the definitions and groupings already made.

For each gender, the relative distribution of socio-economic groups in 2001 is displayed in table 8.

Table 8: The Danish population in 2001 by socio-economic group and gender, ages 15 years+ (%)

	Men	Women
Self-employed	8	2
Employed by spouse	-	1
Top-level managers	2	1
Employees, high level	8	7
Employees, medium level	8	12
Employees, basic level	26	24
Other employees	8	4
Employees, not otherwise specified	6	5
Unemployed	2	2
Pensioners	21	29
Other people outside the labour force	11	14

Source: Statistics Denmark 2003a.

Regarding the occupationally active part of the population, a consistent trend towards a higher share of salaried employees at the expense of (primarily) manual workers is obvious for both genders (tables 4-5).

A. People outside the Labour Market

Some people cannot, for somatic or mental reasons, live up to the labour market's demands. Being expelled from the labour force, these people typically find that their socio-economic positions deteriorate.

People who are classified as inactive do not, however, constitute a homogeneous group, but belong to a number of distinct sub-populations, including students and trainees, housewives and domestic helps, early-retired people, disability pensioners, and people on social benefit. Apart from the fact that these groups are not active on the labour market, they differ in most respects, including health behaviour. In the literature, however, the occupationally inactive groups are usually merged into a single category.

B. *Conclusion*

The socio-economic grouping applied in this paper is based on present labour market association. Among occupationally active people, a time trend towards a higher share of salaried employees is obvious.

4. Social Security

The Danish tax-financed welfare system provides the inhabitants with such social benefits as retirement pension, disability pension, sickness benefit, maternity leave benefit, social benefit, health care, and old-age care. Further, a partly tax-financed unemployment benefit is available to members of an unemployment fund, and to the same people, an early retirement benefit may also be available.

For people of occupationally active ages, the benefits and pensions are independent of previous income level, and most of the welfare payments compare in terms of amount paid per month. In 2002, the maximum welfare payments constituted 45% of the average earned income (Statistics Denmark 2003a). (Old-age pensions are considerably lower)

Formally, the welfare payments should be continuously regulated to keep up with the development in salaries and wages, but for many years, the regulation has been based on discretion, not on factual data. In consequence, the regulation has been defective, and the pensions and benefits have not followed the salaries and wages.

Living costs are high in Denmark: taxes/duties are high, and housing, transportation, kindergarten fees, and consumer goods are expensive. In consequence, the budget of most families is based on both parents earning a full-time income.

Compared with people who are occupationally active, people with no other earnings than the welfare payments may maintain only a humble standard of living. Recently, charity-based relief agencies, municipal social services departments, and cooperative housing societies have reported that a number of families living on social benefit are experiencing serious financial difficulties.

A. Retirement

From the age of ordinary retirement, everybody is paid a tax-financed retirement pension. In addition, many people have a supplementary private pension insurance scheme.

In 1979, early retirement from the age of 60 was made optional. From the start, the early retirement benefit was income-related and tax-financed, but this has been altered so that today the benefit is insurance-based, and for all practical purposes unrelated to previous income level.

B. Childbirth, Illness, and Disability

People, who are occupationally active, may receive a tax-financed sickness benefit when falling ill. Further, a tax-financed maternity/paternity leave benefit is available for occupationally active people. For most people, the benefit paid is unrelated to the person's ordinary income. However, many salaried employees receive full compensation during maternity or sick leave, the difference between the tax-financed benefit and the person's ordinary salary being financed by the employer.

People who develop diseases that prevent them from returning to their job may be referred to rehabilitation. However, for many years the resources for rehabilitation have been scarce, and recent legal changes mean that the present poor situation is likely to become worse. There are no public incentives for employers to organise rehabilitation.

People suffering from diseases that make them permanently incapable of working may be awarded a tax-financed disability pension. Recently, the legal acts that define the financing of disability pensions have been altered to the effect that disabled people have become less likely to be awarded a pension.

C. Social Benefit

People having no other earnings may receive a tax-financed social benefit to cover their basic needs. Recently, however, the Government has introduced a ceiling for the social benefit, which has meant that some impoverished families have had difficulties in paying their rent.

People on social benefit may have to accept working for a private entrepreneur or for the public sector, without being paid a wage and without being able to qualify for the right to unemployment benefit.

D. Unemployment

Unemployed people looking for a job may receive unemployment benefit, provided that they have been employed, have been members of an unemployment fund for a certain period, and have lost their job through no fault of their own.

The unemployment benefit is financed by the unemployment fund as well as by a particular tax. In 2002, the maximal compensation was DKK 157,040 (about USD 24,900) per year, while the average earned income was DKK 345,200 (about USD 54,700) per year (Statistics Denmark 2003a).

Unemployment benefit can only be obtained for a limited period, and only if the person is actively looking for a job and willing to accept a job far from home or within a trade with which he or she is not familiar.

Recent governmental initiatives aiming at restricting the right to unemployment benefit have prompted private insurance companies to launch supplementary unemployment insurance schemes, an initiative that is also based on the fact that for many employees, the compensation level is quite low.

E. Conclusion

The Danish welfare system provides people with a tax-financed social security net, but the system is becoming undermined because welfare payments have not followed salaries and wages. In consequence, many occupationally active people have opted to pay for supplementary private insurance.

5. Social Inequality in Health

The Danish life expectancy figures have been stagnant for some decades, a phenomenon that has received much political attention. The stagnating development in life expectancy was first observed for males in the early 1950s and for females in the early 1980s (Ingerslev *et al.* 1994); i.e. for both genders, the trend of stagnation appeared 30-35 years after the start of the smoking epidemic, which, roughly speaking, commenced after World War I in males, and after World War II in females, with an increasing prevalence of smokers in successive birth cohorts until recently.

An unhealthy lifestyle in terms of leisure time activity, diet, and smoking tends to be more prevalent in the lower socio-economic groups than in the higher ones, and the same seems to be true also for other types of risk-taking behaviour.

While smoking is one of the major causes of chronic disease and premature death in Denmark today, the very high overall frequency of people with a smoking history implies that the social gradient in smoking-related morbidity is played out against a high background level. For smoking-related diseases, relative morbidity measures are therefore rather insensitive in terms of detecting social or occupational heterogeneity.

A. Mortality

In general, age-specific death rates are much lower for women than for men, the male/female ratio being about 3 among young adults (20-34 years of age) and about 1.5 for people older than 35 years (Johansen and Jacobsen 2001).

In both genders, the mortality differs significantly by socio-economic status (figures 2-4) (standard of comparison: all occupationally active males/females).

Figure 2: Mortality (SMR), males, by period and socio-economic group

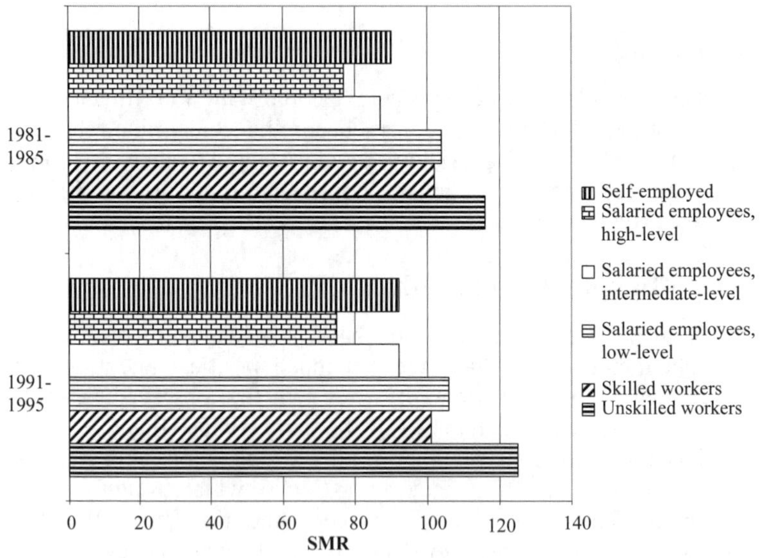

Source: Andersen et al. *2001.*

Figure 3: Mortality (SMR), females, by period and socio-economic group

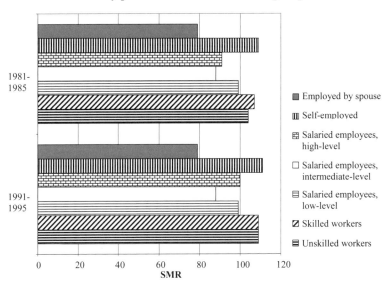

Source: Andersen et al. *2001.*

Figure 4: Mortality (SMR), occupationally inactive people, by period and gender

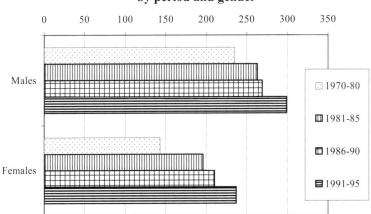

Source: Andersen 1985, Andersen et al. *2001.*

Among occupationally active men, data on standardised mortality ratio (SMR) during the period 1970-1995 (Andersen 1985, Andersen *et al.* 2001) (data not shown) indicate a time trend of increasing SMR for unskilled workers who also experience the highest SMR of all active groups. For skilled workers, the SMR has decreased slightly over time, while for the other active socio-economic groups, no time trend is seen. Within the group of salaried employees, a marked and stable social gradient is seen, with high-level salaried employees experiencing the lowest mortality of all the socio-economic groups considered. The general pattern is that the mortality is higher for manual workers (skilled or unskilled) and low-level salaried employees than for the rest of the occupationally active male population.

For occupationally active women, the mortality pattern for 1970-1995 is somewhat different and no time trend is seen (Andersen 1985, Andersen *et al.* 2001) (data not shown). While salaried employees in intermediate-level jobs and women employed by their spouse experience the lowest mortality of all active groups, self-employed women tend to experience the highest mortality.

People outside the labour market (figure 4) experience a much higher mortality than those who are occupationally active, a difference that seems to be increasing over time. However, the steep time trend seen for inactive women partly reflects the fact that in 1970, most (83%) of the 'inactive' women were housewives – a low-risk social category, which in 1991 had become almost non-existent. Danish women of today are expected and expect to hold a full-time job, and at present, inactive women constitute an extremely selected group.

It is worth noting that mortality is associated not only with labour market activity but also with educational background (table 9), a feature indicating that educational background reflects a person's underlying socio-economic 'priming' and indicates his or her real resources and options.

Table 9: Mortality during the period 1981-1995 among people aged 20-64 years, by labour market activity, educational background, and gender: standardised mortality ratio (SMR) for comparison with the total occupationally active population

		SMR	
		Active	Inactive
Basic school	Males	110	309
	Females	107	242
Vocational training	Males	100	296
	Females	95	224
Short-cycle higher education	Males	94	283
	Females	89	229
Medium-cycle higher education	Males	72	201
	Females	90	202
University	Males	73	182
	Females	87	172

(Absolute rates not available).
Source: Andersen et al. 2001.

Figure 5: Cause-specific mortality (SMR), males, 1970-1980

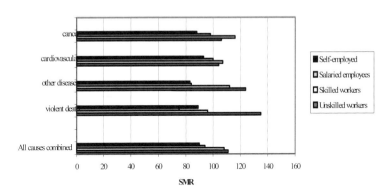

Source: Andersen 1985.

The major causes of premature death, including external causes, cancer, cardiovascular diseases, and 'other diseases', all contribute to the social heterogeneity seen for the years 1970-1980 (figures 5-7). Regrettably, comparable data (cause-specific mortality by socio-economic group) are not available for more recent years.

Figure 6: Cause-specific mortality (SMR), females, 1970-1980

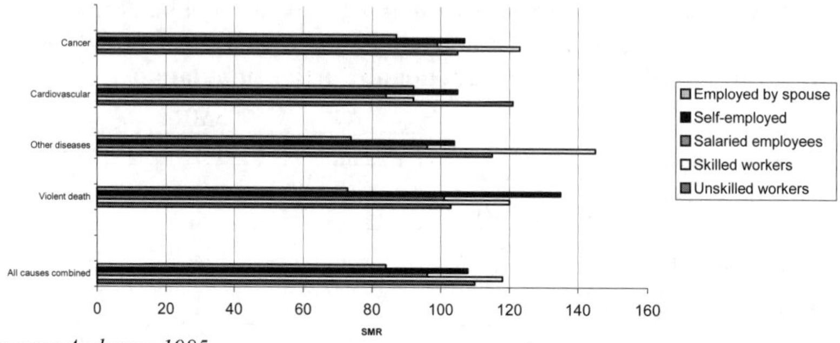

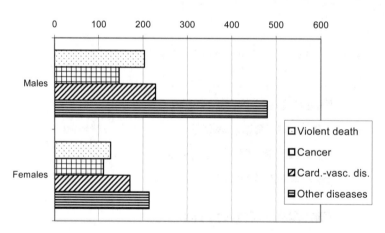

Source: Andersen 1985.

Figure 7: Cause-specific mortality (SMR) 1970-1980, occupationally inactive people in occupationally active ages

Source: Andersen 1985.

B. Cancer

The data on cancer mortality 1970-1980 (figures 5-7) indicate the presence of a social gradient for males, but not for females.

Regarding the mortality from respiratory cancer, manual workers (both genders) suffer a higher mortality than salaried employees do, while self-employed people (both genders) and women employed by their spouse display the lowest mortality from respiratory cancer (Andersen 1985).

For lung cancer, the incidence among people with low social status is 2-3 times that seen among people with high social status, even after control for smoking history (Engholm *et al.* 2003, Hein *et al.* 1992a). So, despite the fact that smoking is a strong causal factor for most types of lung cancer, the social disparity in lung cancer incidence can hardly be explained by differences in smoking habits between the groups compared.

C. Cardiovascular Diseases

For cardiovascular diseases, a social gradient resembling that seen for the total mortality appears, with the most marked disparity seen between people who are occupationally active and people who are not, a disparity that is seen in both genders (figures 5-7).

Within the occupationally active groups, the data on cardiovascular mortality 1970-1980 indicate a weak social gradient among males, with manual workers (skilled or unskilled) suffering the highest mortality, and self-employed people the lowest mortality (figure 5). Among occupationally active women, a rather high mortality from cardiovascular diseases is seen for unskilled workers, while otherwise no social gradient appears (figure 6). Ischaemic heart disease (IHD) is reported to stand for most of the social heterogeneity seen in women (Andersen 1985).

Mortality and incidence data from cohort studies on middle-aged males living in the Copenhagen region indicate the existence of a social gradient, even after controlling for a number of well-established risk factors including age, blood pressure, body mass index, physical activities during leisure time, and smoking and drinking habits (Hein *et al.* 1992b, Suadicani *et al.* 1997).

D. Mortality Due to Other Diseases

The mortality from diseases other than cancer and cardiovascular disease, 1970-1980, is much lower among people who are occupationally active than among those who are not (figures 5-7). Among occupationally active males, a marked social gradient appears with a lower SMR for self-employed and salaried employees than for skilled and unskilled workers (figure 5). Among occupationally active women, a gradient is seen for women employed by their spouse, salaried employees, and manual workers (skilled or unskilled), while self-employed women stand out with a relatively high SMR (figure 6).

E. Violent Death

Among males, a high SMR is seen among occupationally inactive people, 1970-1980, while among the occupationally active groups, unskilled male workers stand out with a high mortality (figures 5,7). No social gradient is seen among females (figures 6-7).

F. Self-Rated Health (SRH)

People who are occupationally active tend to rate their health as good or very good, and no marked social disparities are seen within this group, while almost 70% of the disability pensioners rate their health as less than good (table 10).

The overall time trend in 1994-2000 indicates a slight decrease in self-rated health, a decrease that is most marked among occupationally active people with low socio-economic status (table 10). Males generally rate their health slightly better than females do, but this difference seems to decrease over time.

Table 10: Prevalence of 'self-rated health less than good',
by year and socio-economic group, ages 16 years+,
both genders combined (%)

	1994	2000
Self-employed with no employees	19.9	19.6
Self-employed with employees	11.0	14.8
Higher-level salaried employees	9.0	8.0
Intermediate-level salaried employees	9.9	9.6
Lower-level salaried employees	11.5	14.1
Manual skilled workers	8.8	14.9
Manual unskilled workers	14.5	18.4
Students	8.2	10.7
Old-age pensioners	44.3	41.4
Disability pensioners	68.4	67.0
Housewives	26.1	(No data)
Unemployed	18.5	28.4
Early-retired people	(No data)	25.1
Other	28.9	44.4
Total	20.9	22.1
Males	17.1	20.5
Females	24.4	23.7

(Gender-specific data by socio-economic group not available).
Source: Kjøller et al. 1995, Kjøller and Rasmussen 2002.

The data indicate a weak tendency for unskilled manual workers to report sub-optimal health more often than other employees do (table 10), a finding that matches observations made in a 5-year panel study of Danish employees. The latter study indicated a social gradient in odds ratio for deteriorating self-rated health from "good" or "very good" to less than good within a 5-year period. About 10% of the sample deteriorated in SRH, while about 6% improved, but no social gradient was seen for improvement (Borg and Kristensen 2000).

G. Self-reported Long-standing Illness

Long-standing illness is extremely prevalent (about 90%) among disability pensioners, but it is also rather prevalent among people who are occupationally active, particularly among unemployed people (table 11). No social gradient is seen among the other groups of occupationally active people.

Table 11: Self-reported prevalence of long-standing illness, by year and socio-economic group, ages 16 years+, both genders combined (%)

	1994	2000
Self-employed with no employees	34.1	37.9
Self-employed with employees	22.7	30.9
Higher-level salaried employees	25.0	28.8
Intermediate-level salaried employees	27.6	31.7
Lower-level salaried employees	26.2	32.5
Manual skilled workers	25.8	29.7
Manual unskilled workers	28.5	32.9
Students	26.5	30.5
Old-age pensioners	60.5	60.3
Disability pensioners	83.3	87.6
Housewives	47.8	(No data)
Unemployed	40.1	45.1
Early-retired people	(No data)	47.4
Other	51.6	62.4
Total	37.6	41.1
Males	34.9	40.4
Females	40.1	41.7

(Gender-specific data by socio-economic group not available).
Source: Kjøller et al. 1995, Kjøller and Rasmussen 2002.

The time trend indicates an increasing prevalence of long-standing illness in all groups except retirement pensioners.

H. Conclusion

The data available indicate significant social inequalities in such health parameters as overall and cause-specific mortality, self-rated health, and self-reported prevalence of long-standing illness. Within the occupationally active ages, the most marked differences are seen between occupationally active and inactive people. Among people who are occupationally active, the mortality data and data on self-rated health indicate social inequalities, while the data on long-standing illness do not discriminate between the active socio-economic groups – a discrepancy that may partly be explained by a strong health-based selection expelling people of sub-optimal health from the labour market.

6. Working Conditions

Since men and women are typically employed in different trades and jobs, the exposure to most occupational health hazards differs by gender. For example, more males than females are exposed to physical and chemical agents, whereas more women than men are exposed to biomechanical hazards (National Institute of Occupational Health 2003b). As regards psychosocial hazards, no gender disparities are apparent.

Regarding time trends, the prevalence of noise exposure seems to have been increasing within the last decade, and an increase is also seen for self-reported exposure to fixed working postures and repetitive, overspecialised movements. On the other hand, the prevalence of exposure to heavy physical workloads has decreased markedly, in the same way as exposure to chemical agents (National Institute of Occupational Health 2003b).

Among employees, marked social disparities are seen for occupational exposure to physical, chemical, biomechanical, and climatic hazards or inconvenience, the prevalence being much higher among manual workers than among other employees, and the same is true for skin exposure to water and chemical substances (table 12).

Table 12: Self-reported prevalence of classic occupational exposures among Danish employees in 1995, by gender and socio-economic group: Percentage of the socio-economic group that reported the exposure in question (%)

	Salaried employees		Skilled manual workers	Unskilled manual workers		Total	
	Men	*Women*	*Both genders**	*Men*	*Women*	*Men*	*Women*
Fixed postures	28	10	68	59	18	43	14
Repetitive, overspecialised movements	42	8	41	73	18	49	11
Noise	33	24	46	45	19	37	21
Vibrations	39	36	22	58	31	43	35
Draught	20	3	36	41	10	31	6
Heat	24	1	19	45	4	28	2
Dry air	7	3	19	26	7	15	5
Organic solvent vapours	2	1	11	5	3	3	1
Mineral oil mists	16	6	9	29	13	23	12
Skin exposure to detergents or mineral oils	18	8	23	21	25	18	12

* Gender-specific data for skilled workers not available.
Source: Bonke 1997.

As regards psychosocial working conditions, almost one in ten employees work unsocial hours (table 13). Unsocial working hours occur in all groups of employees, but the prevalence is highest among unskilled manual workers. Further, an increasing number of employees report bad or sub-optimal psychosocial working conditions; e.g. the prevalence of high demands, low control, and lack of support seems to have increased significantly from 1900-1995 until 2000 (Borg and Burr 1997, Burr *et al.* 2002, National Institute of Occupational Health 2003b). (However, the questionnaire used in the 2000 survey differs markedly from the previous ones, and the data may not be comparable) While employees with low social status often experience low decision authority and high job insecurity, employees with high social status often experience high psychological demands and conflicts (table 14).

Table 13: Unsocial hours at work (i.e. working outside ordinary working hours) among Danish employees in 1995: Percentage of the socio-economic group that reported the exposure in question (%)

	Shift work	Night work	Other	Total
Salaried employees, high-level	1	1	5	7
Salaried employees, intermediate-level	7	1	4	12
Salaried employees, low-level	4	1	3	8
Skilled manual workers	8	1	1	10
Unskilled manual workers	7	3	4	14
Total	5	1	3	9

(Gender-specific data by socio-economic group not available) Source: Bonke 1997.

Table 14: Self-reported psychosocial work environment of Danish employees 1990, by socio-economic status: Percentage of the socio-economic group that reported the exposure in question (%)

	Socio-economic group				
	I	II	III	IV	V
High psychological demands	37	31	19	23	18
Low decision authority	6	14	22	24	42
Low social support	27	27	25	20	31
Low skill discretion	10	15	24	19	47
High level of conflicts	51	53	38	37	27
High job insecurity	4	8	13	11	14

I Higher salaried employees, II Intermediate salaried employees, III Lower salaried employees, IV Skilled manual workers, V Unskilled manual workers. Gender-specific data not available.
Source: Borg and Kristensen 2000.

Unfortunately, no data are available as to workplace exposure of self-employed people or people employed by their spouse.

A. Job Insecurity

In general, job security is not an issue in Denmark, and there is nei-ther legislation nor a tradition of employers being responsible for the job security of their employees. In fact, most employees can be dis-missed after three months' notice, and people may even be dismissed when they are on sick leave. In periods of increasing unemployment, the risk of losing one's job at short notice is likely to cause mental stress.

B. Commuting between Home and Work

An increasing number of people have to travel long distances be-tween work and home, a time-consuming necessity that is likely to increase the level of mental stress, in particular because most commuters travel by car. In 2000, commuters constituted 46% of the labour force with an average travelling distance of 54 km per working day (Johansen and Jacobsen 2001).

C. The Work Environment Act

At every workplace – except the smallest ones – the legislation requires the presence of a health and safety organisation (HSO). The HSO, which includes employer and employee representatives, is in charge of supervising the work environment and may ask for external expert assistance, e.g. from an occupational health service unit. The HSO representatives have to complete a specific work environment training (a '§9 course') paid for by the employer. The initiatives of the HSO may include e.g. replacement of hazardous substances and procedures with safer ones.

A particular characteristic of the Danish occupational health services (OHS) is that they are focused on occupational hygiene rather than on the medical treatment of individual employees. The OHS units are staffed with engineers, chemists, occupational therapists, physiotherapists, psychologists etc., while only a very few of them employ a medical doctor. By working in an interdisciplinary manner, the OHS units are usually well suited for problem-solving and for the implementation of preventive measures. In 2002, about 40% of Danish employees were covered by the OHS system, the trades covered including the most dangerous, heavy, and dirty ones.

D. Conclusion

A number of traditional work-related hazards still frequently occur in Danish workplaces and in addition, many employees report suboptimal psychosocial conditions. Among employees, marked differences are seen between manual and non-manual workers as regards workplace exposure to inconvenient or hazardous working conditions, including physical, chemical, biomechanical, and climatic exposures. Also, skin exposure to water and chemical substances occurs primarily among manual workers. Regarding psychosocial embarrassment, no social gradient is seen, but the type of problem differs between socioeconomic groups.

7. Work and Health

In view of the heterogeneous social distribution of a number of potentially hazardous occupational exposures (see above), one would expect a social gradient in health outcome related to the exposures in question. Those workplace exposures known to occur with a social gradient may cause hearing loss, musculoskeletal diseases, contact dermatitis, and a number of other diseases, including e.g. lung disease, cardiovascular disease, neurological disease, allergy and cancer. Unfortunately, population data on the social distribution of these adverse health outcomes are scant or non-existing.

A. Health-Based Selection of the Labour Force

People suffering from long-lasting health problems typically experience great difficulty in getting a job, and employed people tend to lose their job when they develop symptoms leading to long-term sick leave. To be active on the Danish labour market, good health is generally required, and people of sub-optimal health are likely to be expelled from the labour force.

People who lose their job for health reasons may be suffering from a work-related disease in the sense that occupational exposures have caused or contributed to the development of the disease in question. For instance, chronic and sub-chronic conditions such as obstructive lung disease, musculoskeletal diseases, and hand eczema may be incompatible with holding a manual job.

A strong health-based selection of the labour force is likely to mask a social gradient in work-related health, and in particular, cross-sectional studies may miss real differences.

B. Mortality

Regarding the overall mortality pattern, a marked occupational heterogeneity is seen, also within socio-economic strata (Andersen 1985).

For cardiovascular diseases, a follow-up study on middle-aged Copenhagen males has demonstrated a smoking-and-work relatedness of fatal IHD attacks: among men employed in jobs involving occasional vigorous physical activity, smoking was associated with a dramatic (six-fold) risk increase, while smoking did not seem to influence the risk in people holding other types of jobs (Suadicani *et al.* 2001). Other data from the same study have indicated an increased IHD mortality among men exposed to soldering fumes or organic solvents (Suadicani *et al.* 1997, Suadicani *et al.* 1995).

C. Cancer Incidence

Cancer registry data indicate an increased incidence of lung cancer among people employed in the production industry, construction, transportation, store and warehouse trades, hotels and restaurants, sailing and fishing (Lynge and Thygesen 1990, Olsen and Jensen 1987,

Andersen *et al.* 1999, Hansen and Meersohn 2003). In most of these trades, manual workers are likely to be exposed to dust and aerosols, many of which may be carcinogenic.

D. Notified Cases of Work-related Injuries

The Danish notification system for work-related injuries covers about half of the casualties due to occupational accidents with a marked trade-related heterogeneity in coverage. As regards work-related diseases, we have no data indicating the level of coverage, but the notified cases are likely to cover a rather small part of the true figures, mainly because most doctors do not notify a case of work-related disease unless the patient is likely to be indemnified.

Unfortunately, the notifications do not include the marine trades that are not under the auspices of the Danish Working Environment Authority.

Nevertheless, the notification figures may provide us with some idea about the predominant types of work-related injuries.

E. Occupational Accidents with Injury

Based on emergency department data, occupational casualties are estimated to cause about 10% of the contacts and to amount to 120,000 casualties per year. For comparison, the annual number of notified occupational casualities amounts to about 60,000 (National Working Environment Authority 2002).

As regards fatal occupational casualties, the incidence has slightly decreased within the last decade, with a present level around 60 deaths per year (figure 8) corresponding to an annual incidence rate of 2.2 per 100,000, or 4-5% of all violent deaths due to external causes among people of occupationally active ages. The male/female ratio is about 13: 1, and young and inexperienced workers are particularly at risk.

Figure 8: Notified occupational casualties: Number of deaths from occupational accidents, by year (both genders combined)

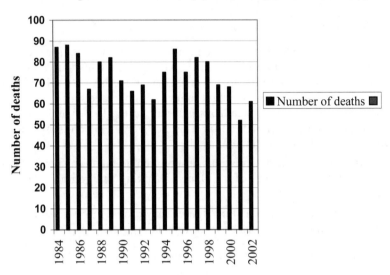

Source: National Working Environment Authority 2002, Autrup et al. *2003.*

Death while at work is primarily related to traffic accidents, work on scaffolds, and work with trucks and tractors etc. High-risk groups include males in a number of manual jobs, and the high-risk trades include agriculture, construction, the metal industry, and transportation.

Further, many people have to travel long distances between home and work, a necessity that increases the risk of death on the road. While death on the road between home and work is related to being occupationally active, commuter accidents are not registered as occupational accidents and we have no data indicating the size of this problem. But the fact that commuters constitute almost half of the labour force leaves much room for commuter-related casualties.

F. Work-related Diseases

According to the national notification data, the three most frequent work-related diseases are musculoskeletal diseases, loss of hearing, and hand eczema (National Working Environment Authority 2002).

Musculoskeletal Diseases

The Danish notification system for work-related diseases points out musculoskeletal disease as the most frequently notified diagnostic group, with an overall notification rate approximating 250 per 100,000 person years (National Working Environment Authority 2002).

A survey on general practioner (GP) contacts indicates that work-related musculoskeletal diseases occur frequently in the primary health sector: a work-relatedness was reported in 23% of the patients seeking medical help for low back pain, and in 40% of the patients presenting with symptoms located to the neck, shoulder, arm, or hand (Kibsgaard *et al*. 1998). These work-related symptoms seem to be particularly prevalent among people working in agriculture, construction, service trades, health care, and social care (Kibsgaard *et al*. 1998).

Further, hospitalisation data indicate that osteoarthritis of the knee occurs in excess among males employed in construction and agriculture, and among females employed in health care and social care; that cox-arthrosis occurs in excess among people employed in agriculture; and that prolapsed intervertebral disc of the cervical spine occurs in excess among people employed in health care and social care, among males employed in construction, transportation and service, and among female industrial workers (National Institute of Occupational Health 2003a).

Noise-induced Hearing Loss

The prevalence of premature loss of hearing is reported to be high among male skilled manual workers and self-employed men with no employees (Rasmussen *et al*. 1988), and screening data indicate that noise-induced hearing loss affects 35-40% of a middle-aged male population (Paving *et al*. 1983, Ostri and Paving 1991). For most people, however, a moderate hearing impairment does not impede occupational activity, and many cases of noise-induced hearing loss may remain undiagnosed.

The notification rate for work-related noise-induced hearing loss approximates 75 per 100,000 person years. A marked gender disparity appears, the male/female ratio being 20: 1. The notification rate is particularly high for people employed in construction and industry (National Working Environment Authority 2002).

Hand Eczema

The notification system identifies hand eczema as the most frequent occupational skin disorder, the overall notification rate being 55 per 100,000 person years (National Working Environment Authority 2002).

A particularly high risk is seen in food manufacturing, cleaning, care, hairdressing, metal industry, wood manufacturing, and construction work (National Working Environment Authority 2002). Hand eczema often forces the patient to find another type of job.

G. Self-rated Health and Self-reported Long-standing Illness

Among occupationally active people, population surveys have revealed no marked social gradient regarding these health parameters (Kjøller *et al.* 1995, Kjøller and Rasmussen 2002) and there seems to be no point in discussing the 'contribution' of work. However, a 5-year panel study over the period 1990-5 has indicated a social gradient in odds ratio for deteriorating self-rated health, and in a separate analysis of the subjects whose health deteriorated, a significant reduction of the social gradient was obtained by controlling for a number of lifestyle and work-related factors noted at baseline. The most important occupational factors seemed to be ergonomic and climatic exposures, repetitive work, skill discretion, and job insecurity (Borg and Kristensen 2000). Unfortunately, no information is available as to whether the people whose health deteriorated were still occupationally active at the time of the second survey in 1995.

H. Conclusion

Mortality data indicate considerable disparities between occupational groups, also within social strata. Disparities are seen for violent death as well as for cancer, cardiovascular diseases, and other diseases.

Notification data from the National Working Environment Authority indicate that musculoskeletal diseases, hearing loss, and hand eczema are the most frequently occurring work-related diseases; and that occupational accidents cause about 4-5% of the total number of violent deaths occurring among people of occupationally active ages.

Regarding self-rated health, panel data indicate an association of deteriorating self-rated health and certain workplace factors, while survey data display a less marked social gradient among occupationally active people.

Many states of sub-optimal health are incompatible with labour market participation, and the resulting health-based selection of the labour force complicates the study of many work-disease relations.

8. Discussion

Social inequalities in health reflect inequalities in lifelong living conditions, together with the negative socio-economic consequences of disabling disease. Considering the importance of a life-course perspective on health impairment, long-term follow-up data are likely to be much more sensitive than cross-sectional data, particularly when health-based selection is operating.

A. Mortality

Regarding socio-economic disparities in mortality, the most significant finding is that within the occupationally active ages, mortality is much lower among labour force participants than among non-participants. The mortality of the occupationally inactive group is two to three times that of the active group – a mortality gap that seems to be widening over time. For both genders, a marked gradient in mortality is also seen for educational level among occupationally active people as well as among those who are inactive.

Further, among people who are occupationally active, a negative social gradient is seen for both genders: on average, an active man or woman with a low social position dies at a younger age than an active man or woman with a high social position, the only marked exception being self-employed women that seems to experience an overall mortality comparable to that of female manual workers. Data on occupational mortality indicate a considerable disparity within socio-economic strata concerning total mortality as well as violent death, cancer, cardiovascular diseases and other diseases (Andersen 1985).

Among people of occupationally active ages, 4-5% of deaths due to external causes are caused by occupational accidents (Statistics Denmark 2003a, Andersen 1985, National Working Environment Authority 2002), with agriculture, construction, transport services, and the metal industry standing out as involving particularly high risks. The high risk of violent death seen among unskilled male labourers may partly be due to fatal occupational accidents.

B. Non-fatal Diseases, Signs and Symptoms

If emergency department contacts are taken as indicator, occupational accidents account for about 10% of the acute morbidity. Alternatively, if contact with a GP is taken as a measure of sub-acute and chronic morbidity, work-related conditions account for about 16% of the morbidity, with the figure amounting to 35% for contacts related to musculoskeletal diseases (Kibsgaard *et al.* 1998). Further, hospitalisation data indicate that employment in certain trades involves an excess risk of a number of diseases, including musculoskeletal diseases, upper digestive tract ulcers, hernia, and varicose veins (National Institute of Occupational Health 2003a).

Musculoskeletal Diseases

Musculoskeletal diseases, and in particular conditions causing low back pain, are prevalent in the Danish population (National Institute of Occupational Health 2003a, Rasmussen *et al.* 1988, Kjøller *et al.* 1995,

Kjøller and Rasmussen 2002), a feature that makes it difficult to recognise potential differences between socio-economic or occupational subgroups.

Among people who are occupationally active, self-reported prevalence data on musculoskeletal disease do not indicate a social gradient. However, the prevalence seems to be associated with level of education (Kjøller *et al.* 1995), and among salaried employees, a slight social gradient has been described (Kjøller and Rasmussen 2002). For certain diagnoses, such as coxarthrosis of the hip or knee, and prolapsed cervical disc, a more distinct pattern emerges, revealing that particular occupations involve a high risk (National Institute of Occupational Health 2003a). The same is also true for musculoskeletal diseases affecting the smaller muscle groups located to the neck, shoulder, arm, wrist, and hand. For the latter group of diseases, occupational exposures are reported to be involved in almost half of the GP contacts (Kibsgaard *et al.* 1998).

Work-related exposure to various types of biomechanical strain is quite prevalent, but differs between males and females and between occupational groups. Occupational exposures may have contributed to the development of many cases of musculoskeletal disease seen in primary care (Kibsgaard *et al.* 1998), and the heterogeneity of occupational exposure over socio-economic groups is likely to bring about a social inequality in musculoskeletal health.

Hearing Loss

Hearing impairment is prevalent in Denmark, with a particularly high prevalence of self-reported hearing impairment among male skilled workers and self-employed males with no employees (Rasmusen *et al.* 1988). As regards noise-induced hearing impairment, the prevalence among middle-aged men is 35-40% (Parving *et al.* 1983, Ostri and Parving 1991).

About 50% of occupationally active males report exposure to high levels of work-related noise (Parving *et al.* 1983, Bonke 1997). Occupational noise exposure tends to be prevalent among people employed in construction and industry, a feature that is in agreement with the observed high prevalence of self-reported hearing impairment among male skilled workers and self-employed males (Rasmussen *et al.* 1988).

Based on the data available, it seems likely that occupational noise exposure has contributed, and is still contributing, significantly to the development of noise-induced hearing loss – a rather prevalent chronic condition that reduces quality of life. Because of the distribution of occupational noise exposure, it is most likely that work contributes to a social inequality in noise-induced hearing loss.

Work-related Hand Eczema

Skin disorders located to the hand or forearm affect about one in eight occupationally active Danes (National Institute of Occupational Health 2003b) and in most cases, occupational exposures are of major importance. The most widespread environmental risk factors for work-related hand eczema are prevalent in a number of manual jobs, but rare in the upper social strata. Due to the disparity of exposures, the incidence of hand eczema is likely to display a marked social gradient. Since hand eczema often forces the patient to find another type of job, prevalence data are likely to underestimate the magnitude of this health problem.

Self-rated Health and Self-reported Long-standing Illness

Among people who are occupationally active, a parallel to the social gradient seen for mortality does not appear in the survey data on long-standing illness and is not as pronounced as one might assume for self-rated health (Rasmussen *et al.* 1988, Kjøller *et al.* 1995, Kjøller and Rasmussen 2002).

This discrepancy seems intriguing, since it is a well-known fact that self-reported poor health is a superior prognostic indicator of approaching death. However, as long as they are not seriously ill, most people will tend to state their health as good when asked about their general health status. (This may in fact explain the superior predictive value – in terms of individual life expectancy – of people's answer to the question: "Is your health very good, good, fair, poor, or very poor?")

Next, health perception and behaviour is likely to differ between people belonging to different socio-economic groups, as most people tend to compare their health with that of their peers, i.e. with people sharing their living conditions, lifestyle, and standard of health. In addition, people with little or no education beyond basic school may not report signs of sub-optimal health unless they are asked very specific questions. For example, asking a group of unskilled manual workers whether they have 'respiratory symptoms' is likely to be unproductive, while asking the same people specific questions about the frequency of cough, expectoration, difficulty in breathing etc. may reveal a high prevalence of symptoms.

Further, a survey, with its cross-sectional design, is extremely vulnerable to health-based selection, a selection that may totally blur a real work-health relation.

C. Occupationally Inactive People

Within the occupationally active ages, an excess mortality is seen for occupationally inactive males and females at any educational level. In like manner, the occupationally inactive group stands out with a high prevalence of long-standing illness and low self-rated health. The excess morbidity and mortality seen among people outside the labour force indicates that those who are occupationally inactive generally have serious health problems.

D. Health-based Selection of the Labour Force

The significant health gap between people who are occupationally active and people who are not, indicates that the Danish labour force is subject to a rather effective health-based selection, resulting in people of sub-optimal health being squeezed out of the labour market.

Among people who have no education beyond basic school, the in-activity rate is high, and those who are occupationally active typically have unskilled manual jobs or low-level salaried jobs. In other words, these people are employed in jobs that often involve low control, high demands, unsocial working hours, heavy workloads, fixed postures, noise, and inhalation of, or skin contact with chemical and biological components – exposures that may cause chronic disease.

The general lack of job security characterising the Danish labour market facilitates the expulsion of people with sub-optimal health. Having no legal or informal obligation to guarantee their employees an earned living, many employers do not hesitate to dismiss a person on long-term sick leave, and most employers avoid taking on people with sub-optimal health.

At present, the Danish labour market in general is not for people with sub-optimal health, particularly not if they have no educational qualifications. A large part of those who are occupationally inactive have been expelled from the labour market for health reasons, and some of these people have become worn out early in life because of their work.

We lack reliable population data on the work-and-health relatedness of labour market expulsion. However, it is beyond any doubt that – due to the health-based selection of the active labour force – a considerable part of the burden of disease seen among occupationally inactive people should be ascribed to prior occupational exposures.

The existence of an efficient social security net has undoubtedly influenced the incentives and conduct of employers, labour unions, and people suffering from sub-optimal health. The tough health-based selection of the labour force and the general job insecurity would hardly be tolerable – morally and politically – if it were not for the tax-financed welfare system that provides people outside the labour market with a living. The delicate balance between job insecurity, health-based selection, and availability of welfare benefits is vulnerable to political changes, and disturbances are likely to cause social instability as long as people of sub-optimal health are being squeezed out of the very selective and highly competitive labour market.

E. Conclusion

Occupational exposures may play a role in the aetiology and pathogenesis of most chronic and sub-chronic diseases, and because of the marked social disparity in working conditions, the risk of work-related diseases is likely to be much higher in lower socio-economic groups than in the higher ones – an inequality contributing to the social inequality in health. However, the major part of this work-related inequality is likely to go undetected because of the health-based selection of the labour force – a selection that is generally most restrictive for low-status jobs. Thus, those who have been expelled from the labour market are likely to carry a major part of the burden of work-related disease.

9. Perspectives for the Next Decades

A. Unemployment and Job Insecurity

According to the 'European Round Table', the overvalued US dollar presents an imminent threat to the world economy: a devaluation of the US dollar will weaken the competitive position of most other economies, including those of the 'Euro zone', and will most likely result in increasing unemployment. (The Danish currency is tied to the Euro, and will follow any *de facto* revaluation of the Euro).

Further, the advance of technology is likely to go on increasing the percentage of jobs that require certain theoretical skills, while the number of jobs for people with no qualifications beyond basic school is likely to decrease.

In consequence, many people may lose their job – a process that is facilitated by the very low level of job security in the Danish labour market. Further, unemployed people may be more willing to accept a low-paid and inconvenient job far from home, and those who still have a job may become anxious about losing it.

As regards health issues, a high risk of becoming unemployed is likely to increase the level of mental stress and increase the incidence of a number of stress-associated mental and somatic disorders.

B. Wages under Pressure

Compared with many other European countries, Danish salaries and wages are high, and many industrial plants employing unskilled manual workers are now transferring their production to low-wage countries.

Another trend is that labourers from Eastern European countries are being hired by a local or Danish entrepreneur to work in Denmark for a wage much below the Danish standard. The problem of underpaying is particularly pertinent within the construction sector and in farming, forestry, and gardening. Today (in 2003), this traffic is illegal, but as a consequence of the future expansion of the European Union to also include a number of Eastern European countries, the practice of under-paying labourers from these countries may become legitimate. Obvi-ously, this will put pressure on Danish wages, and it is easy to imagine how this may bring about social animosity towards the underpaid for-eign workers.

C. The Work Environment under Pressure

With increasing unemployment and underpaying, the labour market is getting tougher, and among other things this is likely to reduce the standard of the work environment.

In addition, a side effect of many EU regulations and directives im-proving the conditions for trade and commerce has been a reduction of the protection level for Danish workers and consumers, while the EU legislation on working conditions is dominated by a deregulation trend. Recent examples include the directive on part-time work and the bill on services.

At the national level, the Government recently has cut the budgets for the National Working Environment Authority, reconstructed the labour inspectorate organisation, and reduced the number of unnotified workplace control visits. Further, a recent reform has relaxed the legis-lation on workplace health and safety organisations and occupational health services – the effect being that fewer working people are covered and that the service level is reduced.

D. Social Security and Health: From Welfare to Insurance

Being a member of the EU, Denmark must adapt to the so-called in-ternal EU market. One major consequence of this adaptation is that we cannot retain our tax-financed welfare system, because in the near future any EU citizen may claim for welfare payments financed by Danish tax payers.

As described previously in this chapter, the compensation level of our welfare payments is now so low that many people have opted to pay for a supplementary private insurance scheme. A similar process from tax-financed welfare towards private insurance is seen for the health services, mainly due to political incentives that put strict limitations on public expenditure at the county and municipal level – limitations that affect the resources allotted to the public health care system.

E. Conclusion

If the trends seen during the last three decades continue for another decade or two, a future scenario may be depicted in which the Danish society is becoming still more segregated and polarised, to the effect that people outside the labour force become further marginalised and impoverished. In short: unless the prevailing trends are reversed, all kinds of social inequalities, including inequality in health are likely to increase significantly.

References

ANDERSEN A., BARLOW L., ENGELAND A., KJAERHEIM K., LYNGE E., PUKKALA E. 1999. "Work-related cancer in the Nordic countries", *Scand. J. Work Environ. Health* 25 Suppl 2: 1-116.

ANDERSEN O. 1985. *Occupational Mortality 1970-80. Statistical Studies* 41. Copenhagen: Statistics Denmark.

ANDERSEN O., LAURSEN L., PETERSEN J.K. 2001. *Occupational Mortality 1981-1995.* Copenhagen: Statistics Denmark.

AUTRUP H., BONDE J.P., RASMUSSEN K., SIGSGAARD T. (eds.). 2003. *Occupational and Environmental Medicine.* Copenhagen: FADL.

BACH E., BORG V., HANNERZ H., MIKKELSEN K.L., POULSEN O., TÜCHSEN F. 2002. *Work Environment and Health.* Copenhagen: National Institute of Occupational Health.

BONKE J. (ed.). 1997. *Living conditions in Denmark: Compendium of Statistics 1997.* Copenhagen: Statistics Denmark and the National Institute of Social Research.

BORG V., KRISTENSEN T.S. 2000. "Social Class and Self-Rated Health: Can the Gradient Be Explained by Differences in Life Style or Work Environment?", *Soc Sci Med* 51: 1019-30.

BORG V., BURR H. (eds.). 1997. *Work Environment and Health of Danish Employees 1990-95.* Copenhagen, National Institute of Occupational Health.

BURR H., BACH E., BORG V., VILLADSEN E. 2002. *Work Environment in Denmark 2000.* Copenhagen: National Institute of Occupational Health.

ENGHOLM G., PALMGREN F., LYNGE E. 1996. "Lung Cancer, Smoking, and Environment: A cohort study of the Danish population", *BMJ* 312: 1259-63.

HANSEN J., MEERSOHN A. 2003. *Cancer incidence (1970-97) among Danish employees*. Copenhagen: National Working Environment Authority.

HEIN H.O., SUADICANI P., GYNTELBERG F. 1992. "Lung Cancer Risk and Social Class. The Copenhagen Male Study, 17-years' follow up", *Dan. Med. Bull.* 39: 173-6.

HEIN H.O., SUADICANI P., GYNTELBERG F. 1992. "Ischemic heart disease incidence by social class and form of smoking: the Copenhagen Male Study, 17 years' follow-up", *J. Intern. Med.* 231: 477-83.

INGERSLEV O., MADSEN M., ANDERSEN M. 1994. *Social Mortality Disparities in Denmark*. Copenhagen: Report to the Ministry of Health.

JOHANSEN B., JACOBSEN L. (eds.). 2001. *Statistical Ten-Year Review*. Copenhagen: Statistics Denmark.

KIBSGAARD K.A., ANDERSEN J.H., RASMUSSEN K. 1998. "Occupational Medicine in General Practice. A study of the extent and nature of occupational injuries in the county of Ringkjobing". *Ugeskr Laeger* 160: 4863-7.

KJØLLER M., RASMUSSEN N.K., KEIDING L., PETERSEN H.C., NIELSEN G.A. 1995. *Danish Health and Morbidity Survey 1994, and Trends since 1987*. Copenhagen: Danish Institute of Clinical Epidemiology.

KJØLLER M., RASMUSSEN N.K. 2002. *Danish Health and Morbidity Survey 2000, and Trends since 1987*. Copenhagen: National Institute of Public Health.

LYNGE E., THYGESEN L. 1990. "Occupational Cancer in Denmark. Cancer incidence in the 1970 census population". *Scand. J. Work Environ. Health* 16 Suppl 2: 3-35.

NATIONAL INSTITUTE OF OCCUPATIONAL HEALTH: *National Population Data on Hospitalization and Trade*. http://www.ami.dk/nationaledata/1.html. National Institute of Occupational Health, Copenhagen 2003a.

NATIONAL INSTITUTE OF OCCUPATIONAL HEALTH: *The National Work Environment Cohort, Work Environment in Denmark 2000*. http://www.ami.dk /nationale%20data/den%20nationale%20arbejdsmiljøkohorte%20%20nak.as px. National Institute of Occupational Health, Copenhagen 2003b.

NATIONAL WORKING ENVIRONMENT AUTHORITY: *Notified Occupational Injuries 2001*. National Working Environment Authority, Copenhagen 2002.

OLSEN J.H., JENSEN O.M. 1987. "Occupation and Risk of Cancer in Denmark. An analysis of 93,810 cancer cases, 1970-1979", *Scand. J. Work Environ. Health* 13 Suppl 1: 1-91.

OSTRI B., PARVING A. 1991. "A longitudinal study of hearing impairment in male subjects, an 8-year follow-up", *Br. J. Audiol.* 25: 41-8.

PARVING A., OSTRI B., POULSEN J., GYNTELBERG F. 1983. "Epidemiology of Hearing Impairment in Male Adult Subjects at 49-69 Years of Age", *Scand. Audiol.* 12: 191-6.

RASMUSSEN N.K., GROTH M.V., BREDKJÆR S., MADSEN M., KAMPER-JØRGENSEN F. 1988. *Danish Health and Morbidity Survey 1987*. Copenhagen: Danish Institute of Clinical Epidemiology.

STATISTICS DENMARK: *Statistical Yearbook 2003*. Statistics Denmark, Copenhagen 2003a.

STATISTICS DENMARK: *Denmark in Numbers 2003*. Statistics Denmark, Copenhagen 2003b.

STATISTICS DENMARK: *The Danish Bank of Statistics http://www.statistikbanken.dk/statbank*, Statistics Denmark, Copenhagen 2003c.

SUADICANI P., HEIN H.O., GYNTELBERG F. 1997. "Strong Mediators of Social Inequalities in Risk of Ischemic Heart Disease: A six-year follow-up in the Copenhagen Male Study", *Int. J. Epidemiol.* 26: 516-22.

SUADICANI P., HEIN H.O., GYNTELBERG F. 1995. "Do Physical and Chemical Working Conditions Explain the Association of Social Class with Ischemic Heart Disease?", *Atherosclerosis* 113: 63-9.

SUADICANI P., HEIN H.O., GYNTELBERG F. 2001. "Socioeconomic status and ischemic heart disease mortality in middle-aged men: importance of the duration of follow-up. The Copenhagen Male Study", *Int. J. Epidemiol.* 30: 248-55.

TÜCHSEN F., BACH E., MARMOT M. 1992. "Occupation and Hospitalization with Ischemic Heart Diseases: A new nationwide surveillance system based on hospital admissions", *Int. J. Epidemiol.* 21: 450-9.

France

Isabelle NIEDHAMMER & Annette LECLERC

Introduction

This chapter presents the French situation regarding the labour market, employment, working conditions, social inequalities in health and the contribution of work to these inequalities.

Health at work has only recently been considered as a public health concern in France. In the same way, social inequalities in health have been considered as a public health priority since the mid-1990s (Haut comité de la Santé Publique 2002). Until recently, research efforts on social inequalities in health have been almost non-existent.

Social inequalities in health in France have been described in a collective book (Leclerc *et al.* 2000), and may be more pronounced in France than in other European countries, especially for premature mortality among men. Despite this fact, little research has been conducted until now to gain a better understanding of social inequalities in health, and try to evaluate the contribution of work to these inequalities. It should be noted that national data are available either on work and working conditions, or on health, and to our knowledge no available data would enable the simultaneous study of work and health among a large representative sample of the French population. Cohort studies have been conducted for example among specific sectors of activity, and could provide some insights into the questions treated in this chapter. Consequently, research has begun and we can look forward to the presentation of results later on.

The first section in this chapter describes the labour market, employment, working conditions, and how they have evolved over the last two decades. This section also underlines the social differences regarding employment and working conditions. A second section is about social inequalities in health, in terms of morbidity and mortality. A third section tackles the contribution of work to social inequalities in health; as French data on this subject are almost non-existent, an attempt has been made to explain social differences in self-reported health by some indicators of working conditions from the data of a prospective study among a cohort of workers employed by the national company for gas and electricity. A fourth section deals with social policies and their potential contribution to the reduction of social inequalities in health. Finally, the last section provides some conclusions and prospects for future research.

1. The Labour Market, Employment and Working Conditions in France: Description, Developments over the Past Twenty Years and Social Differences

A. The Total Population, the Working Population, Rates of Activity and Situations of Inactivity

According to the French population census of 1999, the population aged 15 years or more, i.e. more than 23 million men and nearly 25 million women, is distributed as follows: 56% of the men and 41% of the women are employed, 7% of the men and women are unemployed, 22% of the men and women are retired, 11% of the men and women are students, and 4% of the men and 19% of the women are in other situations of inactivity. According to the 1999 population census, the working population in France therefore comprises 26.5 million persons, 12.2 million of them women, and 14.3 million, men. This total includes 23.1 million actively employed persons and 3.4 million self-reported as unemployed. According to the figures supplied by the censuses conducted in 1982, 1990 and 1999, the working population has grown, but the growth slowed down during the 1990s. Since 1982, the rate of activity according to age group, i.e. the size of the working population in relation to that of the total population, has remained practically unchanged for men, but has continued to increase for women of all age groups between 25 and 59 years, thus confirming the trend observed since the 1960s. Note, too, that the rate of activity has declined for the youngest age groups (24 years or less) and for the oldest (60 years or more). The decline in the latter group is due to the lowering of the full retirement age to 60 years in 1982. In 1999, women constituted 46% of the working population, but in 1990, only 44% (Bourlès and Courson 2000). In 2002, the rate of activity for persons aged 15 to 64 years was 68%, and the rate for women continued to catch up with the rate for men: it was 62% in 2002 compared with 61% in 1999, as against 74% for men in both 1999 and 2002. It is true that in 2002, women of all age groups still had rates of activity lower than those for men, but the differences between the rates for men and women have decreased considerably since 1968. For the 20-24, 25-49 and 50-59 age groups, the rates in 2002 were 56, 95 and 81% respectively for men, and 47, 80 and 65% for women (INSEE 2002).

According to the Observatoire de l'Emploi Public (2004), the number of wage earners (with a permanent contract or not) working in the public sector was around 5,000,000 people, who accounted for 22% of all wage earners in 2001.

According to the census of 1999, there were 4,310,000 immigrants in France, defined as any person born outside France who lives in France, whatever his or her nationality. Immigrants represented 7.4% of the total population, a rate that has been stable since 1975 (Boëldieu and Borrel 2000). In 1999, the number of immigrant workers was 2,294,000, i.e. 8.6% of the total working population (Borrel and Boëldieu 2001).

The 'Handicaps, Incapacités, Dépendance' (HID) survey (Mormiche 2003) gives the number of persons in different employment categories in 1999 for the 30 to 65 age groups, with details concerning those who are not employed and who are classified as follows: employed (including self-employed), unemployed (but trying to find work), students, homemakers, retired, and other unoccupied persons, including those who are not working for health reasons. 'Early-retired' and 'retired' persons are grouped together in table 1. The reasons for unwanted early retirement are mostly economic (Such retirement is one of the social repercussions of an employer's economic problems.). For a person who is too young to retire by law but is chronically ill, the only possibilities are either to go on working or to become 'otherwise unoccupied', which means a drastic reduction of income. Those who are not employed are distributed among the different categories as shown in table 2.

Table 1: Percentage of persons not employed
(not employed/number of persons, in each age-sex group)

	30-49	50-59	60-64
Men	10.3	25.5	91.3
Women	27.2	48.7	92.1

Source: HID survey, 1999.

**Table 2: Situation of those not employed (in % of the total
of those not employed in each age-sex group)**

	30-49		50-59		60-65	
	Men	Women	Men	Women	Men	Women
Unemployed	72.2	32.3	19.4	11.2	0.3	4.4
Studying	3.7	0.2	-	-	-	-
Homemakers		56.1		57.2		26.0
Retired	0.5	3.5	44.6	18.2	98.5	67.9
Otherwise unoccupied	23.5	7.9	35.9	13.3	1.2	1.6
Total	100	100	100	100	100	100
Number, unoccupied	851,865	2,370,758	844,825	1,625,716	1,162,717	1,249,820

Source: HID survey, 1999.

B. Educational Levels, Occupational Categories, Sectors of Activity and Earnings

During the past 15 years, the French educational system has under-gone profound changes. In the middle of the 1980s, the objective was to enable 80% of the youngsters to complete their secondary education by 2000 in order to raise their qualifications, prepare them better for the economic transformations and reduce the number of school leavers without any qualifications. In 2000, 70% of the young were able to take the school-leaving exam (*baccalauréat*), compared with 36% in 1986. The proportion of those who passed was 62% in 2000, compared with 31% in 1986, i.e. the figures doubled in 15 years. Thus, according to the census figures, the youngest generations are the highest qualified: 30% of those aged at least 25 years said they had the baccalauréat in 1999, compared with 22% in 1990 and 13% in 1975. It is also noteworthy that today, women have higher university degrees than men (table 3). In addition, the employment surveys show that 38% of young people today leave the education system with a university degree, and 8% without any qualification. In 1980, both these figures were 15% (Esquieu and Poulet-Coulibando 2002). Nevertheless, although the past twenty years have seen a marked rise in the overall educational level of the French population, especially among the youngest, unemployment, the time it takes to find a job, the qualifications needed and job remuneration, are all closely dependent on the level of degrees and qualifications. Fur-thermore, since 1995, the number of unskilled jobs has risen by 14%. This rise, which is linked to a trend towards rising employment, and to measures to reduce the social contributions of the lowest wage earners, has only favoured in part the access to employment of the least qualified unemployed. Taking into account both the qualifications required for jobs and the degrees of those employed in them, this paradox indicates the 'devaluation' of university and other degrees for people in jobs that require lower qualifications (Audric 2002, Chardon 2001). In addition, the general lengthening of the period of schooling has only been accompanied by a partial reduction in social inequalities regarding access to teaching (Goux and Maurin 1997, Thélot and Vallet 2000). It is, in particular, noteworthy that despite the relative democratisation of higher education, the social inequalities of access to France's *élite* establishments – the *Grandes Écoles* – persisted and even increased during the 1980s (Albouy and Wanecq 2003).

Table 3: The French population of 25 years or more, by sex and qualification, according to the 1999 census

Men	Studies in progress	No qualification Primary	School-leaving certificate	University degree	Total
25-29 years	120,410	302,858	1,077,522	590,583	2,091,373
%	5.8	14.5	51.5	28.2	100
30-39 years	20,965	789,198	2,446,132	1,004,137	4,260,432
%	0.5	18.5	57.4	23.6	100
40-59 years	-	2,240,760	3,892,549	1,415,376	7,548,685
%	-	29.7	51.6	18.7	100
60 years or more	-	3,226,469	1,566,705	490,886	5,284,060
%	-	61.1	29.6	9.3	100
Women					
25-29 years	124,329	275,554	948,308	738,212	2,086,403
%	6.0	13.2	45.4	35.4	100
30-39 years	20,349	793,077	2,340,290	1,164,268	4,317,984
%	0.5	18.4	54.2	26.9	100
40-59 years	-	2,676,796	3,596,018	1,371,882	7,644,696
%	-	35.0	47.0	18.0	100
60 years or more	-	5,034,022	1,785,936	374,109	7,194,067
%	-	70.0	24.8	5.2	100

Source: Census, INSEE, 1999.

The French classification by INSEE (National Institute for Statistics and Economic Studies) of occupations is generally used in national surveys designed to describe the working population (Nomenclature des professions et catégories socio-professionnelles 2003). The present authors will deal here with six main categories which are close to the international standard classification of occupations (1990). These categories comprise: farmers; self-employed workers (including craft trades workers, business agents and company managers, etc.); managers (including departmental managers, engineers, as well as teaching, health and science professionals, etc.): associate professionals (including technicians, foremen, as well as administrative, health, social work and teaching associate professionals, etc.); clerks and service workers; and blue-collar workers. In this chapter, the occupational categories will refer to this classification. The distribution of the working population among the six main INSEE categories, according to the population censuses of 1982 and 1999 (excluding the military and the unemployed who had never worked), is presented in table 4 (Amossé 2001, Amossé and Chardon 2002). The distribution for men and women is shown in table 5, and shows that more women than men are employed as clerks or service workers and as associate professionals (Grcic and Morer 2002, Djider 2002). Note also that immigrants are more likely to be employed as blue-collar workers and service workers (Borrel and Boëldieu 2001, Thave 2000). Table 6 presents the distribution of immigrants according to occupational category for men and women.

Table 4: Distribution of the actively employed population among occupational categories in 1982 and 1999

	1982		1999		Change 1982-1999
	N	%	N	%	%
Farmers	1,466,000	6.8	627,000	2.7	-57
Self-employed	1,815,000	8.5	1,525,000	6.6	-16
Managers	1,860,000	8.7	3,023,000	13.1	+63
Associate professionals	3,784,000	17.6	5,318,000	23.1	+40
Clerks and service workers	5,502,000	25.6	6,655,000	28.9	+21
Blue-collar Workers	7,044,000	32.8	5,905,000	25.6	-16
Total	21,472,000	100	23,053,000	100	

Source: Census, INSEE, 1982, 1999 (Amossé 2001).

Table 5: Distribution of the actively employed population among occupational categories for men and women in 2001

	Women		Men		
	N	%	N	%	% women
Farmers	200,000	1.9	414,000	3.2	32.6
Self-employed	429,000	4.0	1,018,000	7.8	29.6
Managers	1,183,000	11.1	2,203,000	16.8	34.9
Associate professionals	2,382,000	22.4	2,662,000	20.3	47.2
Clerks and service workers	5,189,000	48.7	1,695,000	12.9	75.4
Blue-collar workers	1,272,000	11.9	5,087,000	38.8	20.0
Military	1,000	0.0	26,000	0.2	3.7
Total	10,653,000		13,105,000		

Source: Employment survey, INSEE, 2001 (Djider 2002).

Table 6: Distribution of immigrants (%) according to occupational categories for men and women in 1999

	Men		Women	
	Total population	Immigrants	Total population	Immigrants
Farmers	3	1	2	1
Self-employed	8	9	4	4
Managers	14	11	9	8
Associate professionals	21	13	23	13
Clerks and service workers	13	11	49	50
Blue-collar workers	39	53	12	19
Unemployed who had never worked	2	2	2	5
Total	100	100	100	100

Source: Census, INSEE, 1999 (Borrel and Boëldieu 2001).

From 1982 to 1999, among the total working population, the numbers of farmers, self-employed workers, and those of blue-collar workers, have diminished, whereas the numbers of managers, of associate professionals, and of clerks and service workers, have increased. Between 1982 and 1999, the number of farmers fell by 57%, and there have indeed been profound changes in the agricultural sector over the past twenty years: agriculture has become more concentrated and specialised, as small farms have been replaced by intensive specialised agricultural activities. The numbers of self-employed workers also dropped, by 16%, between 1982 and 1999 (Amossé 2001, Amossé and Chardon 2002). During this period, the craft trades sector underwent reorganisation, and the different trades tended to conform to developments in consumer behaviour. Business is also undergoing far-reaching changes, due to competition with supermarkets and hypermarkets, which has led to the closing down of many small businesses. The respective transformations in agriculture and business partly explain the decrease in the number of self-employed. The switch from self-employed work to wage-earning jobs has been in progress since 1975: 88% of those in jobs were wage earners in 1999 compared with 86% in 1990. This increase has been steady since 1975 (Bourlès and Courson 2000). Between 1982 and 1999, the numbers employed in the public sector, as well as in public services such as health, education and administration, have risen considerably. Consequently, the numbers of doctors, nurses, hospital auxiliaries, teachers, specialised instructors and social workers have greatly increased. Note that large numbers of women are employed in most of these activities. Between 1982 and 1999, there was also a large rise, of 62%, in the numbers of managers. This growth resulted from the development of advisory activities in job recruitment, training, strategies, organisation, auditing, etc., of research and development, and computer skills. The numbers of associate professionals grew by 40% between 1982 and 1999, thanks to the development of business activities among administrative associate professionals, as well as of information technology, the chemicals sector, and agribusiness. The general rise in the level of education has also contributed to the replacement of traditional secretaries and clerks by managerial assistants and administrative experts. Nevertheless, the numbers of clerks and service workers increased by 21% between 1982 and 1999, whereas the number of blue-collar workers dropped by 16% during this period. These developments in fact reflect great changes in unskilled employment. The numbers of blue-collar workers dropped because of the reduction in the number of jobs in many industrial sectors, including mainly textiles, clothing, metallurgy, mechanics and timber. At the same time, the demand for services has increased considerably, especially for home helps, babysitters and restaurant staff. Unskilled labour has therefore moved from industry to services and business. There has been a notable rise in the numbers of babysitters, family workers, service employees, maintenance workers, shop cashiers, waiters and self-service workers, activities that mainly employ women, and for those employing men, in the numbers of safety workers, sorters, packers, dispatchers, etc. Only the numbers of clerks diminished, by 15%, between 1982 and 1999. The development of office and information technology has reduced the need for administrative staff, except for activities involving business or human relations such as those of hostesses and commercial staff in transport and tourism.

The different sectors of activity are classified here according to the French classification system (Nomenclature d'activités et produits 2003). The data available for the distribution of the working population by sector of activity show that the number of jobs in services has increased rapidly since the middle of the 1970s, whereas the numbers in industry and agriculture are diminishing (Dumartin and Tomasini 1993, Trogan 1993, Fouquin *et al.* 2000). Industry, which employed 32% of wage earners in 1978, only employed 21% in 1996. The corresponding fraction for agriculture, which at 2% was already small in 1978, diminished to 1% in 1996. For the building industry, the figure dropped from 8 to 6% during the period from 1978 to 1996. For services, it rose from 58 to 72% during the same period (Fouquin *et al.* 2000).

The 1998 employment survey provides recent information about the earnings of men and women in France. Among wage earners as a whole, the distribution of wages was more favourable for men than for women. Table 7 shows the median wage, and the 1st and 9th deciles. The average difference between the earnings of men and women in 1998 was 25% and has remained stable ever since. Part of the difference is due to the large proportion of women who work part-time. For the population with full-time jobs, the gaps between the earnings of men and women are diminishing but are still marked (see table 7). Although there are other factors which explain why women are paid less than men for full-time jobs, including the type of degree and the occupation or sector of activity, they do not entirely account for the difference, part of which can therefore be attributed to discrimination against women (Meurs and Ponthieux 1999, Meurs and Ponthieux 2000). On the basis of observations made in monographs, some authors have suggested that the unexplained gap between the wages of men and women reflects systems of promotion and bonuses which are more favourable to men (Barrat and Meurs 2003). Wage levels are closely dependent on the occupational category: thus, in 2000, a manager earned 2.6 to 2.7 times as much as a blue-collar worker or clerk. This manager-blue-collar worker wage ratio has decreased since 1967, when it was 4.6. This decrease is due to a drop in the age of managers and a rise in that of blue-collar workers. However, at an identical age, the gap between managers and blue-collar workers has increased (Bayet and Demailly 1996). In 2000, the average monthly net wages for men and women by occupational categories are shown in table 7. Social differences in wages are less marked in the public sector. In addition, note that most of the information given here regarding wages concerns full-time work and the main occupational categories, and therefore masks part of the occupational wage hierarchy, i.e. the lowest wages, mostly earned by part-time unskilled workers, and the highest wages earned by company directors who are included in the manager category (Bihr and Pfefferkorn 1999). However, earnings are only one of the items that make up initial household income, as this also includes inherited estate income, unemployment benefits and retirement pensions. In addition, the sociofiscal system affects initial income in such a way that available income reflects a reduction in inequalities, because the lowest income groups enjoy more benefits than the highest, and the taxes are greater for the highest incomes than for the lowest. Thus, in 2001, inequalities in the standard of living decreased markedly for working households, on account of the differences between initial income and available income (Gini's Index decreased from 0.362 to 0.279). When the overall shifts are taken into account, the 50% of households with the highest incomes received 69% of the total available income, whereas for initial income, this proportion was 75%. Note that benefits reduced inequalities of income more than taxes, as they accounted for 58% of this reduction, compared with 42% for taxes (INSEE 2002). Data concerning average available incomes show that the inequality of incomes increased between 1984 and 1994: thus, the ratio of incomes of self-employed workers to those of unskilled workers rose from 2.9 to 4.2, and that for the incomes of managers to those of unskilled workers, from 2.5 to 3.0 (Bihr and Pfefferkorn 2000). Lastly, part of the working population was considered to be poor. If poor workers are defined as workers who either have a job, or are unemployed for six months of the year or more but have worked at least one month of the year, and are part of a household whose standard of living is below 50% of the median standard (i.e. 534 euros a month for one person, and 1,120 euros for a couple with two children), there were 1,305,000 poor workers in France (60% of them men and 40%, women) in 1996, which corresponds to 6% of the working population (Lagarenne and Legendre 2000a; 2000b).

**Table 7: Monthly net wages in 1998 (2000 for the public sector)
and distribution of average monthly net wages
by occupational categories in 2000**

Euros	Among all wage earners in the private sector		Wage earners Working full-time in the private sector		Wage earners working full-time in the public sector	
	Men	Women	Men	Women	Men	Women
1998						
1st decile	838	427	899	810	1,195	1,128
Median	1,288	1,031	1,316	1,220	1,913	1,710
9th decile	2,313	1,829	2,345	1,982	3,259	2,584
2000						
Managers	-	-	3,495	2,641	2,675	2,193
Associate professionals	-	-	1,685	1,608	1,734	1,637
Clerks and service workers	-	-	1,314	1,202	} 1,519	} 1,337
Blue-collar workers	-	-	1,282	1,045		

Sources: Employment survey, INSEE, 1998 (Meurs and Ponthieux 1999), DADS, INSEE, 2000 (Rasolofoarison and Seroussi 2002), and Fichier de paye des agents de l'Etat, INSEE, 2000 (Cornuau and Quarré 2001).

C. Unemployment, Precariousness and Part-time Work

In 1999, 11% of the male working population, and 15% of the female population, was unemployed, according to the census conducted that year. Note, however, that these figures include all persons who said they were unemployed, except for those who explicitly stated that they were not looking for work. The employment survey used the International Labour Office (ILO) definition of the unemployed, which includes anyone of working age (15 years or more) who (i) is actively looking for work, is available, and was not employed during the reference week, or (ii) is available but has found a job which is due to start at some future time. The definition of unemployment used in the 1999 census is therefore broader than that used in the employment survey. According to this survey, conducted in 2002, the number of unemployed, based on the ILO definition, was 2,341,000, or about 9% of the working population, 8% for men and 10% for women. Since 2001, the unemployment rate has risen slightly, especially for men, after decreasing substantially since 1997. The period from 1975 to 1997 was characterised by a large increase in the number of unemployed, which rose from 808,000 in 1975 to 3,152,000 in 1997 (Bihr and Pfefferkorn

1999). Unemployment especially affects the youngest age groups; thus, for those aged from 15 to 24 years, the rate in 2002 was 18% for men and 23% for women. It also affects immigrants; their rate of unemployment was 20% and 23% for men and women respectively in 1999, compared with 10% and 14% for men and women in the total working population at the same time (Thave 2000). Unemployment is higher for the least qualified, and for the lowest occupational grades. For instance, the unemployment rate was 4% for managers, 5% for associate professionals, 10% for clerks and service workers and 11% for blue-collar workers in 2002. Since 1982, the gaps between the occupational categories have widened (figure 1). Note that 32% of the unemployed (30% of the men and 33% of the women) had not had a job for a year or more (Aerts and Bigot 2002, INSEE 2002). Clerks and service workers, and blue-collar workers were more likely to be long-term unemployed (Bihr and Pfefferkorn 1999).

**Figure 1: Unemployment rate by occupational categories
from 1982 to 1998**

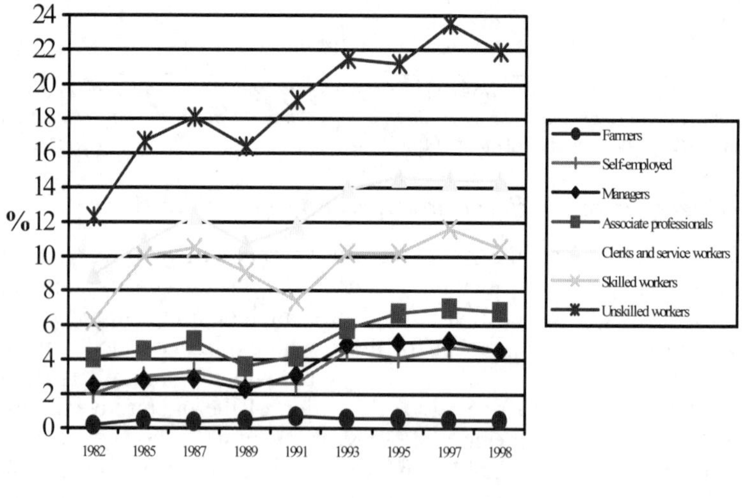

Source: Employment surveys, INSEE.

According to Castel (Castel 1995), unemployment, and more especially the increasing precariousness of employment, are the two main factors that have transformed the labour market during the last few decades in France. The employment contract of unlimited duration (*contrat de travail à durée indéterminée – CDI*) is on the decline and is often replaced by contracts for 'special types of employment', which include a host of heterogeneous jobs. The term 'special type of employment' applies to all work contracts other than the CDI, including those of limited duration (*contrats à durée déterminée – CDD*), temporary work, occupational training schemes and contracts to assist employment, i.e. those supported by the authorities as part of the campaign against unemployment. According to the census, special types of employment concerned 8% of the men and 10% of the women in the working population with a job in 1990, and 12% of the men and 15% of the women in 1999 (Bourlès and Courson 2000). Among immigrants, these rates were 15% and 17% for men and women respectively (Borrel and Boëldieu 2001). Between 1990 and 1999, especially striking increases were observed in the numbers of temporary workers and of those with a CDD, which increased by 83 and 67% respectively (Bourlès and Courson 2000). The employment surveys for the years 1992 and 2000 also provide indications about the developments in the numbers engaged in special types of employment, which concerned 6% of the total French population in 2000 as against 4% in 1992. Young people starting their working life, i.e. those who had left the educational system less than 5 years previously, were the most affected by these types of employment, which concerned 20% of them in 2000 as against 14% in 1992 (Martin-Houssart 2001). The precariousness of employment increased as the occupational level decreased, and affected clerks and service workers, and blue-collar workers more than managers and associate professionals; and unskilled workers more than skilled workers (Bihr and Pfefferkorn 1999). Note that since 2001, the proportion of temporary jobs (CDDs, interim posts, apprenticeships and state-supported contracts) has decreased, no doubt owing to the slowdown of activity in all economic sectors. The decrease is chiefly due to the reduced number of interim jobs and CDDs (Aerts and Bigot 2002, INSEE 2002).

Another major transformation of the labour market during the past twenty years is due to the development of part-time work. In 1975, 8% of the working population with a job (except for those doing military service) were on part-time work, and in 1998 the figure was 17%, according to the employment surveys. Many more women than men were doing part-time work: thus, in 1975 and 1998, the figures for men were 3 and 6% compared with 16 and 32% for women (figure 2). Consequently, in 1995, women accounted for 80% of part-time workers. In particular, part-time work also concerned young people under 25 years of age and the working population aged 60 years or more. Part-time work also affects immigrants (Borrel and Boëldieu 2001, Thave 2000). The proportion of part-time workers varied according to occupation, and was larger for the least qualified, mainly consisting of clerks or service workers and unskilled workers. Part-time work concerned over 35% of the women in these two categories. The five categories with the most part-time workers were cleaning women and domestic workers, other cleaners, cashiers, babysitters and home helps, most of whom are women. The service sector is the one where there is most part-time work. This work includes very different situations, which in fact arise from various individual requirements: on the one hand, part-time work may be the worker's choice, and on the other, it may be imposed by firms aiming for greater flexibility. During the last few decades, imposed part-time employment has increased; thus, in 1995, 54% of the men and 36% of the women doing part-time work would have liked to work more, compared with 33 and 34% in 1990. The young were also more affected by imposed part-time work, and more than half of both the men and women under 25 years of age would have liked to work more (Bisault *et al.* 1996). The employment survey conducted in 1995 among wage earners in the private sector showed that compared with full-time workers, those doing part-time work were subject to four types of disadvantage as regards working conditions (Galtier 1999):

1) They were more likely to have irregular working hours, and to work on Saturdays and Sundays, their work schedules were imposed by their company, and absence was less tolerated than for full-time workers;

2) Time work was more often temporary, and therefore precarious: 22% of the women working part-time who would have liked to work more were temporarily employed (interim, CDD, training schemes or state supported contracts) compared with 8 and 7% respectively of those working full-time or working part-time by choice. For men, 11% of those on imposed part-time work were temporarily employed, as were 37% of those working part-time by choice, compared with 6% of full-time workers;

3) In 1995, the average net monthly wage for part-time work was 579 euros compared with 1,392 euros for full-time work. The difference was partly due to differences in the duration of work and in qualifications. Nevertheless, all other things being equal, men on part-time work, especially when it was imposed, were paid a lower hourly wage than those working full-time;

4) Lastly, training was less easily available for part-time workers.

Note that although the growth of part-time work was stimulated by the lowering of social contributions in 1993, it has decreased since 1999, when it concerned 15% of the working population with a job, compared with 14% in 2002, according to the employment surveys. The decrease coincided with the introduction of regulations concerning exemption from social contributions, which have become less favourable since the passing of laws on the reduction of working hours. At the same time, the proportion of those with imposed part-time jobs diminished between 1997 and 2002 to 34% of those on part-time work who would have liked to work more (INSEE 2002).

Today, the difficulties of finding employment, and stable full-time employment at that, are not equally distributed amongst all occupational categories. In addition, these difficulties tend to accumulate in the case of those in the least qualified categories, for whom precarious and part-time employment often go hand in hand. These social inequalities of access to work can therefore be considered as an initial barrier limiting the access to income, and constitute favourable ground for the development of poverty.

Figure 2: Percentage of part time workers among the occupied active population from 1975 to 1998

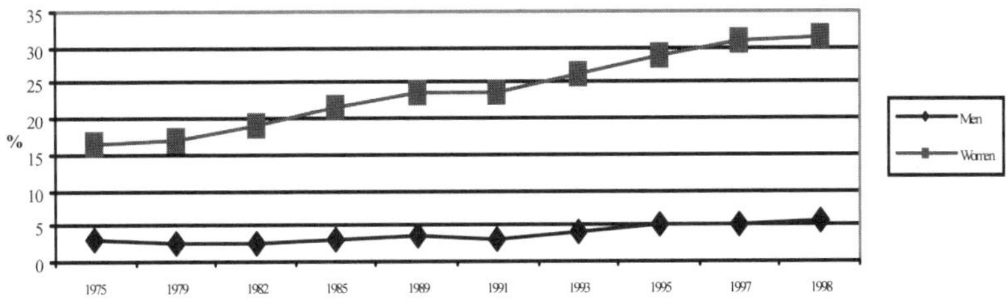

Source: Employment surveys, INSEE (Bihr and Pfefferkorn 1999).

D. *Working Conditions: Physical, Chemical, and Ergonomic Exposures, Psychosocial Work Factors, Working Hours and Atypical Work Schedules*

Working conditions in France are described in the periodical surveys, chiefly in the working conditions section of the employment surveys conducted in 1984, 1991 and 1998 and in the SUMER surveys conducted in 1987, 1994 and 2003. The data provided by these surveys concern the chemical, physical, biological, ergonomic, and psychosocial risks at work.

According to the working conditions surveys, overall physical effort and occupational risks rose between 1984 and 1998. In 1984, 64% of wage earners stated that their work involved at least one type of physical effort, as against 72% in 1998. There was a large increase in the numbers stating that their work involved physical constraints such as carrying heavy loads, working in difficult and perhaps tiring positions, or frequently having to walk long distances. Similarly, exposure to at least one occupational risk rose, as it concerned 62% of wage earners in 1984 but 74% in 1998. The rise concerned risks such as exposure to dust, smoke, road accidents and infectious or toxic agents, the risk of wounds, burns, falls or being hit, etc. The occupations most affected by physical effort and risks were those employing blue-collar workers and also those connected with health, the police and army, and business and service employees (Cézard and Hamon-Cholet 1999a, Bué and Guignon 2002). The SUMER survey, conducted by occupational physicians, is known for its reliable information on the different forms of occupational exposure. According to data collected in 1994, 27% of wage earners are exposed to noise (more than 85 dbA or to impacts or impulses exceeding 135 dbA); 19% to excess heat or cold (temperatures below 15°C or above 25°C, damp and bad weather); and 8% to carcinogenic agents (specified in List I of the International Agency for Research on Cancer – IARC). Most of the physical and chemical exposures, the most frequent and intense form, concern blue-collar workers (table 8). The sectors concerned were mainly agriculture and the building and other industries. Ergonomic exposure is also common; thus, 20% of wage earners have to perform repetitive actions at a fast rhythm, 9% are exposed to vibrations, and 28%, to standing for more than 20 hours a week. Exposure affected more blue-collar workers than others (table 8) (Héran-Le Roy and Sandret 1996, Héran-Le Roy and Sandret 1997b, Héran-Le Roy 1999).

Of the sample of wage earners investigated in the SUMER survey of 1994, 38% were exposed to manual materials handling, and 7% to handling for over 20 hours a week. In agriculture and building, 56 and 58% of wage earners respectively were engaged in handling, and in industry and the services the figures were 38 and 33%. The industrial sectors involving the most exposure were the timber and paper industries, agrobusiness, and among the services, the retail and wholesale trades, and transportation. Handling was very common amongst blue-collar workers, as 60% were involved in it, 13% for more than 20 hours a week. On the other hand, handling only concerned 28% of clerks and service workers, 27% of associate professionals and 8% of managers. However, blue-collar workers were not the only ones subject to high exposure, as it also affected the business and health sectors. Note that handling was often associated with other occupational risk factors of a physical or ergonomic type (exposure to cold, constraints of movement and posture, and repetitive actions), and with psychosocial factors (dependence on colleagues or clients, and irregular hours) (Héran-Le Roy and Sandret 1997a, Héran-Le Roy *et al.* 1999).

Table 8: Occupational risk factors
and occupational categories among wage earners

% exposed	Managers	Associate professionals	Clerks and service workers	Blue-collar workers
Noise	10	22	13	47
Excess heat or cold	6	14	8	35
Repetitive actions at a fast rhythm	2	7	17	35
Vibrations	0	4	1	22
Standing more than 20 hours a week	6	19	25	42
Manual materials handling	8	27	28	60

Source: SUMER survey, DARES, 1994 (Héran-Le Roy 1999).

Here is an example of chemical exposure at work. It concerns the way in which exposure to asbestos has evolved. Occupational exposure to asbestos is responsible for mesothelioma and for a substantial proportion of lung cancer cases. Since the 1950s, a large and regular increase in the number of cancer cases due to asbestos has accompanied the massive development of the use of asbestos in industrialised countries, although this increase has been delayed on account of the long latency period between exposure and the development of cancer. In France, as in other countries, the use of asbestos has been reduced. The changes in exposure with time, at the individual level, according to birth cohort, were studied in a sample of 4,700 men with a detailed job history. This cohort was derived from 11 case-referent studies (Goldberg *et al.* 2000). The highest levels of exposure were observed during the period from 1960 to 1970. Those born between 1920 and 1929 were the most severely exposed.

As far as we know, no French national figures are available which would make it possible to evaluate exposure to the factors defined by Karasek (Karasek and Theorell 1990) in the Demand-Control-Support model. The latest SUMER survey, conducted during 2003, included, for the first time, an evaluation of psychological demands, decision latitude and social support at work, and will shortly make it possible to provide data for a large sample of wage earners on a national scale. Consequently, the information given by the present authors is not based on this model, but data on psychosocial risks at work are available (table 9). Surveys of working conditions show that wage earners' autonomy rose during the years between 1991 and 1998, and even though it still exhibits a marked social gradient (see table 10: managers always have greater autonomy than associate professionals, clerks and service workers, and blue-collar workers), the different occupational categories as a whole have, with time, acquired greater freedom of action. As a result, increasing numbers of wage earners solve problems personally, do not apply orders strictly, and change time limits. This autonomy sometimes goes with greater job satisfaction, although the frequency of repetitive work remained stable from 1991 to 1998 (table 9, see the question of continuous repetition of the same series of actions), and even progressed among blue-collar workers and some other categories. In particular, conveyor-belt work concerned 15% of skilled workers and 30% of unskilled workers in 1998. Autonomy was also accompanied by greater responsibility towards the firm; thus, in 1998, half the wage earners considered that faulty work could cost the firm a great deal, and 35% that it could seriously affect the quality of products or services. Overall, the factors connected with the psychological demands of work progressed between 1991 and 1998 (table 9), as did interruptions and shortage of time – which chiefly concerned managers and associate professionals – and also the demand for vigilance and constraints concerning the speed of work, mainly affecting blue-collar workers and certain categories of clerks or service workers (table 10). Tensions among colleagues or between higher and lower grades, which concerned 21 and 30% of wage earners in 1998, were more frequently reported by those with executive responsibilities than by others, whatever their occupation. Tension with clients or the public, which in 1991 mainly concerned those in the business and health sectors, the police and social workers, had risen by 1998 in all occupational categories, especially among teachers (Hamon-Cholet and Rougerie 2000, Cézard and Hamon-Cholet 1999b, Bué and Rougerie 1999). The proportion of wage earners in contact with the public remained stable, at 62%, from 1991 to 1998. It varied depending on the sector of activity: in the service sector it was 72%; in the building industry, 56%; in industry, 34%; and in agriculture, 32%. It also varied depending on occupational category. Thus, among the managerial echelons, those most concerned were teachers and scientists, technical and financial managers, and business administrators; among associate professionals, workers in the health and social sectors, and instructors; among clerks and service workers, those employed in business and the health and social sectors; and among workers, drivers. The working conditions of the wage earners in services who are in contact with the public were characterised by particular constraints as regards working hours, high pressure from external demands, and more frequent tensions, both with the public and with their colleagues and their superior (Guignon and Hamon-Cholet 2003).

Table 9: Developments in psychosocial conditions at work
for wage earners, between 1991 and 1998

% exposed	1991	1998
Factors relating to autonomy		
You are only told the objective of the task	82	86
You solve problems personally	65	72
You do not apply orders strictly	58	63
You can change deadlines	63	67
Factors relating to psychological demands		
Faulty work can lead to:		
– serious consequences for product quality or services	60	65
– large financial costs for the firm	44	50
– dangerous consequences for your safety or that of others	31	38
– personal sanctions (risk of losing the job, large reduction of pay)	46	59
You often have to leave a task to perform another unforeseen one	48	56
To do your work properly, you do not usually have the following:		
– enough time	23	25
– clear and sufficient information	18	21
– the possibility of cooperating	13	14
– a sufficient number of collaborators	21	24
You often have tense relations with the public	22	30
You have to repeat the same series of actions continuously	30	29
Performance of your task makes it necessary:		
– to keep your eyes constantly on your work	26	32
– to read letters or figures in small type, and/or badly printed or written	22	30
– to scrutinise very small objects and/or details	12	16
– to look out for very brief visual signals that may be unpredictable or hard to detect	12	13
– to look out for very brief sound signals that may be unpredictable or hard to detect	12	13
The speed of your work is imposed by:		
– a demand calling for immediate satisfaction	46	54
– production norms or deadlines to be fulfilled in one hour or more	16	23
– specific speeds of task performance*	8	10
– permanent checking or supervision by superiors	23	29
– immediate dependence on the work of one or several colleagues	23	27

* *Conveyor-belt work or speed imposed by the automatic movement of a product or part, or by the automatic speed of a machine.*
Source: Working conditions surveys, DARES, 1991, 1998 (Hamon-Cholet and Rougerie 2000, Cézard and Hamon-Cholet 1999b, Bué and Rougerie 1999).

Table 10: Psychosocial conditions at work
and occupational categories for wage earners in 1998

% exposed	Managers	Associate professionals	Clerks and service workers	Blue-collar workers
Factors relating to autonomy				
You are only told the objective of the task	97	93	84	77
You solve problems personally	90	82	68	60
You do not apply orders strictly	82	71	57	55
You can change deadlines	76	73	68	56
Number of constraints on the speed of work (see table 9 for details)				
0	30	24	27	22
1	41	36	35	26
2 or more	29	40	38	52

Source: Working conditions survey, DARES, 1998 (Hamon-Cholet and Rougerie 2000).

The surveys referred to above, especially those called working conditions surveys, deserve some comments. Firstly, although they were conducted by professional investigators, they were based on wage earners' statements, and it therefore seems difficult to assign the correct weight to the actual developments in working conditions and to changes in subjective perceptiveness and statements. Secondly, as regards the part concerning psychosocial risks at work, the questionnaire used in the working conditions surveys may have been more appropriate for the industrial sector than for other sectors. Consequently, wage earners outside industry may have found it hard to answer certain questions, concerning, for instance, the speed of task performance, and the degree of exposure may thus have been underestimated for certain non-industrial occupations.

We have data mainly based on French national surveys. In addition, a few epidemiological studies on psychosocial factors at work have been conducted during recent years in France. Among these studies, those concerning the GAZEL cohort (Goldberg *et al.* 2001) give information about exposure to psychosocial factors at work in a large cohort of wage earners with various occupations but in the same sector of activity, i.e. Electricité de France-Gaz de France (EDF-GDF), the national gas and electricity utility. On the basis of the models of Karasek and Siegrist, the results showed the existence of a marked occupational gradient for exposure to psychosocial factors at work (Niedhammer *et al.* 2000b, Niedhammer *et al.* 2000a, Niedhammer 2002). In this respect, decision latitude, psychological demands, social support and reward were all the higher as the occupational category is also high (table 11). Consequently, exposure to job strain and the imbalance between effort and reward rose as the level of the occupational category diminished, especially for clerks.

Table 11: Percentages exposed to working conditions as defined by the four dimensions of the Job Content Questionnaire by Karasek according to occupational categories in the GAZEL cohort in 1997

	N	Low levels of decision latitude[1] (%)	High levels of psychological demands[1] (%)	Low levels of social support[1] (%)	High levels of physical demands[1] (%)
Men	*8,277*				
Managers, engineers	3,580	25.9	59.8	43.5	30.6
Administrative associate professionals	969	46.4	53.5	55.6	45.2
Technicians	464	62.7	42.2	57.2	64.8
Foremen	2,414	46.8	43.5	52.9	58.2
Clerks	223	78.2	44.4	57.8	56.3
Skilled industrial workers	300	70.1	25.0	51.4	87.6
Craftsmen	302	67.2	34.2	57.1	83.8
Women	*3,170*				
Managers, engineers	476	31.1	63.9	48.7	35.7
Administrative associate professionals	1,739	62.3	52.1	52.6	47.5
Foremen	367	62.9	44.9	53.6	50.1
Clerks	579	80.8	49.0	60.0	54.8

[1] *Each score was dichotomised at the median of the total sample of men and women.*

One other important aspect of working conditions concerns working hours and schedules. In France, the laws have gradually been altered so as to reduce working hours, resulting in the measures to reduce working hours passed in 1996 and 1998, and the limitation of legal working hours to 35 hours a week. In firms employing more than 20 wage earners, the 35-hour limit came into force at the beginning of the year 2000, but only as from January 1st, 2002 for firms with fewer than 20 wage earners and for workers in the public sector. Since then, new measures have been introduced to mitigate the consequences for firms, of the law on the reduction of working hours. In 1995, a survey on duration of work showed that the average weekly duration of full-time work was 41 h 5 m. For managers, the duration was markedly longer than for other categories, at 44 h 45 m. For blue-collar workers, it was close to that for clerks and service workers (40 h 17 m. and 40 h 20 m. respectively) and for associate professionals, it was a little longer (41 h 2 m.). Note that men worked an average of 1 h 52 m. longer than women, partly because of the different distributions for men and women according to occupational category (Fermanian and Baesa 1997). Between 1995 and 2001, the weekly duration of work diminished by 1 h 20 m. for full-time wage earners working regular hours. The reduction was a little more marked for men than for women (1 h 30 m. versus 1 h 15 m.). Whereas the duration of work remained unchanged for managers between 1995 and 2001, it diminished by 1 h 20 m. for clerks and service workers, 1 h 30 m. for associate professionals and 2 h for blue-collar workers (Afsa *et al.* 2003). Note that 2001 was a year of transition in the process of reducing the number of working hours. However, although the duration of work diminished, the constraints regarding work schedules grew stronger. Thus, the data collected during the working conditions surveys indicate that working hours became less regular and more diversified between 1984 and 1998. Among wage earners, 50% had the same daily work schedules in 1998, as against 59% in 1984. During the same period, there were increases in work on Saturdays (44% in 1984 and 47% in 1998), work on Sundays (18% in 1984 and 25% in 1998), night work (12% in 1984 and 14% in 1998), and in work by alternating shifts (8% in 1984 and 9% in 1998). In 1998, 6% of female blue-collar workers and 21% of male blue-collar workers were on night shifts (Bué and Guignon 2002). In addition, the reduction of working hours introduced by the different laws passed since 1996 was accompanied by radical measures to reorganise working hours, such as their annualization, the individualisation of work schedules and the introduction of a calendar of production targets. In particular, shorter working hours led to more variable and less predictable hours for unskilled workers, especially women. And as these wage earners, more than others, had already been subject to variable and unpredictable work schedules, the shorter hours seem to have increased the differences between wage earners as regards the organisation of working hours (Estrade and Ulrich 2002). Similarly, Bué *et al.* (2003) showed that the working conditions of blue-collar workers, clerks and service workers deteriorated when the shorter working hours were introduced. These categories had already been subject to stringent restrictions as regards working hours and work organisation, and the shorter hours involved additional organisational transformations such as changes in procedure, additional polyvalence and the imposition of new tasks, with little or no new recruitment in compensation. These organisational shocks have increased the intensity of work and are often accompanied by loss of autonomy.

Working conditions are unequally distributed amongst occupational categories. Blue-collar workers are more likely to be exposed to physical, chemical, and ergonomic risk factors at work. These risks may also concern some groups of service workers. Psychosocial risk factors also have a greater effect on the two categories of blue-collar workers, and of clerks and service workers than the others, especially for low levels of decision latitude and low levels of reward. To summarise, these occupational categories seem to accumulate unfavourable working conditions, with the exception of psychological demands and working hours, which are more likely to be elevated among managers.

E. Changes in the Accident Rate at Work as a Possible Marker of Developments in Working Conditions

The above data on working conditions in France and the way in which they have changed are necessarily incomplete. Employment surveys have been conducted for several years, but are based on reports by wage earners, and therefore do not correctly assess the importance of changes in perception and its effect on those reports on the one hand, and the actual developments in working conditions on the other. The SUMER surveys, based on data that are collected, as already stated, by occupational physicians, give a more objective picture of the working conditions of French wage earners. However, the only figures so far available are those for 1987 and 1994, so it is not very clear how these conditions are changing. The accident rate and its development over time may constitute an indirect marker of working conditions and the way in which they are changing. For accidents involving at least one day's sick leave, the census is done by the health insurance authorities. The accident rate, defined by the number of accidents per million of hours worked, has the advantage of giving the number of accidents occurring during the time of workers' exposure to risks. Since 1970, a reduction in the total rate has been observed, although this reduction seems to have slowed down very much since the end of the 1980s. And indeed, for industry and building activities, the rate decreased twice as slowly between 1988 and 1998 as between 1970 and 1987. In the services, the decrease has been virtually at a standstill since 1987. There are various possible explanations for these trends: during the period from 1970 to 1987, efforts to prevent accidents, and the widespread automation of production systems, certainly helped to lower the risk of accidents, but from 1988 to 1998, technological and organisational innovations, and new methods of organising work, may have raised that risk (Bouvet and Yahou 2001, Coutrot 1996).

2. Social Inequalities in Health

Data for social inequalities of mortality, based on the results for co-horts followed up after a census, have been available since 1965 (Calot and Febvray 1965, Desplanques 1984, Mesrine 1999, Desplanques 2001). Other results, especially those dealing with causes of death, are issued from cross-sectional analyses (Jougla *et al.* 2000). For morbidity, at least two national surveys are available, but comparisons between the situation in France and other countries are difficult.

A. General Mortality

The data on mortality given below are based on the results from cen-sus cohorts reported by Mesrine in 1999. Table 12 shows the mortality for occupied men and women for the period from 1982 to 1996. Large differences were observed according to occupational category and also gender. For men, a manager aged 35 years could expect to live 7.5 years longer than an unskilled worker of the same age. For women, the corre-sponding difference was smaller (4 years). Comparisons with other countries indicate that for middle-aged men, social inequalities as regards mortality are greater in France than in other European countries (Kunst *et al.* 1998, 2000).

Table 12: Risk of death and life expectancy for the period from 1982 to 1996 according to occupational category in 1982 (active population)

	Men		Women	
	Risk of death between 35 and 65 (%)	Life expectancy at 35 (years)	Risk of death between 35 and 65 (%)	Life expectancy at 35 (years)
Managers	13.0	44.5	6.5	49.5
Farmers	15.5	43.0	8.0	47.5
Associate professionals	17.0	42.0	7.0	49.0
Self-employed	18.5	41.5	7.5	48.5
Clerks and service workers	23.0	40.0	8.5	47.5
Skilled workers	24.5	38.5	10.0	46.5
Unskilled workers	29.0	37.0	11.0	45.5

Source: Echantillon de mortalité de 1982, INSEE (Mesrine 1999) Men and women aged 30-64 years old in 1982.

The links between mortality and unemployment were studied in three categories, in the light of their employment status (Mesrine 2000, Desplanques 2001): employed, unemployed looking for a job, and other unemployed, including those unemployed for health reasons.

During the 5 years of follow-up, mortality was higher among unemployed men and women looking for a job than among the employed, irrespective of period, i.e. 1975-1980, 1982-1987 or 1990-1995 (table 13). The fact that those looking for a job had a lower occupational category and a lower educational level only explains the excess mortality in part, and only for men. For the period from 1990 to 1995, the relative risk of mortality among men being 'unemployed, looking for a job' diminished from 3.1 to 2.7 when adjusted for occupational and educational levels, and to 2.3 when adjusted for marital status as well. For women, the same adjustments did not affect the results much, as the relative risk of mortality among women 'unemployed, looking for a job' was 1.9, and 1.8 after adjustment for occupational and educational levels, and marital status. There might be at least two explanations for the excess mortality among those looking for a job: firstly, as in the category of 'other unemployed', a selection according to health may have an effect; and secondly, unemployment has a negative effect on health. If the first explanation is correct, the relative risk of mortality among the unemployed can be expected to decrease if this group is large. If unemployment increases, the risk of being unemployed remains very high for those in poor health, and also rises for the healthier categories. For men, the decrease of the relative risk from 3.2 to 2.7 between the periods from 1975 to 1980 and from 1982 to 1987 is consistent with a health selection. Thus, during this period, the proportion of those looking for work rose from 1.5 to 3.5%, which may have reduced the health selection effect in this group. However, from 1985 to 1995, the proportion of those looking for a job rose from 3.5 to 5.5%, and the relative risk did not decrease. This might have been due to another effect of health selection: especially for physically demanding work, more workers with health problems were excluded from the labour market than during previous periods. This may have raised the average level of health of those employed. The increase in the relative risk of mortality from 1985 to 1995 might also reflect the effects on health of unfavourable living conditions over a relatively long period among those who were, at least temporarily, excluded from the labour market. For women, the significance of the changes in the relative risk of mortality among those having to look for a job during the three periods is difficult to define, because it differs according to socio-economic category (Mesrine 2000).

Table 13: Relative risk of mortality according to employment status

	Mortality 1975-1980, according to the situation in 1975	Mortality 1982-1987 according to the situation in 1982	Mortality 1990-1995 according to the situation in 1990
Men			
Employed	1	1	1
Unemployed, looking for a job	3.2	2.7	3.1
Other unemployed	3.5	4.3	5.1
Women			
Employed	1	1	1
Unemployed, looking for a job	1.5	1.9	1.9
Other unemployed	1.4	2.0	2.5

Source: Echantillon démographique permanent, INSEE (Desplanques 2001, Mesrine 2000). Men and women aged 30-64 years old at baseline.

Mortality among those classified as 'other unemployed', which includes those unable to work on account of a disease or disability, was very high, especially among men, although in 1990 only 3.5% of the men were in this category. Women were classified in this category for health or other reasons, such as personal choice. The proportion of women thus classified depended on the birth cohort, period, level of qualifications and also marital status. Among married women, the highest level of inactivity (49%) was found at the top and bottom of the social scale (managers and workers). To study the link between unemployment and mortality for women, it was necessary to take into account various confounding factors. One important conclusion, based on various models, was that for those with low qualifications, inactivity seems to have a negative effect on mortality (Mesrine 2000).

For men, the differences between occupational categories as regards mortality were comparable for the three 5-year periods that followed the censuses of 1975, 1982 and 1990. However, from the figures in table 14, it would be difficult to conclude that the social inequalities in this respect have either increased or diminished, because of the changes in the size of each category. Thus, during the first period, from 1975 to 1980, the reference category, i.e. managers, comprised 11% of the population, but 17% during the third and most recent period, from 1990 to 1995, which means that in terms of relative social position, it is now closer to the average. Consequently, a decrease in the relative risk of mortality for all categories could have been expected. However, for skilled workers, who comprise 24 to 26% of the population, this risk increased during the period from 1990 to 1995, and the same applied to clerks and service workers. For unskilled workers, the relative risk has since decreased, but comparison with the reference category is difficult, because the proportion of unskilled workers also decreased during this period.

Table 14: Relative risk of mortality by occupational categories, comparisons between three periods (Men, active population)

	1975-1980	1982-1987	1990-1995
Managers	1	1	1
Farmers	1.3	1.2	1.3
Self-employed	1.4	1.3	1.3
Associate professionals	1.2	1.2	1.3
Clerks and service workers	2.0	1.9	2.2
Skilled workers	1.9	1.8	2.0
Unskilled workers	2.6	2.5	2.4

Source: Echantillon démographique permanent, INSEE (Mesrine 1999). Men aged 30-64 years old at baseline.

B. Mortality According to Cause of Death

The data available concerning mortality according to cause of death are cross-sectional data. They have made it possible to quantify the relative contribution of each cause to the excess premature mortality in the low occupational categories (Jougla *et al.* 2000, Kunst *et al.* 1998, 2000). For men, the excess number of deaths was due to first neoplasms, especially lung cancer and cancer of the upper respiratory and digestive tracts, and to accidents and suicides. These causes of death together accounted for 63% of the excess deaths in the group broadly classified as 'blue-collar workers, and clerks and service workers', compared with the manager group. The figure for cardiovascular diseases was lower (14%) (Jougla *et al.* 2000). As in European countries further south, cardiovascular diseases, especially ischaemic heart disease, made a limited contribution to social inequalities in mortality among men (Kunst *et al.* 1998, 2000). For women, the situation was more complicated, as a large proportion of the premature deaths were due to breast cancer, which, in France as in other developed countries, is more frequent among upper-class women (Herbert and Launoy 2000). For most causes of death, the social distribution over time was fairly stable. One exception was AIDS, for which the risk for men was higher in the upper classes during the period from 1979 to 1985. Subsequently, however, the high risk categories were reported to be the blue-collar workers and those with no occupation (Calvez 2000). For cardiovascular diseases, changes over time have also been observed. Until the end of the 1960s, the risk was no higher for several categories of blue-collar workers and for clerks and service workers than for the manager category (Lang and Ribet 2000).

C. Cardiovascular Diseases

Social differences in mortality due to coronary heart diseases may be attributable to differences either in their incidence or in survival rates. The data from cardiovascular disease registries give more details about social inequalities for incidence of acute myocardial infarction or other coronary event, and also for survival in the 28-day period after the coronary heart disease episode (Lang and Ribet 2000). The data given in table 15 indicate that for men 30-59 years old both differences in incidence and survival contribute to social inequalities. However, the relative importance of each type of difference varies according to occupational category. For unskilled workers, the survival rate is the main factor responsible for mortality from coronary heart diseases. This is also the case for farmers, but the incidence of such diseases among them is low. The opposite is the case for clerks and service workers, whose survival rate is relatively favourable but among whom the incidence of coronary heart diseases is high. Among managers, this incidence and survival rates are both favourable.

Social inequalities have been documented for conventional risk factors such as smoking and obesity, which in turn contribute to inequalities in the incidence of cardiovascular diseases (Brixi and Lang 2000). This is presented in the next paragraph. Social inequalities as regards knowledge about the prevention of cardiovascular diseases have also been observed (Lang and Ribet 2000).

Occupational factors may partly explain the social inequalities in the incidence of these diseases, and the links between psychosocial factors at work and cardiovascular risk factors have been studied in a large cohort of workers in France (Niedhammer *et al.* 1998c). Psychosocial factors at work were found to be associated with cardiovascular risk factors, but the pattern of these associations was different for men and women. These findings are in agreement with those of other studies in various countries. However, the specific effect of psychosocial factors at work on socio-economic inequalities as regards the incidence of cardiovascular diseases and mortality cannot yet be evaluated in France.

The data for lifestyle risk factors presented in table 16 are issued from a representative sample of about 3,500 subjects aged 35-64 years old in three regions in France. They are consistent with other results in France for this age group (Brixi and Lang 2000). Among men, the frequency of smoking is the highest for blue-collar workers, and the lowest for farmers. The frequency of smoking is lower in general among women; in the 1980s, the highest frequency of smoking was among fcmale managers; however, in the following decade there was an important increase in the frequency of smoking for lower categories. As a consequence, smoking is now associated with the lowest occupational categories among the youngest women. Several studies indicate that the lowest alcohol consumption is found among managers, especially for men. This category is also in the best situation regarding practice of regular physical exercise as a leisure activity. For body mass index, the data in table 16 are consistent with eating habits according to occupational categories: farmers have a high calory intake, and a high level of education is associated with a low calory intake.

Table 15: Incidence and case fatality of coronary events according to occupational categories for men aged 30-59 years old, period 1985-1989, Monica study

	Percentage of the studied sample	Incidence of all coronary events Odds ratio	Case fatality Odds ratio
Farmers	2.2	0.8	1.4
Self-employed			
Craftsmen	4.1	0.7	1.2
Salesmen	2.9	1.1	1.1
Managers			
Public sector	5.3	0.7	1.0
Private sector	9.0	0.6	0.6
Associate professionals			
Education, health, civil service	5.1	1.0	0.9
Private sector	5.5	1.2	1.2
Technicians	4.7	0.7	0.9
Foremen	4.6	0.9	1.1
Clerks and service workers			
Public service	5.3	1.8	0.8
Private sector	3.2	1.7	1.0
Blue-collar workers			
Skilled workers (reference)	23.6	1	1
Unskilled workers	12.2	1.2	1.4
Retired	2.6	2.1	1.7
Other inactive	4.8	2.5	1.7

Source: (Lang et al. 1997, Lang and Ribet 2000).
Odds ratio adjusted for age Occupational categories comprising less than 2% of the sample not included in the table.

Table 16: Smoking, alcohol consumption, physical exercise, body mass index, by occupational categories, men and women 35-64 years old, 1996-1997

	N	Smokers (%)		Alcohol consumption (g/day)		Regular physical exercise as a leisure activity (%)		Body Mass Index (kg/m^2)	
		Men	Women	Men	Women	Men	Women	Men	Women
Farmers	72	18	0	32.6	7.2	26	19	27.7	28.0
Self-employed	243	30	14	35.8	10.8	30	18	27.3	26.3
Managers	426	24	23	24.9	10.9	41	21	25.8	23.8
Associate professionals	866	26	18	30.2	9.3	39	29	26.8	24.7
Clerks and Service workers	911	29	16	32.7	9.3	31	16	26.6	26.5
Blue-collar workers	730	37	14	36.6	10.9	28	12	26.9	27.6

Source: Random sample of men and women aged 35-64 years old (Haute Garonne, Bas-Rhin, communauté urbaine de Lille), 1996-1997 (Brixi and Lang 2000).

D. Self-reported Health

France has been compared with other European countries for differences in perceived general health, for men and women, according to educational level (Cavelaars *et al.* 1998). The health variable was the question "Do you consider your present state of health less than good?", and the population studied included 21,586 respondents, aged 25 to 69 years, to a national survey on health and the use of medical care conducted in 1991 and 1992. The Relative Inequality Index (RII) was used to quantify social differences and was interpreted as the odds for considering their state of health 'less than good' for those at the bottom of the educational ladder compared with those at the top. Among the eleven European countries surveyed, France was ranked fifth (Rank 1 being the best position), with an RII of 4.23 for men (95% CI, 2.55 to 7.03). For women, the rank was not as good (8/11), with an RII of 4.18 (95% CI, 2.82 to 6.21). These results suggest that France occupies the least favourable position in Europe for social inequalities in premature mortality amongst men, but a fairly average position for social inequalities in perceived health. In this survey, however, the specific question on perceived health was part of a questionnaire that laid much stress on diagnosed diseases and the use of health care. If the same question had been part of a survey focused on disabilities in general, the results might have been different.

E. Impairment and Disability

In 1999, a national survey entitled *Handicaps, Incapacités, Dépendance* (handicap, disability and impairment) was conducted in France. It was based on a representative sample of 16,900 persons of all ages, and provided an estimate of the importance of impairments and disabilities, as well as of the magnitude of social differences in this field of health (Mormiche 2002, Haut comité de la Santé Publique 2002). In this survey, subjects were classified according to the social position of the head of the household. The results indicated the existence of a cumulative disadvantage among the lower social classes: the level of impairment, whether physical or mental, was higher, and the impairments had more negative consequences for the ability to function in daily life (i.e. caused greater disability). When the head of the household was a blue-collar worker, the proportion of persons suffering from one or several impairments was multiplied by 1.6, compared with persons belonging to households whose head was in the managerial class, after the results of the comparison were adjusted for age and gender. The same was observed, at all ages, when social position was assessed according to the occupational category of the father of the person included in the survey. Therefore the relationships observed cannot be interpreted as the result of a selection effect (i.e. of the socio-economic position resulting from health problems). In this survey, social inequalities were greater for disabilities than for impairments. Thus, the ratio that quantified the difference between blue-collar workers and the managerial class was 3, for the presence of at least one disability. There are several possible explanations for these results, one of them being that in blue-collar workers' families, impairments are greater, and/or more difficulties in coping with them are encountered.

For mortality and self-reported health, the limitations of the available data include the lack of information about the period around the year 2000. Additional studies are also needed in order to compare the magnitude of social inequalities for different periods.

F. Accidents at Work

The 1998 survey of working conditions provided information about the link between occupational category and accidents at work in a broad sample of wage earners (Hamon-Cholet 2002). Of the subjects questioned, 8% reported an accident at work during the previous 12 months (11% of the men and 5% of the women). Of the accidents, 55% gave rise to sick leave. The accident rate was 15% among blue-collar workers compared with 6% for associate professionals, and clerks and service workers, and 3% for managers. In addition to having the largest accident rate, blue-collar workers had the longest sick leave after accidents (Hamon-Cholet 2002). Note that this study was based on self-reported accidents, consequently a reporting bias cannot be excluded.

3. The Contribution of Working Conditions to Social Inequalities in Health in France: a Prospective Study in an Occupational Cohort

Currently, no information is available regarding the contribution of working conditions to social inequalities in health in France. In addition, there is no national survey that could provide data useful for such an analysis. However, some data from other surveys could help in this issue; they will be described in the discussion section regarding forthcoming studies. For this chapter, an attempt has been made to study the contribution of working conditions to social inequalities in self-reported health, using the data of a large cohort of workers employed by the national company for gas and electricity, the GAZEL cohort (Goldberg *et al.* 2001). A reanalysis of the data has been performed regarding psychosocial factors at work and self-reported health. A paper has been recently published using the same data (Niedhammer and Chea 2003).

A. Objective

The objective here was to evaluate the contribution of working conditions, defined by the four dimensions of psychological demands, decision latitude, social support, and physical demands elaborated by Karasek (Karasek and Theorell 1990), and stressful occupational events, in the relationship between occupational grade and self-reported health in a one-year prospective study. The previous paper has already shown that (1) occupational grade predicted poor self-reported health one year later, and (2) working conditions also had predictive effects on self-reported health (Niedhammer and Chea 2003). A comparison with a cross-sectional analysis of these data has also been made, in order to compare the results obtained in prospective and cross-sectional approaches.

B. Population, Materials, and Methods

The GAZEL cohort was established in 1989 and originally included 20,624 subjects working at Electricité de France – Gaz de France (EDF-GDF), comprising men aged 40-50 and women aged 35-50 at baseline (Goldberg *et al.* 2001). Since 1989, this cohort has been followed up by means of yearly self-administered questionnaires and by data collection from the company's personnel and medical departments. Research on psychosocial factors at work and health has been conducted in this cohort since 1995 (Niedhammer *et al.* 1998a, 1998b, 1998c, 2000a,

2000b, Niedhammer 2002, Niedhammer and Chea 2003, Niedhammer *et al.* 2004).

The scales of decision latitude, psychological demands, social support, and physical demands were included in the self-administered questionnaire of the GAZEL cohort for the year 1997. The French version used here has already been used and/or validated elsewhere (Brisson *et al.* 1998, Houtman *et al.* 1999, Niedhammer 2002, Larocque *et al.* 1998). Decision latitude and psychological demands each comprised 9 items, social support, 8 items, and physical demands, 5 items. Answers were graded according to the following Likert-type scale: 'totally disagree', 'disagree', 'agree', and 'totally agree'. The scores for each scale were constructed according to Karasek's recommendations and were dichotomised at the median of the total sample of men and women, for use in the analyses. The number of stressful occupational events within the previous 12 months (job change, transfer, reconversion, and department restructuring) was also studied as a potential contributor of social inequalities in self-reported health.

Occupational grade included 7 categories for men, and 4 for women. Data for this variable were supplied by the EDF-GDF personnel department. Occupational grade in 1997 was used in this study.

Self-reported health was based on an 8-level scale ranging from 'very good' (coded 1) to 'very poor' (coded 8). The question was formulated as follows: 'How do you rate your general health status?'. Poor self-reported health was defined by levels ranging from 5 to 8, i.e. with a cut-off in the middle. Self-reported health was included in the questionnaires for 1997 and 1998.

Several covariates were used as potential confounding variables. They were the number of chronic conditions within the 12 previous months (including chronic bronchitis, asthma, hypertension, angina pectoris, myocardial infarction, claudication, osteoarthritis, diabetes, hyperlipidaemia, and cancer), age (in 5-year groups), marital status (6 categories), the number of stressful personal events occurring during the previous 12 months (the 12 events included: death of a spouse, death of a close relative, divorce, marital separation, etc.), educational level (6 categories), smoking (non-smokers versus smokers), overweight (defined by Body Mass Index, calculated as weight/height^2 exceeding 27.2 kg/m^2 for men and 26.9 for women), and alcohol consumption, graded according to the frequency (number of days/week), the quantity (glasses/day) and the type consumed (wine, beer or spirits). Drinkers were classified as: abstainers, light drinkers (1-13 drinks/week for men and 1-6 drinks/ week for women), intermediate drinkers (14-27 drinks/ week for men and 7-20 drinks/week for women), and heavy drinkers

(28 drinks/week or more for men and 21 drinks/week or more for women). Data for these variables were obtained in 1997.

The cross-sectional analysis of the data was designed to explore the associations between occupational grade in 1997 and self-reported health at the same time. The prospective analysis was designed to establish whether occupational grade considered in 1997 was predictive of poor self-reported health one year later among the sub-group of the study population who rated their health as good at baseline, i.e. in 1997. Furthermore, the analysis was performed before and after adjustment for working conditions, to evaluate their contribution in the relationship between occupational grade and self-reported health. Adjustments were also made for covariates measured at baseline and analysis was made using the logistic regression model. Poor self-reported health was used as the dependent variable. Three models were constructed. First, a model (model 1) was constructed including occupational grade and age as independent variables. Second (model 2), adjustment was made for occupational grade, chronic conditions, personal characteristics (age, marital status, stressful personal events, and education), and behavioural risk factors (smoking, alcohol consumption, and overweight). Third (model 3), additional adjustment was made for the variables of working conditions. Each variable of working conditions was added separately to the model, and only those which contributed to diminishing the relationship between occupational grade and self-reported health were retained in model 3. The contribution of working conditions to the explanation of social inequalities in self-reported health was estimated by the change in OR between model 2 and model 3. Men and women were studied separately to explore potential gender-specific associations. Statistical analysis was performed with the SAS statistical software package (SAS Institute 1999).

C. Results

The cross-sectional analysis was based on 11,447 subjects, comprising 8,277 men and 3,170 women, who were working in 1997 and answered the questionnaire that year. The prospective analysis was based on 7,664 subjects, 5,575 men and 2,089 women, who rated their health as good in 1997, were working, and responded to both the 1997 and 1998 questionnaires. Details regarding the number and situation of losses of follow-up, the rate of participation, and the comparison between the respondents and non-respondents may be found in the previous paper (Niedhammer and Chea 2003). Table 17 gives a description of the studied population in 1997 and 1998, by occupational grade and self-reported health, for men and women.

The relationships between occupational grade and working conditions have been described in a previous paper (Niedhammer 2002). To summarise these results, for the variables of decision latitude and physical demands, the lower the level of occupational grade, the higher the prevalence of harmful conditions (low decision latitude and high physical demands). For psychological demands, the opposite trend was observed, the higher the occupational grade, the higher the levels of psychological demands. Social support at work was not clearly associated with occupational grade, especially among men (table 11). The association between occupational grade and stressful occupational events was significant for men (p<0.001) and women (p<0.05), and showed that managers and engineers for men and women, administrative associate professionals for men, and forewomen were more likely to be exposed to these events.

Table 18 presents the results of the three models for the cross-sectional analysis. Model 1 presents the association between occupational grade and poor self-reported health after adjustment for age. Significant odds ratios were observed for administrative associate professionals, and clerks for men and women, and for foremen, skilled industrial workers and craftsmen for men. After additional adjustment for personal, behavioural, and health-related variables (model 2), these associations diminished, but remained significant for clerks for women, and for administrative associate professionals and craftsmen for men. Additional adjustment for working conditions still diminished these associations, which remained significant for clerks for women, and for craftsmen for men (model 3). Note that model 3 included decision latitude and physical demands only, as adjustment for social support resulted in very small changes of the odds ratios for some occupational categories, and adjustment for psychological demands and stressful occupational events resulted in an increase of the odds ratios for all categories. The percentage changes in odds ratios between model 2 and model 3 ranged from 36% to 100% for men, and from 12% to 75% for women (table 20).

Table 19 shows the results of the three models for the prospective analysis. Model 1 presents the predictive effects of occupational grade on poor self-reported health one year later, after adjustment for age only. For men, being a foreman or a skilled industrial worker increased the risk of poor health. For women, this risk was increased for the category of clerks. Model 2 included adjustment for personal, behavioural, and health-related variables. This model shows the same associations as previously, since foremen, male skilled industrial workers, and female clerks were more likely to report poor health one year later. Note that the odds ratios increased a little from model 1 to model 2. Model 3 included additional adjustment for working conditions. As previously, this model retained the variables of decision latitude and physical demands, which both contributed to diminishing the odds ratios for all occupational categories. The percentage changes in odds ratios between model 2 and model 3 ranged from 14% to 70% for men, and from 9% to 17% for women (table 20).

Note that craftsmen were more likely to report poor health in the cross-sectional analysis, but not in the prospective one. This occupational category had the highest prevalence of poor health in 1997; consequently those in poor health were dropped from the prospective analysis leading to a potential selection bias, which could explain the fact that this category was no longer at risk in the prospective analysis (table 17).

Table 17: Description of the GAZEL cohort in 1997 and 1998

| | Respondents to the 1997 questionnaire and working in 1997 | | | Respondents to the 1998 questionnaire and still working in 1998 | | | | | |
| | Total | Prevalence of poor health in 1997 | | Total | | In good health in 1997 | | Incidence of poor health in 1998 | |
	N (1)	N (2)	% (2)/(1)*	N (3)	% (3)/(1)	N (4)	% (4)/(3)*	N (5)	% (5)/(4)*
Total	11,447	2,262	19.9	9 559	83.5	7,664	80.7	959	12.6
Men	8,277	1,532	18.6	6,853	82.8	5,575	81.9	643	11.6
Managers, engineers	3,580	570	16.0	3,018	84.3	2,517	83.8	255	10.2
Administrative associate professionals	969	207	21.6	799	82.5	630	79.6	70	11.2
Technicians	464	89	19.4	395	85.1	319	81.4	38	12.0
Foremen	2,414	460	19.2	1,953	80.9	1,584	81.4	206	13.1
Clerks	223	50	22.6	177	79.4	138	78.4	19	13.9
Skilled industrial workers	300	66	22.4	252	84.0	192	78.0	32	16.9
Craftsmen	302	88	29.6	239	79.1	175	74.2	21	12.1
Women	3,170	730	23.2	2,706	85.4	2,089	77.8	316	15.3
Managers, engineers	476	85	18.1	414	87.0	338	82.8	45	13.4
Administrative associate professionals	1,739	388	22.4	1,484	85.3	1,161	78.6	172	14.9
Foremen	367	74	20.3	317	86.4	251	79.7	30	12.0
Clerks	579	181	31.6	482	83.2	332	69.6	69	21.2

Missing values may explain that direct calculation does not exactly provide the same %.

Table 18: Contribution of working conditions to social inequalities in self-reported health: cross-sectional results of the GAZEL cohort

	Men		Women	
	OR	95% CI	OR	95% CI
Model 1	(N=8,191)		(N=3,137)	
Managers, engineers	1		1	
Administrative associate professionals	1.44	1.20-1.72	1.30	1.00-1.69
Technicians	1.24	0.96-1.59	-	
Foremen	1.22	1.06-1.40	1.16	0.82-1.63
Clerks	1.53	1.10-2.12	2.10	1.56-2.81
Skilled industrial workers	1.49	1.12-1.99	-	
Craftsmen	2.16	1.66-2.82	-	
Model 2	(N=8,084)		(N=3,063)	
Managers, engineers	1		1	
Administrative associate professionals	1.33	1.09-1.62	1.26	0.90-1.75
Technicians	1.15	0.88-1.50	-	
Foremen	1.13	0.96-1.33	1.16	0.78-1.74
Clerks	1.22	0.85-1.73	1.91	1.31-2.77
Skilled industrial workers	1.30	0.94-1.79	-	
Craftsmen	1.88	1.40-2.52	-	
Model 3	(N=7,742)		(N=2,831)	
Managers, engineers	1		1	
Administrative associate professionals	1.21	0.99-1.48	1.23	0.86-1.75
Technicians	0.94	0.71-1.24	-	
Foremen	1.00	0.84-1.18	1.04	0.68-1.60
Clerks	0.96	0.66-1.39	1.59	1.06-2.39
Skilled industrial workers	0.96	0.68-1.35	-	
Craftsmen	1.43	1.05-1.96	-	

Model 1: adjusted for age Model 2: additionally adjusted for marital status, stressful personal events, education, chronic conditions, smoking, alcohol, and overweight Model 3: additionally adjusted for decision latitude and physical demands.

Table 19: Contribution of working conditions to social inequalities in self-reported health: prospective results of the GAZEL cohort

	Men		Women	
	OR	95% CI	OR	95% CI
Model 1	(N=5515)		(N=2061)	
Managers, engineers	1		1	
Administrative associate professionals	1.12	0.84-1.48	1.12	0.78-1.59
Technicians	1.21	0.84-1.75	-	
Foremen	1.34	1.10-1.64	0.86	0.53-1.42
Clerks	1.43	0.86-2.36	1.71	1.13-2.58
Skilled industrial workers	1.82	1.21-2.72	-	
Craftsmen	1.23	0.77-1.99	-	
Model 2	(N=5457)		(N=2016)	
Managers, engineers	1		1	
Administrative associate professionals	1.12	0.82-1.52	1.22	0.76-1.97
Technicians	1.27	0.87-1.87	-	
Foremen	1.36	1.08-1.72	0.98	0.55-1.76
Clerks	1.23	0.72-2.11	1.90	1.11-3.26
Skilled industrial workers	1.95	1.27-3.02	-	
Craftsmen	1.30	0.79-2.14	-	
Model 3	(N=5244)		(N=1875)	
Managers, engineers	1		1	
Administrative associate professionals	1.04	0.76-1.43	1.20	0.72-1.99
Technicians	1.14	0.76-1.70	-	
Foremen	1.28	1.00-1.63	0.97	0.53-1.78
Clerks	1.07	0.60-1.89	1.75	0.98-3.10
Skilled industrial workers	1.82	1.15-2.86	-	
Craftsmen	1.25	0.75-2.10	-	

Model 1: adjusted for age Model 2: additionally adjusted for marital status, stressful personal events, education, chronic conditions, smoking, alcohol, and overweight Model 3: additionally adjusted for decision latitude and physical demands.

Table 20: Contribution of working conditions to social inequalities in self-reported health: cross-sectional and prospective results of the GAZEL cohort

Change in OR* (%)	Cross-sectional study		Prospective study	
	Men	Women	Men	Women
Managers, engineers (reference category)				
Administrative associate professionals	36.4	11.5	66.7	9.1
Technicians	100.0	-	48.1	-
Foremen	100.0	75.0	22.2	-50.0
Clerks	100.0	35.2	69.6	16.7
Skilled industrial workers	100.0	-	13.7	-
Craftsmen	51.1	-	16.7	-

* *Calculated as: (OR model 2 – OR model 3)/(OR model 2 – 1) Model 2: adjusted for age, marital status, stressful personal events, education, chronic conditions, smoking, alcohol, and overweight Model 3: additionally adjusted for decision latitude and physical demands.*

D. *Discussion*

This study showed that a substantial part of the association between occupational grade and self-reported health could be explained by poor working conditions, that is low levels of decision latitude, and high levels of physical demands. This finding was observed both in the cross-sectional and prospective analyses, although the contribution of these variables to social inequalities in self-reported health may be somewhat lower in the prospective analysis. In addition, this contribution may be greater for men than for women.

Several potential limitations are worth noting.

The population studied is not representative of the whole French working population, as these employees are working in a public-sector company and benefit from job security. Consequently, they may also work in better working conditions. In addition, they may be healthier than the French working population.

A selection bias cannot be excluded. The rate of participation of the GAZEL cohort was 44% at baseline in 1989. Furthermore, the rate of response to the self-administered questionnaire in 1997 was 74% and a comparison between the respondents to the 1998 questionnaire and the non-respondents with respect to the study variables in 1997 suggested that non-respondents were more likely to be less educated and exposed to physical demands for men, and to have poorer health for both men and women. These two first limitations may lead to an underestimation of the relationship between occupational grade and self-reported health on one hand, and of the contribution of working conditions to social class differences in health on the other.

Our study is based on a one-year prospective analysis. This follow-up period may be too short to allow the evaluation of the impact of occupational category and working conditions on self-reported health. In the same way, only one evaluation of working conditions was used in this study, and not history or duration of exposures. In this connection, the GAZEL cohort was initially composed of middle-aged people. In 1997, they were aged at least 48 years for men and 43 for women. As this prospective study is here restricted to the subgroup who rated their health as good in 1997, a part of the studied population is excluded because of poor health. Consequently, a selection bias may have operated before 1997, leading to underestimation of the effects of occupational grade on health and of the contribution of working conditions.

The measures of working conditions and health may have limitations. Self-reported health is strongly related to more objective measures of morbidity and mortality, but is a general indicator of health status, which covers various aspects of health. Working conditions were measured using the scales elaborated by Karasek, which include psychosocial factors at work and ergonomic exposures, but not other occupational risk factors such as chemical or physical exposures. Furthermore, as both working conditions and health were measured by self-report, our results may be affected by a reporting bias. This bias connected with 'common method variance', for example through social desirability or negative affectivity, can lead to inflated associations between exposure and health. Note that such bias has not been demonstrated in a previous study (Schrijvers *et al.* 1998).

In spite of these potential limitations, this is the first attempt to study the contribution of working conditions to social inequalities in self-reported health in a French working population. This is also a prospective study in a large sample of men and women. There are only a few international studies that have been performed so far on this topic. Note for example the study by Schrijvers *et al.* (1998) which showed that a substantial part of the association between occupational class and perceived health could be attributed to a differential distribution of hazardous physical working conditions and low job control across occupational classes. However, this study had a cross-sectional design. A prospective study was performed by Borg and Kristensen (2000), and showed also that a large part of the social gradient for self-rated health could be explained by a set of work environment factors, which were ergonomic exposures, repetitive work, skill discretion, climatic exposures, and job insecurity. Further studies are needed in the GAZEL cohort, but also in other French study populations, to evaluate whether and to what extent working conditions contribute to the explanation of the relationship between occupational grade and health. This present study is a first demonstration that in France working conditions may contribute to social inequalities in health. In conclusion, improving working conditions would lead not only to better health for workers, but also to reduced social inequalities in health.

4. The Contribution of Social Policies to the Reduction of Social Inequalities in Health in France

Social policies affect fields as varied as employment, work, precariousness, unemployment, education and training, income, housing and access to health care, and may, directly or indirectly, help to reduce social inequalities in the field of health. In this section, the authors review the most important social policies that may be capable of helping to do this in France. The subjects dealt with comprise (A) social security, with its three domains, covering health insurance, the compensation and prevention of occupational risks, and retirement pensions, (B) social policies dealing with employment and unemployment, and (C) in connection with these social policies, the role of institutions representing company workers, especially trade unions.

A. Social Security

The French Social Security was founded in 1945, in order to "guarantee workers and their families against any risk, of any kind, liable to reduce or abolish their earning capacity, and to cover the maternity expenses and family expenses incumbent on them". The system is based on four general principles: universal coverage (all risks and all workers), the same administration and organisation for all (the general system), the same benefits and contributions for all, and autonomy of the different social security organisations. However, these praiseworthy aims have only been achieved in part. The social security system covers various risks: illness (including maternity and disability), accidents at work and occupational diseases, old age, and family expenses.

Concurrently, complementary insurance systems, i.e. mutual funds and private insurance, are developing because of the insufficient coverage of retirement and illness provided by the social security. These systems rely on optional affiliation, which increases the differences between the coverage among various sectors of the population, as it is harder for the poorest to obtain the benefits provided by these systems because they cannot afford the contributions necessary to obtain them. Nevertheless, the effects of these inequalities, especially as regards health care, are now less severe, thanks to the existence of universal medical coverage.

Health Insurance

To assess the contribution of health insurance to the reduction of social inequalities in the field of health, it is necessary to examine access to care and the standard of care management. Since the Second World War, there has been a trend towards the generalisation of the coverage of illness, which is now practically complete. The proportion of 50% of the population covered by health insurance in 1946 has now risen to more than 99%. The health insurance system initially conceived for wage earners was extended to non wage earners and inactive persons as from the 1960s. Subsequently, the generalisation of protection against the risk of illness, regardless of occupation, came to be accepted as a priority of social protection, as certain categories of unemployed and other inactive persons were still insufficiently or poorly covered. Thus, successive laws increased the State's contribution to health insurance for groups entitled to welfare allocations. Nevertheless, despite this increase, 150,000 persons, mainly young people under 25 years of age, were not entitled to any protection at the end of the 1990s. In addition to this absence of coverage, 14% of those with social security insurance gave up applying for health care, for financial reasons. This proportion reached 28% for those not covered by complementary health insurance, and 30% for the unemployed in 1998 (Bocognano *et al.* 1999).

The introduction of universal health insurance coverage (Couverture Maladie Universelle – CMU) in 1999 enabled these shortcomings to be rectified. All persons residing regularly and permanently in France are obligatorily affiliated to this system. Affiliation is automatic, immediate and free for those whose maximum annual resources amount to 6,744 euros or less for single persons. In addition, the CMU provides complementary free health insurance under the same conditions to almost 5 million beneficiaries. This additional benefit permits equal access to health care and means that many of those insured no longer refrain from being treated because of the cost of their share of the expenses.

As a result of all this, considerable progress has been made over the past few years as regards equality of access to health care, especially since the introduction of universal coverage. Nevertheless, it seems desirable to evaluate this progress more precisely, in order to determine the final impact of the recent new measures, especially regarding social inequalities in health. Moreover, the CMU can be considered to have had at least two kinds of negative effect. Firstly, the very low maximum limit of the expenses to which its beneficiaries are entitled creates problems concerning refusal to be treated and the possibly poor quality of the care they receive. Secondly, there is a 'threshold effect', whose arbitrary nature may deprive certain people of complementary coverage because their resources are slightly above the required limit.

Prevention of and Compensation for Occupational Risks

In France, the prevention of occupational risks is chiefly the responsibility of occupational physicians, who are independent of the employers. Most of their time is spent carrying out compulsory medical checkups, which are performed at recruitment, annually, and after sick leave. In addition, one third of their time is spent studying job functions and working conditions. Thus, by exerting preventive action on health and safety at work, these occupational physicians could help to reduce social inequalities in the field of health, by giving special attention to categories of wage earners who otherwise have little or no contact with medical doctors. Since 1946, all employers have been required to allow inspections by occupational physicians, whatever the size of their company.

Compensation for accidents at work and occupational illnesses constitutes a separate part of the social security system. It comprises a form of protection, which automatically calls into play the responsibility of the employer, whether or not the wage earner is at fault, and institutes lump sum compensation. Damages to wage earners are thus automatically compensated, whereas employers enjoy immunity from Civil Law liability, except in cases of inexcusable or intentional error. Nevertheless, problems still remain:

– the system of compensation for occupational risks is more like a form of insurance for employers and seems inadequate for inculcating employers with a sense of responsibility and inciting them to take preventive measures;

– the restrictive and complex compensation procedure, its extreme slowness and the small compensation obtained dissuade certain victims from claiming compensation, thus accounting for the under-declaration of occupational diseases;

– the system of compensation for occupational risks makes no provision for the re-employment of victims, and

– the means and personnel allocated to company inspection are limited.

As shown above, occupational risks are unequally distributed among the occupational categories. The prevention and compensation systems carry considerable weight to prevent occupational exposures on the one hand and to compensate the effects of occupational risks on the other.

However, no evaluation has been made to measure their impact on the reduction of social inequalities in health.

Retirement Pensions

The basis of a real retirement pension system was established with the founding of the social security system in 1945. The pension system is distributive, i.e. the active population pays for the pensions of the retired. In the private sector, the retirement age is generally 60 years but in the public sector, it may be lower (55 or even 50 years). A full retirement pension of 75% requires 40 years of contributions in the private sector and 37.5 years in the public sector. A new reform will extend the period of contribution to 40 years for all in 2008, and to 41 years in 2012. Lastly, efforts are being made in favour of those earning the lowest wages, with the aim of achieving, in 2008, an initial pension rate of 85% of the last wage, for workers who have completed their period of contribution and been paid the minimum wage.

However, social inequalities still persist regarding pensions, and three differences may be stressed in this connection:

– the special system of the public sector has advantages as regards retirement age, the method of pension calculation, and the amount paid;

– taking into account the establishment of a single rate of contributions, and the differences between life expectancy after 65 years in the different occupations, income is mainly redistributed from the poorest, who have the shortest life expectancy, to the richest, who have higher pensions because these are proportional to their former earnings, and

– supplementary systems increase these inequalities of income still further, because firstly, all workers cannot afford the additional contributions required, and secondly, these systems are essentially designed for rich companies or sectors, or for various managerial categories.

In conclusion, the part played by old-age insurance in reducing social inequalities still seems to be insufficient, even though in principle, it is an instrument for the redistribution of income. In that sense, the new reform in progress tends to reduce the inequalities between the different systems and to increase the pensions of workers earning low wages. However, no information is currently available regarding the role of the pension system in reducing social inequalities in health.

B. Social Policies Regarding Employment and Unemployment

The object of employment policy is not to deal with social inequalities in health. Nevertheless, its actions may, in theory, help to reduce these inequalities. As shown above, there is indeed a link between health and activity or inactivity, as the health of inactive persons is not as good as that of active persons, and the risk of mortality is higher for the inactive. Effects of selection such as the 'healthy worker' effect may explain this relationship. Employers may prefer to recruit persons in good health, and in addition, a process of selection may be applied during activity, by eliminating those who fall ill. Nevertheless, certain authors (Bouvier-Colle 1983, Mesrine 2000) have shown that these effects only explain the relationship between health and activity in part, as work can also play a protective role in relation to health, by means of various mechanisms, including the reduction of risky types of behaviour such as alcohol abuse, and the presence of a social support or network. On the other hand, inactivity, especially unemployment, has a negative effect on health. Most important, access to employment means access to income, the chief protection against poverty. In addition, as also shown above, unemployment, and consequently the difficulty of finding a job, is unevenly distributed among the different occupational categories. Employment policy can therefore help to reduce social inequalities as regards health, by its action on employment and the labour market, and by its attempts to improve the lot of the poorest.

Employment Policy

In France, employment policies have only recently acquired importance, as they date back to the end of the 1970s and the slowing down of economic growth. Two periods can be distinguished: during the first, from 1945 to 1974, employment policies had to cope with a shortage of manpower. During the second period, from 1974 onwards, the aim was to arrest the rise of unemployment and attenuate its consequences at a time of economic crisis.

French employment policy has recourse to very diverse means of action, but two main objectives predominate:

1) To act on the level of employment, i.e. of unemployment, by creating and preserving jobs.

2) To act on the structure of unemployment, i.e. on long-term unemployment, to combat market selectivity of employment, and take account of certain target groups.

Employment policy in France is characterised by a plethora of measures, some of them focusing on the specific problems of the poorest, but lacks an overall strategy and a vision for the medium term. In addition, the impact of these measures to reduce social inequalities in health is unknown.

Unemployment Insurance

The French unemployment insurance system dates back to 1958, and is separate from the other social protection systems. Unemployment compensation depends on two distinct branches: conventional insurance, and a system of solidarity. The latter has a far less important role than the former. Unemployment insurance concerns private-sector wage earners as a whole and certain public-sector wage earners, i.e. some of those who are not government employees. The maximum allocation is 75% of the last wage, and the minimum 24.76 euros a day. The duration of allocation varies from 7 to 42 months. In 2001, 60% of the unemployed received compensation. After a substantial decrease between 1992 and 1998 due to restrictive measures, this rate has now returned to its 1992 level (Pommier 2003). However, unemployment in France is still high and is only compensated in part. The long-term unemployed are virtually excluded from compensation, even though they constitute one third of the total.

As from 1992, the minimal reinstatement income (*Revenu Minimum d'Insertion – RMI*), instituted in 1988, emerged as the third component of the compensation system, as it compensated those excluded from the two branches described above. The institution of a minimum reinstatement income was the first step towards remedying these deficiencies by its emphasis on reinstatement in order to avoid the process of exclusion, and to foster the return to, or the entry into, employment. The maximum monthly reinstatement income is 411.70 euros for single persons, on three conditions: permanent residence on French territory, age over 25 years (except for those with family responsibilities) and resources below the reinstatement income. This income also carries other rights, especially the right to social security. Recipients of this income are committed to take part in activities to encourage reinstatement. In 2000, these recipients totalled more than one million persons. However, despite the positive results of the system, it did not greatly favour reinstatement and was completed in 1998 by the law to combat exclusion. The impact of this minimal reinstatement income on social inequalities in health has not yet been evaluated.

The Programme to Prevent and Combat Poverty and Social Exclusion

A programme to prevent and fight poverty and social exclusion was instituted in 2001 and constituted a step forward in the fight against exclusion, which had begun in 1998. This programme had a very ambitious aim: to restore equal opportunities for all, and the prospect of social and occupational reinstatement for the poorest. It was oriented in two main directions:

– the return to employment of those furthest away from it, including those with the smallest social allowances, long-term unemployed and young people in difficulty.

– the access to fundamental rights: these include the right to financial resources, to housing and shelter, to health care, to education and participation in social life, and the right to justice. These rights must become realities for all those in a situation of precariousness.

Note that this plan for national action against poverty and social exclusion is part of a European strategy designed to fight all forms of exclusion. No evaluation has been performed regarding social inequalities in health.

C. Representative Workers' Organisations and Trade Unions

Organisations representing the workers may be capable of helping to reduce social inequalities as regards health, by ensuring observance of the labour laws, providing a means of worker-employer communication, and fostering prevention and the improvement of working conditions. It is therefore of interest to examine their contribution in this respect. The French system is characterised by a large number of in-house representative workers' organisations. In addition to the Trade Unions, two bodies represent wage earners: Staff Delegates, and the Company Committee. In addition, there is a special organism within the framework of health at work: the Hygiene, Safety and Working Conditions Committee. There are, however, several limits to this representative system. Firstly, there is the threshold effect: firms employing fewer than 10 wage earners have no obligations as regards representative workers' organisations. Therefore representation varies, depending on company size. Secondly, these organisations are mainly consultative, which means that their role is limited.

According to a survey entitled Occupational Relations and Negotiations with Companies (Relations Professionnelles et Négociations d'Entreprises) conducted in 1998 among various firms and workers' representatives, Trade Union Delegates are only present in 37% of the establishments employing 20 or more wage earners. They are more firmly implanted in large and in long-established companies. There are fewer of them in certain sectors of activity, including business, the building industry, services to individuals and services to companies. The primary cause of this uneven distribution stems from the labour laws, and also from the history of the trade union movement in France, particularly the constitution of large concentrations of industrial workers. Nearly one third of employers state that there is not a single trade union member among those they employ. This absence of membership concerns 42% of firms employing less than 50 wage earners. On the other hand, for firms employing 200 to 500 wage earners, the corresponding figure is only 6%, and for those employing more than 500, it is virtually nil (Furjot 2000). These figures confirm the low trade union membership in France. According to the International Labour Organisation, it was 9% in 1995.

A visit to the website of four of the main French trade union shows how problems concerning work and social inequalities in health are considered. Rather than having a general policy in these respects, all four unions define, in their website statements, their attitudes to the relationships between health and working conditions, and to social inequalities in health care. As regards health and working conditions, several points are dealt with, including the following:

– the importance of primary risk prevention in the workplace, and also of systematic assessment of work-related risks at the regional level. The aspects of health discussed are stress at work and its effects on health, and cancer, as well as the prevention of industrial accidents, and their effects on both workers and the environment;

– medical surveillance in the workplace. The benefits for workers of the particular French system are listed, including compulsory medical examinations and the importance of independence for occupational physicians;

– the consequences of work accidents or occupational diseases in terms of disability and handicaps, and the need to improve tertiary prevention, i.e. to find suitable jobs for the handicapped, and lastly,

– compensation for occupational diseases, and two of the main problems involved: the low number of compensations in relation to the number of work-related diseases, and inequalities as regards the difficulty of obtaining compensation (including regional inequalities). The aspects of health considered are mainly work-related upper limb disorders and occupational forms of cancer, especially those following exposure to asbestos.

As regards social inequalities in the field of health, the trade union statements referred to above stress the differences between the access to care of the different social categories, in connection with the current debate in France on the national health insurance system and access to a mutual insurance company for complementary reimbursement. Several unions emphasise the existence of social inequalities in this respect, especially for the reimbursement of spectacles, dental prostheses and hearing aids. Less space is given in these statements to social inequalities in the field of health in general, and their relationships to working conditions.

5. Conclusion

A. Main Results

Using available national data it is possible to describe the situation in France regarding the labour market, employment, and working conditions. The surveys on working conditions conducted by the European Foundation for the improvement of living and working conditions in Dublin have not been described here, but France can be compared with other European countries. For most of the indicators used in the last survey performed in 2000, France is generally close to the mean of the fifteen European countries (Paoli and Merllié 2001). With the available national data it is not possible to determine precisely how working conditions have developed over the past two decades. Despite the limitations mentioned before, some authors agree that psychosocial conditions at work have deteriorated during the last two decades (Gollac and Volkoff 1996, Hamon-Cholet and Rougerie 2000, Bué and Guignon 2002).

The relationship between occupational category and working conditions is well established: the categories of clerks and service workers, and of blue-collar workers, especially those who are unskilled, have the worst working conditions, whatever the type of occupational exposure considered: physical, chemical, ergonomic or psychosocial. People in these occupational categories are also those who are the most concerned by unemployment, precarious work, and part-time work. Consequently, these categories accumulate detrimental conditions at the labour market level, but also as regards working conditions.

Social inequalities in health have been described for a long time in France, both for mortality and various indicators of morbidity. The unfavourable situation of clerks and service workers, and of blue-collar workers compared with managers, is underlined, and also the unfavourable situation of the category of unemployed compared with those who have a job.

Can we conclude that work and working conditions explain social inequalities in health in France? At this stage, in France, everything is speculation. Nevertheless, in this chapter, a study was performed to test this hypothesis among a cohort of workers in a specific sector of activity. This study showed that a part of the relationship between occupational category and self-reported health was explained by certain indicators of working conditions. The hypothesis that working conditions explain at least in part social inequalities in health has to be tested among other study populations in France and for other health outcomes, in order to better understand the mechanisms underlying social inequalities in health, and to provide possible actions which could improve working conditions and health, and also reduce social inequalities in health.

B. *About Social Policies*

In France, to date, no social policy has had the objective of reducing social inequalities in health. Nevertheless, a number of these social policies focus on the specific problems of the poorest segments of the population, aiming to provide them with fundamental rights such as access to health care, and taking account of their specific problems regarding employment, unemployment, or social exclusion. If French social policies do not focus on the reduction of health inequalities in health, some rely on the notion of equality, for example equality in access to health care, which is one of the underlying principles of the French social security. Lastly, as underlined by the French Committee for Public Health (Haut comité de la Santé Publique 2002), as some measures are directed towards the poorest groups, for example to reduce social exclusion, they also contribute to the reduction of social inequalities in general, and especially in income, access to some rights, etc. The question is then whether these measures have an impact on social inequalities in health. Information is missing, and there has been no evaluation so far to evaluate such an impact. Note that some social policies, for example health insurance, directly concern health, and if uncertainty remains about their role in reducing social inequalities in health, there is no doubt that these policies play a great part in the fact that these inequalities do not increase still more. Other social policies do not deal with health, for example the employment policy or the programme to prevent social exclusion, and can only indirectly contribute to the reduction of social inequalities in health. They could act on potential causes of the deterioration of health in certain groups of the population, for example by facilitating return to employment or allowing access to rights or benefits.

An international review of the literature recently published gives information about the contribution of health insurance to the reduction of social inequalities in health, according to studies from the USA, Great Britain, and France (Dourgnon *et al.* 2001). The main conclusions are the following: if health insurance induces an increase in the use of health care, the effect of this use on health is more difficult to evaluate. Nevertheless, health insurance seems to improve the health status of poor populations, especially as regards infantile diseases, eye diseases, and hypertension. In addition, there may be an indirect effect of health insurance: by preventing health expenses from burdening the household budget, health insurance means that non-medical expenses, which could have an impact on health, such as housing, food, or education, do not decrease. The authors of this review (Dourgnon *et al.* 2001) conclude that health insurance could have a protective role on health, especially for the poorest people, confirming the hypothesis that health insurance could contribute to the reduction of social inequality in health.

C. The Future

What about the future? What developments can we expect for working conditions; for the relationship between occupational category, working conditions and health; and for the potential contribution of work to social inequalities in health?

With regard to the developments in working conditions, data are fragmentary for the last few decades in France. It is not certain that working conditions have improved for chemical, physical and ergonomic exposures. For psychosocial factors, the available data would rather indicate a deterioration of working conditions, related to an intensification of work and an increase of mental constraints. According to some authors (Greenan and Hamon-Cholet 2000), this negative change is associated with the introduction of new forms of work organisation and technological innovations. In addition, the economic context, especially globalisation and the increase of competition, may have had negative consequences on working conditions. Concurrently, many changes have occurred during the past decades. Schooling has become longer. The retirement age has been lowered, and despite new measures to extend the period of contributions, the legal age for retirement will remain 60 years. Holidays are longer (at least 30 working days per year for the working population of the private sector) and working hours have never been so short (35 hours per week). All these elements diminish the period of activity for men and women in France and potentially diminish the duration of occupational exposures.

How is the relationship between occupational category and working conditions changing? It seems difficult to predict this relationship, and consequently the development of social inequalities in working conditions. Will these inequalities increase or decrease? It is already difficult to determine how working conditions will evolve in general; it is still more difficult to predict this development by occupational category. To date, available data have not yet been studied in order to evaluate how social inequalities in working conditions have evolved over the past few decades. More details on the development of working conditions according to occupational category could shed some light on this point.

What about developments in the contribution of work to social inequalities in health? Currently, there are no available national data to evaluate this in France. So it seems very difficult to speculate on developments in the contribution of work to these inequalities. Social inequalities in health have been observed in France for a long time. Social inequalities in premature mortality (risk of dying before the age of 65) among men are noticeable in France compared with other European countries, and risky behaviours would contribute to these inequalities in a substantial way, especially with regard to consumption of alcohol and tobacco habits (Brixi and Lang 2000, Kunst *et al*. 2000).

D. *Ongoing Research on Social Class, Working Conditions and Health*

The ongoing research projects are based on cohorts of employed (or formerly employed) subjects, on case-control studies, on large national surveys, and on a regional surveillance study. Several projects have been developed within the GAZEL cohort (http://www.gazel.inserm.fr) with the aim of studying social inequalities in health and evaluating the relative explanatory role of working conditions and other risk factors, especially for social inequalities in mortality and cancer. Another project with the same objective has been developed for upper respiratory and digestive tract cancer, based on a case-control study (Menvielle *et al*. 2004). At least two large national surveys are currently being studied in order to gain a better understanding of the relationships between social inequalities, occupation and health. The first one is the national survey on impairment and disabilities, which contains many details on physical limitations, social situation, labour market situation, and sources of income (Mormiche 2003, Mormiche and Boissonnat 2003). The second one is a large data set from INSEE (in charge of the censuses) covering about 1% of the population living in France, with data (on occupation, social situation, housing conditions, etc.) collected at several censuses. These data have been analysed for general mortality (Mesrine 1999). Two projects in progress are based on an enrichment of these data with mortality by causes of death. Another project, focused on upper limb disorders and low back pain, is a pilot project in a region of France. A part of it, based on medical services in the region, consists in a registration of all the suspected cases of carpal tunnel syndrome, with details on occupation for those affected. The same approach will be applied to back surgery. Another part relies on a network of occupational physicians in various occupational settings; these physicians perform a standardised physical examination for a random sample of the employees they are in charge of, and each worker in the study fills in a questionnaire on symptoms and working conditions (Roquelaure *et al*. 2002).

E. Data that would be Suitable for International and Comparative Analyses of Work-related Inequity in Health

In-depth comparative research dealing with the contribution of personal and occupational risk factors to social inequalities in health can be developed by comparing data issued from cohorts. For example, a first comparison has been performed between the GAZEL and Whitehall cohorts (Fuhrer *et al.* 2002). This kind of collaborative work should be developed. For large cross-sectional surveys in the general population in France, improvements have been made in recent years in order to increase comparability with similar surveys in Europe. A development of comparative analyses would certainly lead to further improvements in comparability of the study design and questionnaires. For example, it would be useful to have a comparable set of questions about present and past occupational exposures, which might be included in national surveys on health. Present studies in France focus on working conditions or on health, but they seldom include both dimensions. This is a limitation to overcome in the future.

Acknowledgements

The authors thank Stéphanie Degioanni and Simone David for their help in compiling the references, and Mathilde Dreyfus for revising the English manuscript. The authors' thanks also go to Tomas Hemmingsson, Christer Hogstedt, and Ingvar Lundberg for their helpful suggestions in the preparation of this chapter.

References

AERTS A.-T., BIGOT J.-F. 2002. "Enquête sur l'emploi de mars 2002. Chômage et emploi en hausse" (Employment survey of March 2002. Increase in unemployment and employment), *INSEE Première* 857.

AFSA C., BISCOURP P., POLLET P. 2003. "La baisse de la durée du travail entre 1995 et 2001" (Working hours lowering between 1995 and 2001), *INSEE Première* 881.

ALBOUY V., WANECQ T. 2003. "Les inégalités sociales d'accès aux grandes écoles" (Social inequalities in access to France's élite establishments), *Économie et Statistique* 361: 27-52.

AMOSSÉ T. 2001. "L'espace des métiers de 1990 à 1999. Recensement de la population de 1999" (Occupations from 1990 to 1999. 1999 population census), *INSEE Première* 790.

AMOSSÉ T., CHARDON O. 2002. "La carte des professions (1982-1999): le marché du travail par le menu" (The map of occupations (1982-1999): an insight into the labour market), in *Données Sociales 2002: la Société Française*, Paris, INSEE : 215-223.

AUDRIC S. 2002. "Qualification et diplôme" (Qualification and degree), in *Données Sociales 2002: la Société Française*, Paris, INSEE: 183-191.

BARRAT O., MEURS D. 2003. "Les écarts de rémunération hommes-femmes: un positionnement défavorable des femmes dans les grilles de conventions collectives" (Male-female wage gaps. Women's unfavourable positioning in the collective wage agreements), *Premières Informations et Premières Synthèses* 11.3.

BAYET A., DEMAILLY D. 1996. "La hiérarchie des salaires" (Wages hierarchy), *INSEE Première* 487.

BIHR A., PFEFFERKORN R. 1999. *Déchiffrer les Inégalités (Understanding inequalities)*, Paris: La Découverte et Syros: p. 420.

BIHR A., PFEFFERKORN R. 2000. "Évolution générale des inégalités sociales: les revenus, le logement, l'école" (The general development of social inequalities: incomes, housing, school). In A. LECLERC, D. FASSIN, H. GRANDJEAN, M. KAMINSKI, T. LANG, *Les Inégalités Sociales de Santé*. Paris: La Découverte et Syros: 333-348.

BISAULT L., BLOCH-LONDON C., LAGARDE S., LE CORRE V. 1996. "Le développement du travail à temps partiel" (Part-time work development). In *Données Sociales 1996: la Société Française*, Paris: INSEE: 225-233.

BOCOGNANO A., DUMESNIL S., FRÉROT L., LE FUR PH., SERMET C. 1999. "Santé, soins et protection sociale en 1998" (Health, care, and social protection in 1998), *Questions d'économie de la santé* 24.

BOËLDIEU J., BORREL C. 2000. "La proportion d'immigrés est stable depuis 25 ans" (The rate of immigrants has been steady for 25 years). *INSEE Première* 748.

BORG V., KRISTENSEN TS. 2000. "Social class and self-rated health: can the gradient be explained by differences in life style or work environment?". *Soc Sci Med* 51: 1019-30.

BORREL C., BOËLDIEU J. 2001. "De plus en plus de femmes immigrées sur le marché du travail" (There are more and more women-immigrants in the labour market), *INSEE Première* 791.

BOURLÈS L., COURSON J.-P. 2000. "12,2 millions d'actives et 14,3 millions d'actifs. Recensement de la population 1999" (12.2 million women and 14.3 million men in the working population. 1999 population census), *INSEE Première* 749.

BOUVET M., YAHOU N. 2001. "Le risque d'accident du travail varie avec la conjoncture économique" (The accident rate at work is associated with the overall economic situation), *Premières Synthèses* 31.1.

BOUVIER-COLLE M.-H. 1983. "Mortalité et activité professionnelle chez les femmes" (Mortality and employment among women), *Population* 1: 107-36.

BRISSON C., BLANCHETTE C., GUIMONT C., DION G., MOISAN J., VÉZINA M., DAGENAIS GR., MÂSSE L. 1998. "Reliability and validity of the French version of the 18-item Karasek Job Content Questionnaire", *Work Stress* 12: 322-36.

BRIXI O., LANG T. 2000. "Comportements" (Behaviour), in A. Leclerc, D. Fassin, H. Grandjean, M. Kaminski, T. Lang, *Les Inégalités Sociales de Santé*. Paris: La Découverte et Syros: 391-402.

BUÉ J., GUIGNON N., HAMON-CHOLET S., VINCK L. 2002. "Vingt ans de conditions de travail" (Development of working conditions over 20 years), in *Données Sociales 2002: la Société Française*. Paris: INSEE: 273-279.

BUÉ J., HAMON-CHOLET S., PUECH I. 2003. "Organisation du travail: comment les salariés vivent le changement" (Work organisation: how change is perceived by wage-earners). *Premières Informations et Premières Synthèses* 24.1.

BUÉ J., ROUGERIE C. 1999. "L'organisation du travail: entre contrainte et initiative. Résultats de l'enquête conditions de travail de 1998" (Work organisation: between constraint and initiative. Results of the 1998 working conditions survey), *Premières Synthèses* 32.1.

CALOT C., FEBVRAY M. 1965. "La mortalité différentielle suivant le milieu social" (Differential mortality according to social classes), *Études et Conjonctures* 11: 75-159.

CALVEZ M. 2000. "Le sida" (AIDS). In A. LECLERC, D. FASSIN, H. GRANDJEAN, M. KAMINSKI, T. LANG, *Les Inégalités Sociales de Santé*. Paris: La Découverte et Syros: 283-294.

CASTEL R. 1995. *Les Métamorphoses de la Question Sociale. Une Chronique du Salariat (Metamorphosis of the social question. A wage-earners' chronicle)*. Paris: Fayard: 490.

CAVELAARS AE., KUNST AE., GEURTS JJ., CRIALESI R., GROTVEDT L., HELMERT U., LAHELMA E., LUNDBERG O., MATHESON J., MIELCK A., MIZRAHI A., MIZRAHI A., RASMUSSEN NK., REGIDOR E., SPUHLER T., MACKENBACH JP. 1998. "Differences in self reported morbidity by educational level: a comparison of 11 western European countries". *J Epidemiol Community Health* 52: 219-27.

CÉZARD M., HAMON-CHOLET S. 1999. "Efforts et risques au travail en 1998" (Efforts and risks at work in 1998). *Premières Synthèses* 16.1.

CÉZARD M., HAMON-CHOLET S. 1999. "Travail et charge mentale" (Work and mental load), *Premières Synthèses* 27.1.

CHARDON O. 2001. "Les transformations de l'emploi non qualifié depuis vingt ans" (Unskilled jobs transformations over 20 years), *INSEE Première* 796.

CORNUAU V., QUARRÉ D. 2001. "Les salaires des agents de l'Etat en 2000" (Civil servants' wages in 2000). *INSEE Première* 818.

COUTROT T. 1996. "Les nouveaux modes d'organisation de la production: quels effets sur l'emploi, la formation, l'organisation du travail ?" (New features of production organisation: effects on employment, training, and work organisation). In *Données Sociales 1996: la Société Française*. Paris: INSEE: 209-216.

DESPLANQUES G. 1984. "L'inégalité sociale devant la mort" (Social inequalities in mortality), *Économie et Statistique* 162: 29-50.

DESPLANQUES G. 2001. "Effet de sélection et disparités de mortalité" (Effect of selection and disparity in mortality). In *Travail, Santé, Vieillissement: Relations et Évolutions*. Toulouse: Octares: 33-41.

DJIDER Z. 2004. *Femmes et Hommes – Regards sur la Parité (Women and men – An insight into parity)*. Paris: INSEE: 173.

DOURGNON P., GRIGNON M., JUSOT F. 2001. "L'assurance maladie réduit-elle les inégalités sociales de santé ? Une revue de la littérature" (Does health insurance reduce social inequalities in health ? A review of the literature). *Questions d'économie de la santé* 43.

DUMARTIN S., TOMASINI M. 1993. "Déclin de l'emploi industriel et tertiarisation accrue. L'emploi par secteur d'activité entre 1982 et 1990" (Decline in industry and expansion of services. Employment by sectors of activity between 1982 and 1990). *Économie et Statistique* 261: 33-44.

ESQUIEU P., POULET-COULIBANDO P. 2002. "Vers un enseignement secondaire de masse (1985-2001)" (Towards a mass secondary education (1985-2001)), in *Données Sociales 2002: la Société Française*. Paris: INSEE: 71-80.

ESTRADE M.-A., ULRICH V. 2002. "Réduction du temps de travail et réorganisations des rythmes de travail" (Working hours lowering and re-organisation of working rhythms). In *Données Sociales 2002: la Société Française*. Paris: INSEE: 301-308.

FERMANIAN J.-D., BAESA M.-P. 1997. "La durée du travail à temps complet" (Full-time working hours). *INSEE Première* 545.

FOUQUIN M., JEAN S., SZTULMAN A. 2000. "Le marché du travail britannique vu de France" (The Bristish labour market seen from France). *Économie et Statistique* 332-333: 97-115.

FUHRER R., SHIPLEY M.J., CHASTANG JF., SCHMAUS A., NIEDHAMMER I., STANSFELD SA., GOLDBERG M., MARMOT MG. 2002. "Socioeconomic position, health, and possible explanations: a tale of two cohorts". *Am J Public Health* 92: 1290-1294.

FURJOT D. 2000. "Où sont les délégués syndicaux ?" (Where are the Trade-Unions representatives ?). *Premières Synthèses* 41.2.

GALTIER B. 1999. "Les temps partiels: entre emplois choisis et emplois 'faute de mieux'" (Part-time works: between chosen jobs and 'failing anything better' jobs). *Économie et Statistique* 321-322: 57-77.

GOLDBERG M., BANAEI A., GOLDBERG S., AUVERT B., LUCE D., GUEGUEN A. 2000. "Past occupational exposure to asbestos among men in France". *Scand J Work Environ Health* 26: 52-61.

GOLDBERG M., CHASTANG JF., LECLERC A., ZINS M., BONENFANT S., BUGEL I., KANIEWSKI N., SCHMAUS A., NIEDHAMMER I., PICIOTTI M., CHEVALIER A., GODARD C., IMBERNON E. 2001. "Socioeconomic, demographic, occupational, and health factors associated with participation in a long-term epidemiologic survey: a prospective study of the French GAZEL cohort and its target population", *Am J Epidemiol.* 154: 373-84.

GOLLAC M., VOLKOFF S. 1996. "Citius, altius, fortius. L'intensification du travail" (Citius, altius, fortius. Intensification of work). *Actes de la Recherche en Sciences Sociales* 114.

GOUX D., MAURIN E. 1997. "Démocratisation de l'école et persistance des inégalités" (Democratisation of school and persistence of inequalities), *Économie et Statistique* 306: 27-39.

GRCIC S., MORER N. 2002. "L'activité féminine" (Women's activity) in *Données Sociales 2002: la Société Française*. Paris: INSEE: 199-206.

GREENAN N., HAMON-CHOLET S. 2000. "Les salariés industriels face aux changements organisationnels en 1997" (Industrial wage-earners facing organisational changes in 1997), *Premières Synthèses* 9.

GUIGNON N., HAMON-CHOLET S. 2003. "Au contact avec le public, des conditions de travail particulières" (In contact with the public: specific working conditions), *Premières Informations et Premières Synthèses* 09.3.

HAMON-CHOLET S. 2002. "Accidents, accidentés et organisation du travail: résultats de l'enquête sur les conditions de travail de 1998" (Accidents, injured, and work organisation: results of the 1998 working conditions survey), *Premières Synthèses* 20.1.

HAMON-CHOLET S., ROUGERIE C. 2000. "La charge mentale au travail: des enjeux complexes pour les salariés" (Mental load at work: complex stakes for wage-earners), *Économie et Statistique* 339-340: 243-255.

HAUT COMITÉ DE LA SANTÉ PUBLIQUE. 2002. *La santé en France 2002 (Health in France in 2002)*, Paris: La documentation française 410.

HÉRAN-LE ROY O. 1999. "Les risques professionnels pour la santé" (Occupational risks). In *Données Sociales 1999: la Société Française*. Paris: INSEE: 264-271.

HÉRAN-LE ROY O. HÉRAN-LE ROY O., NIEDHAMMER I., SANDRET N., LECLERC A. 1999. "Manual materials handling and related occupational hazards: a national survey in France". *International Journal of Industrial Ergonomics* 24: 365-77.

HÉRAN-LE ROY O., SANDRET N. 1996. "Expositions aux contraintes et nuisances dans le travail" (Exposure to constraints and risks at work). *Premières Informations et Premières Synthèses* 42.1.

HÉRAN-LE ROY O., SANDRET N. 1997. "La manutention manuelle de charges. Résultats de l'enquête SUMER 1994" (Manual materials handling: results of the 1994 SUMER survey). *Premières Informations et Premières Synthèses* 39.1.

HÉRAN-LE ROY O., SANDRET N. 1997. "SUMER 1994: l'état des lieux" (1994 SUMER survey: an assessment of the situation). *Santé et Travail* 20: 13-17.

HERBERT C., LAUNOY G. 2000. "Les cancers" (Cancers). In A. LECLERC, D. FASSIN, H. GRANDJEAN, M. KAMINSKI, T. Lang. *Les Inégalités Sociales de Santé*, Paris: La Découverte et Syros: 239-250.

HOUTMAN I., KORNITZER M., DE SMET P., KOYUNCU R., DE BACKER G., PELFRENE E., ROMON M., BOULENGUEZ C., FERRARIO M., ORIGGI G., SANS S., PEREZ I., WILHELMSEN L., ROSENGREN A., ISACSSON SO., ÖSTER-

GREN PO. 1999. "Job stress, absenteeism and coronary heart disease European cooperative study (the JACE study): design of a multicentre prospective study". *Eur J Public Health* 9: 52-57.

INSEE. 2002. *France, Portrait Social (France, social description)*. Paris: INSEE: 242.

INTERNATIONAL STANDARD CLASSIFICATION OF OCCUPATIONS (ISCO-88). 1990. Geneva: International Labour Office: 457.

OUGLA E.J., RICAN S., PÉQUIGNOT F., LE TOULLEC A. 2000. "La mortalité" (Mortality), in A. Leclerc, D. Fassin, H. Grandjean, M. Kaminski, T. Lang, *Les Inégalités Sociales de Santé*. Paris: La Découverte et Syros: 147-162.

KARASEK R., THEORELL T. 1990. *Healthy Work: Stress, Productivity, and the Reconstruction of Working Life*. New York: Basic Books: 381.

KUNST AE., GROENHOF F., MACKENBACH J.-P. 2000. Le groupe de travail de l'Union européenne sur les inégalités socio-économiques de santé, "Inégalités sociales de mortalité prématurée: la France comparée aux autres pays européens" (Social inequalities in premature mortality: France compared with the other European countries). In A. LECLERC, D. FASSIN, H. GRANDJEAN, M. KAMINSKI, T. LANG, *Les Inégalités Sociales de Santé*. Paris: La Découverte et Syros: 53-68.

KUNST AE., GROENHOF F., MACKENBACH JP., HEALTH EW. 1998. "Occupational class and cause specific mortality in middle aged men in 11 European countries: comparison of population based studies. EU Working Group on Socioeconomic Inequalities in Health". *BMJ* 316: 1636-42.

LAGARENNE C., LEGENDRE N. 2000. "Les travailleurs pauvres" (The poor workers). *INSEE Première* 745.

LAGARENNE C., LEGENDRE N. 2000. "Les travailleurs pauvres en France: facteurs individuels et familiaux" (The poor workers in France: personal and domestic factors). *Économie et Statistique* 335: 3-25.

LANG T., DUCIMETIERE P., ARVEILER D., AMOUYEL P., CAMBOU J.P., RUIDAVETS JB., MONTAYE M., MEYER V., BINGHAM A. 1997. "Incidence, case fatality, risk factors of acute coronary heart disease and occupational categories in men aged 30-59 in France". *Int J Epidemiol* 26: 47-57.

LANG T., RIBET C. 2000. "Les maladies cardio-vasculaires" (Cardiovascular diseases). In A. LECLERC, D. FASSIN, H. GRANDJEAN, M. KAMINSKI, T. LANG, *Les Inégalités Sociales de Santé*. Paris: La Découverte et Syros: 223-238.

LAROCQUE B., BRISSON C., BLANCHETTE C. 1998. "Internal consistency, factorial validity and discriminant validity of the French version of the psychological demands and decision latitude scales of the Karasek 'Job Content Questionnaire'". *Rev Epidemiol Sante Publique* 46: 371-81.

LECLERC A., FASSIN D., GRANDJEAN H., KAMINSKI M., LANG T. 2000. *Les Inégalités Sociales de Santé (Social inequalities in health*. Paris: La Découverte et Syros: 448.

MARTIN-HOUSSART G. 2001. "De plus en plus de passages vers un emploi stable" (Increasing access to stable employment). *INSEE Première*: 769.

MENVIELLE G., LUCE D., GOLDBERG P., LECLERC A. 2004. "Smoking, alcohol drinking, occupational exposures and social inequalities in hypopharyngeal and laryngeal cancer". *Int J Epidemiology* 33: 799-805.

MESRINE A. 1999. "Les différences de mortalité par milieu social restent fortes" (Mortality differences by social classes have remained strong). In *Données Sociales 1999: la Société Française*. Paris: INSEE: 228-235.

MESRINE A. 2000. "La surmortalité des chômeurs: un effet catalyseur du chômage ?" (Overmortality of the unemployed: a catalyst effect of unemployment ?). *Économie et Statistique* 334: 33-48.

MEURS D., PONTHIEUX S. 1999. "Emploi et salaires: les inégalités entre femmes et hommes en mars 1998" (Employment and wages: inequalities between men and women in March 1998). *Premières Synthèses* 32.2.

MEURS D., PONTHIEUX S. 2000. "Une mesure de la discrimination dans l'écart de salaire entre hommes et femmes" (A measurement of discrimination in the wage gap between men and women). *Économie et Statistique*: 337-338: 135-58.

MORMICHE P. 2002. *Handicap et Inégalités Sociales (Handicap and social inequalities)*. Paris: Colloque Handicaps, Incapacités, Dépendance.

MORMICHE P. 2003. "L'enquête 'Handicaps, incapacités, dépendance': apports et limites" (The 'Handicaps, incapacités, dépendance' survey: contributions and limits). *Revue Française des Affaires Sociales* 1-2: 13-30.

MORMICHE P., BOISSONNAT V. 2003. "Handicap et inégalités sociales: premiers apports de l'enquête 'Handicaps, incapacités, dépendance'" (Handicap and social inequalities: first contributions of the 'Handicaps, incapacités, dépendance' survey). *Revue Française des Affaires Sociales* 1-2: 267-86.

NIEDHAMMER I. 2002. "Psychometric properties of the French version of the Karasek Job Content Questionnaire: a study of the scales of decision latitude, psychological demands, social support, and physical demands in the GAZEL cohort". *Int Arch Occup Environ Health* 75: 129-44.

NIEDHAMMER I., BUGEL I., GOLDBERG M., LECLERC A., GUEGUEN A. 1998. "Psychosocial factors at work and sickness absence in the Gazel cohort: a prospective study". *Occup Environ Med.* 55: 735-41.

NIEDHAMMER I., CHEA M. 2003. "Psychosocial factors at work and self reported health: comparative results of cross sectional and prospective analyses of the French GAZEL cohort". *Occup Environ Med.* 60: 509-15.

NIEDHAMMER I., DAVID S., BUGEL I., CHEA M. 2000. "Catégorie socioprofessionnelle et exposition aux facteurs psychosociaux au travail dans une cohorte professionnelle" (Occupational categories and exposure to psychosocial factors at work in an occupational cohort). *Travailler* 5: 23-45.

NIEDHAMMER I., GOLDBERG M., LECLERC A., BUGEL I., DAVID S. 1998. "Psychosocial factors at work and subsequent depressive symptoms in the Gazel cohort". *Scand J Work Environ Health* 24: 197-205.

NIEDHAMMER I., GOLDBERG M., LECLERC A., DAVID S., BUGEL I., LANDRE MF. 1998. "Psychosocial work environment and cardiovascular risk factors in an occupational cohort in France". *J Epidemiol Community Health* 52: 93-100.

NIEDHAMMER I., SIEGRIST J., LANDRE MF., GOLDBERG M., LECLERC A. 2000. "Étude des qualités psychométriques de la version française du modèle du Déséquilibre Efforts/Récompenses" (Psychometric properties of the French version of the Effort-Reward Imbalance model). *Rev Epidemiol Sante Publique* 48: 419-37.

NIEDHAMMER I., TEK ML., STARKE D., SIEGRIST J. 2004. "Effort-reward imbalance model and self-reported health: cross-sectional and prospective findings from the GAZEL cohort". *Soc Sci Med* 58: 1531-41.

NOMENCLATURE D'ACTIVITÉS ET DE PRODUITS NAF REV. 1 – CPF REV. 1 EDITION 2003, Paris, INSEE, 2003, p. 882.

NOMENCLATURE DES PROFESSIONS ET CATÉGORIES SOCIO-PROFESSIONNELLES (PCS) 2003, Paris, INSEE, 2003, p. 665.

OBSERVATOIRE DE L'EMPLOI PUBLIC. 2004. *Rapport Annuel 9 décembre 2003 (Annual report, December 9th, 2003)*. Paris: La Documentation Française: 138.

PAOLI P., MERLLIÉ D. 2001. *Third European Survey on Working Conditions 2000*, Dublin: European Foundation for the Improvement of Living and Working Conditions: 72.

POMMIER P. 2003. "Forte croissance du chômage indemnisé en 2001" (Strong increase in compensated unemployment in 2001). *Premières Informations et Premières Synthèses* 02.2.

RASOLOFOARISON J., SEROUSSI G. 2002. "Les salaires dans les entreprises en 2000. Des salaires horaires toujours dynamiques" (Companies wages in 2000. Hourly wages are still dynamic). *INSEE Première* 833.

ROQUELAURE Y. 2002. *Surveillance Epidémiologique des Troubles Musculo-squelettiques: une Expérience Pilote dans les Pays de la Loire (Epidemiological surveillance of musculoskeletal disorders: a pilot experiment in the Loire's region)*. Grenoble: Congrès National de Médecine et Santé au Travail.

SAS INSTITUTE. 1999. *SAS/STAT user's guide Version 8*. CARY: NC: SAS INSTITUTE INC.

SCHRIJVERS C.T., VAN DE MHEEN HD., STRONKS K., MACKENBACH JP. 1998. "Socioeconomic inequalities in health in the working population: the contribution of working conditions". *Int J Epidemiol.* 27: 1011-1018.

THAVE S. 2000. "L'emploi des immigrés en 1999" (Immigrants' employment in 1999). *INSEE Première* 717.

THÉLOT C., VALLET L.-A. 2000. "La réduction des inégalités sociales devant l'école depuis le début du siècle" (Decrease in social inequalities in access to teaching since the beginning of the century). *Économie et Statistique* 334: 3-32.

TROGAN P. 1993. "Services marchands: un million d'emplois créés en huit ans" (Services: one million jobs created in eight years). *Économie et Statistique* 261: 45-53.

Germany

Richard PETER

Introduction

The present chapter begins with the introduction of changes in the social structure in Germany during the past 12 years. This time window was chosen since Germany – in contrast to other Western European countries – was faced with basic changes. In October 1989 the reunification of Germany started. Two countries, which had developed in different directions economically, politically and socially for more than 40 years, melted together again. The reunification basically influenced the social structure of Germany and, probably, social inequalities in health (Mielck 2000). Over the years the social gap between eastern and western Germany has become more and more obvious.

Therefore the present chapter concentrates on the time after the reunification process had begun. Data are derived from eastern and western Germany but the two parts of the country are not analysed separately and compared regarding social inequality. This is done in other publications (for overview see Mielck 2000). Much information used – particularly referring to the social structure – is derived from official statistics based on the microcensus that is conducted every year. Information displayed and discussed in this chapter is based on the years 1991, 1996, and 2001, the most recent year when all the required data for this chapter were available.

Furthermore, findings from studies on social inequality in health and on the impact of work stress on health are presented. In contrast to other countries, Germany has no official registrar data on these topics. Therefore examples of findings from epidemiological studies in these fields are presented.

1. The Core Data

A. Microcensus

Most information on social status indicators presented in the German chapter is derived from the microcensus. The microcensus is the basis for the official German statistics. Information is collected from a repre-sentative randomised sample consisting of 1% of all households (Mielck 2000). The microcensus is conducted once a year. Information is de-rived from standardised questionnaires and includes among other things a specification of household members in terms of the socio-demographic variables: age, marital status, education and training, occupation, income, and employment/unemployment status. Income is specified as net household income and given in categories. The defini-tion of the occupational group follows the international classification of occupations (ILO 1990). In 1995 and 1998, additional information on health-related factors, i.e. cigarette smoking (current smoker status, age of starting, duration), hospital admissions and duration, visit of a doctor, accidents during the past four weeks and duration of the injury, sick leave, was assessed. Information on health-related factors is derived from a 50% random sample of the above-mentioned 1% sample of all households. The average response rate of the microcensus is 97%. For instance, the rate of refusers for the 1995 microcensus was 10%, under-lining the high grade of representativity of these data (Hein 1996).

B. *Statutory Health Insurance Data*

One of the available data sources for analyses of social inequality in health are statutory health insurance routine data. The data presented in this chapter were collected from one statutory health insurance company between 1987 and 1996 in a region in Northrhine-Westfalia, Germany and actually determined for accounting purposes. The entire study population consists of all insured persons during this time-period (n=414 801, aged 0-102 years) (for details see Geyer & Peter 2000).

The data include information on socio-demographic variables (edu-cation and training, occupation, income, age, gender); diagnosis of hospital admissions according to the ICD 9 classification; all-cause mortality without specification of the cause of death; and information on the duration of membership in the health insurance system, which is identical with the individual observation period. The data represent an open cohort. Reasons for leaving the cohort are death, changing to a different health insurance company, and moving to another area (for details see Geyer and Peter 2000).

Some specific characteristics of the health insurance data need to be mentioned to enable the reader to adequately interpret the findings presented in this chapter. The catchment area is the district of Mett-mann, an urban or urbanised area, west of the city of Duesseldorf. The study population was employed either in the production industry or in the service sector with an over-representation of the 'old' industries. The clientele of local health insurance companies does not correspond to the status distribution of the German population. Due to peculiarities of the German health insurance system, lower socio-economic groups are over-represented, while relatively few people with higher occupational status are included. This may result in an overestimation of risk according to social status. It must also be noticed that officials are not members of the statutory health insurance system in Germany. Officials need private health insurance and are therefore not included in the data under discussion here.

It is planned to calculate post-stratification weights for the social status indicators using the social status information from the microcensus in 1995 to redress representativity of the health insurance data. Respective weighted findings on social class and morbidity/mortality rates will be published in the future, allowing a direct comparison of results with figures based on representative samples.

C. National Survey Data

As mentioned, there is very little data on associations between socio-economic status and health in Germany. One of the most frequently used sources of data for investigation of the association between social status and health is the German Cardiovascular Prevention Study (Deutsche Herz-Kreislauf-Präventionsstudie, DHP) (Mielck 2000). The DHP is a representative sample of the population aged 25 to 69 years living in western German households. People with non-German nationality are not included. Cross-sectional information on socio-economic status and subjective health was collected with the help of standardised questionnaires in 1984/85, 1987/88 and 1990/91 and includes about 5000 persons per year. Biological cardiovascular risk factors (e.g. blood pressure, blood lipids) were assessed in clinical screenings.

A similar study, the Health Survey East, was conducted in 1991/92. It contains information on a representative sample of 2200 inhabitants of East Germany aged 18 to 79 years (Mielck 2000).

Whereas the data described above are cross-sectional, the Socio-economic Panel (SOEP) is a prospective investigation in about 12,000 persons at baseline in 1984 (Hanefeld 1987). Standardised questionnaire information is collected on a yearly basis. Accordingly, information on socio-demographic variables and on health is self-reported. An advantage of these data as compared to those mentioned above is the fact that all inhabitants of Germany (German and foreign) at a specific time are included. The DHP and the Health Survey East are restricted to German households (Mielck 2000).

2. Social Groups – Proportion and Changes over Time

In this section, the proportion of core social status indicators (i.e. education, occupation, and income) in the German population is described. Moreover, changes of these indicators during the past 10 years are discussed. All data are based on the microcensus and respective figures from the official Statistical Yearbook for Germany. All numbers presented in tables were calculated from these figures by the author of this chapter.

A. *Education*

The German school system is somewhat different from school systems in other European countries, particularly so since the reunification. Firstly, the final examination can be taken after 13 years, as compared to 12 years in most other countries. Secondly, a new type of school was added to the school system after the reunification. In former East Germany so-called 'Polytechnical schools' were widely spread. Finishing a polytechnical school was comparable with the 10-year study programme in West Germany but restricted to the technical field.

Table 1 shows levels of education by gender and age. Among men, the overall prevalence of less than 10 years of education is most frequent between 1991 and 2001, followed by 10 years and 13 years in the third position. Between 1991 and 2001 a slight change of this distribution can be observed. There is an increase in the proportion of men with 13 years of education, whereas the percentage of those with less than 10 years has declined. This development characterises an increase in the average educational level. No information about those who have not taken a final examination is available for 1991. Between 1996 and 2001 the rates decreased.

In general, women have fewer years of education as compared with men. The proportion of women with 13 years is smaller, whereas the proportion of those with 10 years and less is higher in comparison with men. Regarding the changes of educational years over time the same trends can be observed in women as were discussed in men, i.e. an increase in the percentage of women with 10 years and more, and a decrease in the proportion of women with less than 10 years.

In sum, the educational level among the male and female German population has increased during the past 10 years. Particularly those of a younger age have more years of education. Among both sexes the youngest age groups (< 20 years) are underrepresented due to the fact that most people in Germany with 13 years of education finish their education after the age of 20.

Table 1: Education by age[1] and gender
(percentages, numbers in brackets)

Men	1991	1996	2001
13 years of education	19.4	21.3	23.7
Age <20	(5,316,000)	(6,375,000)	(7,200,000)
20-34	1.0	1.0	0.9
35-49	42.0	38.3	33.9
50-64	29.7	32.4	34.9
> 64	18.8	18.8	20.5
	8.5	9.5	9.8
10 years[2] of education	25.4	35.8	26.2
Age <20	(6,976,000)	(7,405,000)	(7,966,000)
20-34	6.7	5.3	5.0
35-49	42.8	39.2	32.0
50-64	27.7	33.1	37.2
> 64	15.4	15.4	18.3
	7.4	7.0	7.5
< 10 years of education	55.2	51.6	48.1
Age <20	(15,176,000)	(15,427,000)	(14,646,000)
20-34	3.0	2.6	2.7
35-49	21.8	19.5	15.8
50-64	24.3	23.9	24.9
> 64	32.9	32.2	30.8
	18.0	21.8	25.8
No final examination		2.5	2.0
Age <20		(761,000)	(620,000)
20-34	No information	7.4	6.8
35-49	available	29.5	25.3
50-64		25.9	31.0
> 64		27.1	24.3
		10.1	12.6
Sum	100	100	100
	(27,468,000)	(29,968,000)	(30,432,000)

1) Percentage of men and women in the age group
2) Including 'polytechnical school' of former East Germany.
Source: Statistical Yearbook 1993, 1997, 2002 (own calculations).
Database: MC.

Table 1 continued

Women	1991	1996	2001
13 years of education	12.3%	14.9%	18.0%
age < 20	(3,686,000)	(4,770,000)	(5,809,000)
20-34	1.6%	1.5%	1.4%
35-49	51.9%	47.3%	41.8%
50-64	26.8%	31.2%	35.0%
> 64	12.4%	12.7%	14.6%
	7.3%	7.3%	7.2%
10 years[1] of education	29.0%	28.1%	30.0%
age < 20	(8,674,000)	(9,031,000)	(9,650,000)
20-34	5.8%	4.2%	4.3%
35-49	41.8%	37.5%	29.7%
50-64	26.9%	32.3%	37.4%
> 64	14.4%	15.7%	18.5%
	11.1%	10.3%	10.1%
< 10 years of education	58.6%	54.1%	49.8%
age < 20	(17,522,000)	(17,370,000)	(16,025,000)
20-34	1.7%	1.4%	1.5%
35-49	14.5%	12.9%	10.7%
50-64	21.2%	20.5%	19.9%
> 64	30.9%	30.2%	29.7%
	31.7%	35.0%	38.2%
Without final examination		2.9%	2.2%
Age < 20		(919,000)	(714,000)
20-34	No information available	6.0%	3.5%
35-49		25.0%	23.8%
50-64		26.1%	28.1%
> 64		23.6%	24.4%
		19.3%	20.2%
Sum	100%	100%	100%
	(29,882,000)	(32,090,000)	(32,198,000)

1) Percentage of men and women in the age group.
2) Including 'polytechnical school' of former East Germany.
Source: Statistical Yearbook 1993, 1997, 2002 (own calculations).
DataSource: MC.

B. Occupation

In Germany, as in most other economically developed countries, basic changes in the occupational structure have been observed. In sum, these changes are characterised by increasing numbers of jobs in the service sector and decreasing numbers in the traditional industrial production sector (see also 4.B. below). There are many reasons for this development that cannot be discussed here. However, although the distinction between blue- and white-collar as presented by the official statistics in Germany is perhaps quite crude and therefore not optimal to demonstrate these changes, it nevertheless reflects this trend to some extent.

In order to understand the occupational group labels in Germany it is necessary to point to the specific German situation. In Germany, unlike in other countries, there is a differentiation between the total group of civil servants and so-called 'Beamte', who are labelled 'officials' in the following. Whereas the social status and work contracts of civil servants are very much like those of their counterparts in the private sector, officials are in a special position. In a worldwide comparison officials in Germany are a unique occupational group that is employed by the state and cannot be fired. It should also be noticed that the group of officials contains high- as well as low-level jobs. Therefore it might not be optimal to define this group as white-collar. However, the major part of officials can be characterised as white-collar workers in the sense that they have non-manual jobs.

Table 2 shows the proportion of occupational groups by gender. One clear trend among both sexes can be observed: the number of employees in blue-collar jobs has been declining during the past 10 years. At the same time white-collar jobs have become more frequent. The number of self-employed has been increasing among both sexes. Whereas the proportion of male officials has been decreasing over the past ten years, respective figures are quite stable for women. The highest proportion of women has been working in white-collar jobs. Among men this was the case for men in blue-collar occupations until 1996, whereas in 2001 there was a tendency for the proportions of blue- and white-collar workers to become equal. In sum, the proportion of women among the economically active population has been steadily increasing during the past ten years, whereas the male proportion has been quite stable since 1996.

Table 2: Occupational group by gender in relation to the economically active population[1] (percentages, numbers in brackets)

Men	1991	1996	2001
Blue-collar	46.7 (10,222,000)	44.8 (9,273,000)	40.1 (8,264,000)
White-collar	33.7 (7,361,000)	34.2 (7,092,000)	39.4 (8,120,000)
Officials	8.9 (1,951,000)	8.5 (1,769,000)	7.4 (1,526,000)
Self-employed	10.3 (2,257,000)	12.0 (2,492,000)	12.6 (2,620,000)
Other	0.4 (83,000)	0.4 (79,000)	0.5 (100,000)
Sum	100 (21,874,000)	100 (20,706,000)	100 (20,629,000)
Women			
Blue-collar	27.9 (4,346,000)	24.2 (3,702,000)	23.0 (3,720,000)
White-collar	60.7 (9,447,000)	63.2 (9,660,000)	64.1 (10,376,000)
Officials	3.6 (560,000)	4.5 (692,000)	4.5 (737,000)
Self-employed	5.0 (780,000)	6.0 (916,000)	6.3 (1,012,000)
Other	2.8 (438,000)	2.0 (306,000)	2.1 (341,000)
Sum	100 (15,570,000)	100 (15,276,000)	100 (16,187,000)

1) All persons employed with work contracts or self-employed, part-time and full-time, aged 15 to 65 and more years.
Source: Statistical Yearbook 1992, 1996, 2002 (own calculations). Database: MC.

C. Income

Information on income by occupational group is displayed in table 3. In the official German statistics, income is measured as gross income, which is calculated as a product of the average income of specific occupational groups in a defined time-period. For white-collar jobs, income is calculated as the average income in one month (April of years 1991 to 2001). For blue-collar jobs the average income per hour was used in order to calculate the gross income for one month (April 1991 to 2001). The information on the average gross income in table 3 is based on these two occupational groups.

The numbers display the average monthly income in euros. The percentages reflect the relative income by occupational group and by gender in relation to the average income, which is set to 100%. As can be seen, earnings for male and female members of both occupational groups have been increasing since 1991. During the whole time-period, men received higher monthly income as compared with women, no matter which occupational group is taken into account. Income differences are most obvious between white- and blue-collar workers, i.e. the income increase has been more substantial in white- as compared with blue-collar occupations during the past ten years. This trend includes an increasing income gap in Germany according to occupational group membership. Whereas in 1991 male and female blue-collar workers received 96% of the average income of blue- and white-collar employees, these numbers decreased to 89% in 1996 and to 85% in 2001. During the same time-period the relative white-collar income increased from 104% of the average in 1991 to 111% in 1996, and finally to 115% in 2001. Interestingly the income of blue-collar women covers a higher percentage of the average female income than the earnings of blue-collar men, in comparison with the average male income. Among white-collar jobs men earn a higher percentage of the average income as compared with women.

Table 3: Income[1] (in euros) by occupational group and gender (percentage of average income in brackets)

	1991	1996	2001
Blue-collar	1,596 (96)	1,942 (89)	2,353 (85)
Men	1,670 (92)	2,015 (84)	2,443 (82)
Women	1,209 (94)	1,496 (86)	1,799 (83)
White-collar	1,721 (104)	2,421 (111)	3,207 (115)
Men	1,973 (108)	2,771 (116)	3,511 (118)
Women	1,363 (106)	1,973 (114)	2,533 (117)
Average	1,658 (100)	2,181 (100)	2,780 (100)
Men	1,821 (100)	2,393 (100)	2,977 (100)
Women	1,286 (100)	1,734 (100)	2,166 (100)

1) Monthly gross income for production industries, commerce, credit and insurance.
Source: Statistical Yearbook 1993, 1997, 2003 (own calculations). Database: MC.

Workers in the agricultural industry are listed separately in Germany's official statistics. These statistics are restricted to men, since female agricultural workers are quite rare. The figures in table 4 represent skilled and unskilled agricultural workers. Over the whole time-period their income is much lower in comparison with that of male blue-collar workers in the production industries. Whereas the latter has increased constantly during the past 10 years, the wages of agricultural workers have slightly decreased since 1996. In relation to the average blue-collar income, agricultural wages decreased dramatically from

81.5% in 1991 to 57.3% in 2001. There are several plausible explanations for this development. One is that with the opening of former
communist countries, more people from Poland, the Czech Republic,
and Slovakia are now working in the agricultural sector in Germany.
Trade unions are not strong in this sector. As a consequence, people
from Eastern European countries can work for very low wages in the
agricultural sector in Germany.

**Table 4: Income[1] (in euros) among male workers
in the agricultural sector**

	1991	1996	2001
Monthly Income	1,499	1,704	1,534
Average hours per month	191.9	213.8	200.8
Average income per hour	7.81	7.98	7.64
% of income per hour from the average[2]	81.5	66.6	57.3

*1) Gross income calculated as product of average income per hour and average working
hours per month.*
*2) Percentage from the average male blue-collar income per hour in the respective year
(production industries).*
Source: Statistical Yearbook 1993, 1997, 2002 (own calculations). Database MC.

3. Labour Market Conditions

A. Employment

The following section provides basic information on the German labour force and on the development of numbers regarding the economically active in relation to the inactive part of the German population.
During the past 10 years the proportion of economically active persons
among the German population has constantly decreased even more
among men than in women (table 5). The group of economically active
is defined by employment as the main source of income, either working
in part- or full-time jobs or being self-employed. The group of inactive
persons consists of all those who do not have paid work, and who are
not looking for paid work. The group of economically inactive persons
includes pensioners and persons on welfare who are not working and
not seeking employment. It is important to note that the characteristic
'not looking for paid work' excludes the unemployed population from
the group of economically inactive people. People counted as being
unemployed must actively look for a new job (see table 5). This is a
specific characteristic of the official German statistics. The group of
inactive persons has increased during the past 10 years. This development is partly due to demographic development in Germany, particularly to the increasing proportion of elderly people. Women are more

likely to belong to the inactive group because many women are housewives. The remaining group consists of unemployed people looking for
paid work, pensioners and persons on welfare. It must be noted that
pensioners in Germany are allowed to earn up to a specific amount of
money per month without being treated as employed persons.

Overall, these numbers document some of the problems of Germany
with regard to the demographic development (ageing). The figures
further show an increasing participation of women in the labour market.

**Table 5: Proportion of economically active[1], inactive[2] and
not employed[3] persons by gender (total %, percentages
for men/women, numbers in brackets) at April 1**

	1991	1996	2001
Active	44.5	41.3	40.9
	(35,521,000)	(33,813,000)	(33,656,000)
% Men	60.2	57.5	58.8
Women	39.8	42.5	41.2
Not active	49.8	51.1	50.6
	(39,742,000)	(41,847,000)	(41,728,000)
% Men	38.8	40.6	41.9
Women	61.2	59.4	58.1
Other	5.7	7.6	8.3
	(4,566,000)	(6,172,000)	(6,893,000)
Sum	100	100	100
	(79,829,000)	(81,832,000)	(82,277,000)

*1) All persons employed with work contracts or self-employed, part-time and full-time,
employment main source of income.*
*2) No paid work and not looking for paid work. Persons on welfare and pensioners with
additional paid work, relatives working without being paid, unemployed people looking
for paid work.*
Source: Statistical Yearbook 1993, 1997, 2002 (own calculations). Database: MC.

Unemployment rates are given in table 6. Figures are related to the
employed workforce. Soldiers and the self-employed are not included in
the official statistics since they do not pay any unemployment insurance
and therefore do not receive unemployment benefits. As can be seen, the
rates have been increasing since 1991, with a peak in the second half of
the 1990s. The most recent figures for unemployment are more than
4.4 million with rates beyond 10% in 2003. Germany is suffering from
quite high and stable unemployment rates. Men have an increasing risk
of becoming unemployed as compared with women.

Table 6: Unemployment by gender (unemployment rate[1], numbers in brackets, percentages of unemployed males/females)

	1991	1996	2001
Total	7.3	11.5	9.4
	(2,602,203)	(3,965,064)	(3,851,636)
Men	49.2	53.2	53.6
Women	50.8	46.8	46.4

1) *Calculated in relation to the employed workforce, excluding soldiers and self-employees.*
Source: Statistical Yearbook 1993, 1997, 2002 (own calculations). Database: MC.

Table 7 shows the proportion of part-time work among the working population. Since these figures are based on the self-reported income information from the microcensus, those without income information are excluded. As can be seen, the number of part-time jobs has been constantly increasing since 1991 in men and women. There is a clear gender gap concerning part-time work. Women are at least 7 times more often employed on part-time contracts. These numbers can be inter-preted as a decrease in social security and long-term perspectives in the labour market, particularly among women.

Table 7: Full-time and part-time work[1] by occupational group (percentages, numbers in brackets)

Men	1991	1996	2001
Part-time work	3.1	4.5	5.6
	(644,000)	(889,000)	(1,085,000)
Full-time work	96.9	94.5	94.4
	(19,950,000)	(18,679,000)	(18,370,000)
Sum	100	100	100
	(20,549,000)	19,568,000	19,455,000
Women			
Part-time work	31.8	35.2	39.7
	(4,582,000)	(5,084,000)	(6,063,000)
Full-time work	68.2	64.8	50.3
	(9,822,000)	(9,358,000)	(9,215,000)
Sum	100	100	100
	(14,404,000)	(14,442,000)	(15,278,000)

1) *Full-time work including trainees; 1991 part-time work < 36 hours per week, 2001 self-rated; farmers, helping relatives, and those without information on income excluded.*
Source: Statistical Yearbook 1993, 1997, 2002 (own calculations). Database: MC.

Another important development in Germany refers to the increasing proportion of elderly people in the population and accordingly a steadily increasing number of pensioners (see table 8). Whereas the rate of pension due to a reduced ability to work has been relatively stable during the past 10 years, the proportion of pensions due to age has constantly increased from 14.7% in 1992 to 18.9% in 2001, in relation to the entire population. In the same time-window the proportion of economically active people decreased. These numbers are likely to be underestimated rather than overestimated because some specific pensions are not included in the table. In view of these figures, considerable discussion has been initiated on how to finance the social security system in the future.

Table 8: Pensioners[1] and the economically active[2] in relation to the entire population (percentages, numbers in brackets)

Pension due to	1992	1996	2001
Reduced ability to work	2.2 (1,740,000)	2.3 (1,873,000)	2.3 (1,892,000)
Age	14.7 (11,871,000)	16.5 (13,526,000)	18.9 (15,521,000)
Economically active population	44.1 (35,521,000)	41.3 33,813,000	40.9 33,656,000
Other[3]	39.0 (31,462,000)	39.9 (32,684,000)	37.9 (31,208,000)
Entire population	100 (80,594,000)	100 (81,896,000)	100 (82,277,000)

1) Blue- and white-collar, specific pensions (miners' association); farmers not included.
2) All persons employed with work contracts or self-employed, part-time and full-time, main source of income employment.
3) Economically inactive population, not including pensioners plus farmers and specific pensions.
Source: Statistical Yearbook 1993, 1997, 2002 (own calculations). Database: MC.

B. Immigrants

Immigrants are defined as people living in Germany without German nationality. Germans with dual nationality do not belong to the group of immigrants. The proportion of people from foreign countries living in Germany has slowly but constantly increased by about 300,000 since 1991. Accordingly, the proportion of immigrants among the economically active population is also increasing (see table 9). Since 1991 it has risen from 7.0% to 8.3%, with a higher proportion of foreign men as compared with women working in Germany.

**Table 9: Proportion of immigrants among the economically
active population (percentages, numbers in brackets)**

	2001	
	Economically active[1]	Immigrants[2]
Totally	100 (33,656,000)	8.3 (2,808,000)
Men	58.8 (19,793,000)	9.4 (1,850,000)
Women	41.2 (13,864,000)	6.9 (957,000)

*1) All persons employed with work contracts or self-employed, part-time and full-time,
employment main source of income.*
2) Proportion in relation to the economically active population.
Source: Statistical Yearbook 2002 (own calculations). Database: MC.

These trends are also important with regard to health. A longitudinal
study among more than 6,000 German and foreign men and women
observed a decrease in the healthy migrant effect (i.e. physically and
mentally healthy people are more likely to move to foreign countries)
between 1988 and 1992 (Lechner & Mielck 1998). The healthy migrant
effect was mainly observed among the first generations of migrants in
Germany between 1960 and 1990. More recent studies have found
poorer self-reported health among migrants as compared with German
citizens (for overview see Krones 2001). Among other factors these
findings were attributed to migrants having poorer access to the health
system (Razum & Geiger 2003).

C. Sectors

The development of certain sectors during the past 10 years to some
extent reflects the changes observed regarding occupational groups. As
can be seen in tables 10 a + b, the number of men and women working
in the agricultural sector and in major parts of the traditional industrial
production sector has been decreasing, particularly so in mining and
classic processing industries. At the same time the number of jobs in
commerce and in the service sector has increased for both sexes. It is
likely that these changes influence social inequality in health, and
particularly the prevalence and quality of work stress and its impact on
health. Possible consequences are discussed in section 6.

Table 10 a: Sectors, by gender in relation to the economically active population[1] (percentages, numbers in brackets)

Men	1991	1996	2001
Agriculture, fishing	4.4 (928,000)	3.2 (662,000)	2.9 (609,000)
Production industries Mining, processing industries, Energy, water supply	39.3 (8,359,000)	31.9 (6,610,000)	31.6 (6,521,000)
Construction industry	11.2 (2,380,000)	14.7 (3,042,000)	12.3 (2,522 000)
Commerce, tourism	8.4 (1,777,000)	13.8 (2,859,000)	14.2 (2,938,000)
Traffic, information (newscasting)	7.7 (1,650,000)	6.7 (1,394,000)	7.1 (1,464,000)
Service Credit, insurance	2.8 (601,000)	3.0 (623,000)	3.1 (649,000)
Real estate, renting		5.6 (1,171,000)	7.6 (1,573,000)
Public administration	26.2 (5,587,000)[2]	9.7 (1,979,000)	8.7 (1,790,000)
Public and private service		11.4 (2,368,000)	12.5 (2,565,000)
Sum	100 (21,282,000)	100 (20,706,000)	100 (20,631,000)

1) All persons employed with work contracts or self-employed, part-time and full-time.
2) After 1991 the definition of sectors was changed; therefore all service sectors (real estate, public administration, public and private services) are added to one number for 1991.
Source: Statistical Yearbook 1993, 1997, 2002 based on respective microcensus (own calculations). Database: MC.

Table 10 b: Sectors by gender in relation to the economically active population[1] (percentages, numbers in brackets)

Women	1990	1996	2001
Agriculture, fishing	4.2 (646,000)	2.7 (414,000)	2.1 (334,000)
Production industries Mining, processing industries Energy, water supply	23.7 (3,692,000)	16.4 (2,504,000)	15.5 (2,510,000)
Construction industry	2.1 (327,000)	2.8 (427,000)	2.4 (381,000)
Commerce, tourism	16.6 (2,584,000)	22.3 (3,384,000)	21.8 (3,538,000)
Traffic, information (newscasting)	4.2 (656,000)	3.4 (547,000)	3.6 (591,000)
Service Credit, insurance	4.0 (629,000)	4.3 (653,000)	4.3 (697,000)
Real estate, renting		7.3 (1,114,000)	8.9 (1,433,000)
Public administration	45.2 (7,037,000)[2]	9.1 (1,386,000)	8.1 (1,306,000)
Public and private service		31.7 (4,848,000)	33.3 (5,397,000)
Sum	100 (15,571,000)	100 (15,277,000)	100 (16,187,000)

1) *All persons employed with work contracts or self-employed, part-time and full-time.*
2) *After 1991 the definition of sectors was changed; therefore all service sectors (real estate, public administration, public and private services) are added to one number for 1991.*
Source: Statistical Yearbook 1993, 1997, 2002 based on respective microcensus (own calculations). Database: MC.

4. Socio-economic Status and Health

During the past ten years several studies have been conducted analysing associations between socio-economic group membership and different health outcomes. In Germany, some of these investigations have used indices composed of education, occupation and income to determine the socio-economic group, and some have used single socio-economic indicators. Therefore findings of different studies cannot easily be compared. Studies using single indicators may provide information on the relative contribution of specific socio-economic status indicators to increased morbidity and premature mortality (see for instance Geyer & Peter 2000 below).

A. Socio-economic Status and Morbidity

The first part of the studies to be reported investigated associations between socio-economic status and chronic disease, mainly coronary artery disease. In 1993 an analysis with data from the DHP study showed a strong social gradient with regard to myocardial infarction (Helmert *et al.* 1993) (see table 11). The prevalence of disease increased with decreasing social class in both men and women, and in all age groups except women beyond the age of 60 years. The gradient was most pronounced in the age group 40 to 49 years. The average age stratified excess risk in the lowest compared to the highest social group was 2.5 in men and 3.7 in women. Regarding stroke, a social gradient was observed among both sexes. Over all age groups, male and female members of the middle and the lowest class had the highest prevalence rates. The ratio between the lowest and the highest class was 2.7 for men and 2.8 for women. This was one of the first studies in Germany to show the most pronounced social inequalities in health in middle-aged people.

Table 11: Social class and myocardial infarction, stroke

	Prevalence of myocardial infarction[a] (%) Social class[b]			Lower class/ upper class
	Upper class	Middle class	Lower class	
% in sample Men	19.8	21.0	20.7	
Women	12.9	22.5	24.2	
Prevalence: Men				
40-49 Years	0.8	1.7	2.0	2.5
50-59 Years	3.4	6.0	7.4	2.2
60-69 Years	7.5	10.6	11.6	1.5
Prevalence: Women				
40-49 Years	0.1	0.5	1.2	12.0
50-59 Years	0.8	1.7	2.4	3.0
60-69 Years	3.4	2.6	5.3	1.6
Prevalence of stroke [a] (%)				
Prevalence: Men				
40-49 Years	0.1	0.6	0.8	8.0
50-59 Years	1.3	1.2	3.1	2.4
60-69 Years	3.1	2.5	4.0	1.3
Prevalence: Women				
40-49 Years	0.2	0.5	1.2	6.0
50-59 Years	0.4	1.0	1.1	2.8
60-69 Years	1.0	2.2	2.3	2.3

a) Lifetime prevalence / b) Index composed of education, occupational group, and income (only 3 of 5 categories displayed in the table). Sample: 12,445 men and 13,335 women (40-69 years, German natives, western Germany).
Data basis: survey 1984/86, 1987/88 and 1990/91 (DHP Study).
Source: Helmert et al. 1993. Database: DHP.

A prospective cohort study with data from a statutory health insurance company investigated the risk of hospital admissions due to ischaemic heart disease dependent on qualifications and occupational position in more than 150,000 men and women (Peter *et al.* 2003). In men a gradient was observed with regard to social status indicators and ischaemic heart disease risk (see table 12). In women an inverse association between qualifications and ischaemic heart disease morbidity was also found. With regard to occupation, women in the highest positions showed the lowest risk as compared with the lower occupational groups. The odds ratios observed in this study are higher as compared with risk estimates from other countries. Nevertheless, it is unlikely that the associations in this study are overestimated for several reasons. Firstly, the highest (upper 10% of income) as well as the lowest (people on welfare, homeless) social status groups are not included in the study population. Secondly, since this analysis has been restricted to employed men and women, with information on social status being available in the age group 25-65 years, people who did not have a paid job, or for whom there was a lack of information on occupational group and education, or who exceeded the age cut-off points, have been excluded. Additional analysis presented in this study showed that those included in the analyses did not substantially differ from the excluded group in terms of ischaemic heart disease incidence.

Table 12: Multivariate logistic regression analyses: Incident hospital admissions due to ischaemic heart disease (ICD-9 410-414) by education and occupational status (n exposed, multivariate odds ratios, 95% CI[1])

	Men		Women	
	n	Odds ratio (95% CI)	n	Odds ratio (95% CI)
Model 1: Education and training				
≤ 10 years without vocational training	23,189	6.02 (5.75-6.29)	15,267	3.00 (2.64-3.37)
≤ 10 years with vocational training	48,420	4.46 (4.19-4.73)	14,144	1.75 (1.38-2.12)
> 12 years or university degree	7,200	1.00	2,709	1.00
Model 2: Occupational position				
Un-, semi-skilled manual	35,865	2.95 (2.83-3.06)	20,478	1.98 (1.84-2.13)
Skilled manual	25,221	2.66 (2.54-2.78)	2,513	1.97 (1.75-2.19)
White-collar, intermediate positions, and professionals	19,347	1.00	10,215	1.00

1) Main effects of education/training and occupational position adjusted for age and length of observation period. Source: Peter et al. 2003. Database: HI.

Not only manifest coronary heart disease in relation to socio-economic status was studied but also major behavioural and biological coronary risk factors were investigated. Analyses with the representative DHP data, not presented in detail here, showed that occupations with low qualifications (unskilled and skilled blue-collar, unskilled white-collar) had the highest probability of being characterised by behavioural coronary risk factors such as cigarette smoking, lack of physical exercise, and overweight (odds ratios 2.7 to 6.0 among men and 2.0 to 6.8 in women) as compared with professionals (Helmert 1996). Regarding biological coronary risk factors (hypertension, hypercholesterolemia, low HDL-Cholesterol, type II diabetes) these differences between occupational groups were less pronounced (odds ratios 1.4 to 3 in men and 1.4 to 3.9 in women). Male and female white-collar workers were also characterised by an increased risk as compared with the reference group but odds ratios were lower as in blue-collar workers. Concerning the cumulation of cardiovascular risk factors in one person, a social gradient was observed among both sexes, i.e. risk of three and more coronary risk factors increased with decreasing occupational position. An analysis of cardiovascular disease risk-factor changes between 1984 and 1991, also based on the DHP data, showed that the prevalence of the above-mentioned risk factors was quite stable over time (exceptions: increase of obesity in women and of hypercholesterolaemia in men) (Helmert *et al.* 1995). The risk factor prevalence was highest in the lower social classes. Moreover, the social class gradient increased between 1984 and 1991.

Several studies have investigated associations between social class and subjective health. In these investigations subjective health is measured as self-reported health status (Likert scale ranging from good to poor), prevalence of reported symptoms, and impediment to performing daily activities. One study based on the West German DHP data found a deterioration of subjective health between 1984/86 and 1987/88 among men of all social classes (Helmert 1994) (table 13). Yet, the deterioration was most remarkable among the lower social strata. Moreover, a social gradient regarding subjective health, i.e. increasing risk with decreasing social group, was observed among men during both time-periods. Both trends, although less clear, were also found in women, particularly with regard to the subjective health indicators, impediment to performing daily tasks and health complaints.

Table 13: Social class and self-reported health

	%	Odds Ratios[1] Social class[2]				
		Upper class	Upper middle	Middle class	Lower middle	Lower class
Percentage in sample		14.6	21.4	22.1	19.5	22.4
Poor health[3]						
Men 1987/88	15.1	1.0	1.77**	2.23***	2.58***	4.13***
Women 1987/88	14.2	1,0	1.52	1.72*	2.66***	3.32***
Impediment to performing daily activities[4]	10.7	1.0	2.18**	2.95***	4.22***	7.03***
Men 1987/88	8.5	1.0	2.25**	2.61**	3.42***	3.63***
Women 1987/88						
Reported symptoms[5]	16.2	1.0	2.46***	2.80*	3.49**	5.05
Men 1987/88	21.3	1.0	1.27	**	*	***
Women 1987/88				1.84***	2.48***	1.83**

*) $p < 0.05$; **: $p < 0.01$; ***: $p < 0.001$
1) Reference: upper class; adjusted for age.
2) Index of education, occupational position, and income.
3) Self-reported health: less well or poor.
4) Serious impediment to performing daily activities due to poor health.
5) Zerssen-Sum score > 30 (middle to heavy symptoms).
Sample: 2,448 (1984/86) 2,556 (1987/88) men, 2,461 (1984/86) 2,776 (1987/88) women.
(Stichprobe 1984/86 bzw. 1987/88, 25-69 Jahre, Deutsche, alte Bundesländer).
Data basis: survey 1984/86, 1987/88 (DHP Study). Source: Helmert 1994.

Analyses of more recent data show differences in the prevalence of self-reported psychological exhaustion (e.g. headache, fatigue, gastro-intestinal symptoms, depression) according to occupational group (Hasselhorn and Nübling 2004). Information is derived from a representative 0.1% sample of the workforce aged at least 15 and working for at least 10 hours per week in 1998/99. The sample comprises more than 34,000 men and women. As can be seen from figure 1, these results are contrary to what has been found up to now, since the prevalence of psychological exhaustion increased with increasing occupational class. The authors explain this finding by the high prevalence of psychological exhaustion in specific occupational groups such as teachers.

Figure 1: Psychological exhaustion by occupational group

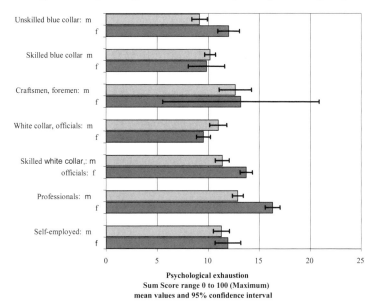

Psychological exhaustion
Sum Score range 0 to 100 (Maximum)
mean values and 95% confidence interval

Source: Hasselhorn and Nübling 2004.

There is very little data comparing the magnitude of social inequality in health between western Germany and the part that was formerly East Germany. One such study using information from the DHP and the Eastern Health Survey found associations between the relative income and indicators of subjective health (Helmert *et al.* 1997) (table 14). Odds ratios for the lowest income group ($\leq 62,5\%$ of the average income) as compared with the highest were higher for men in comparison with women, and higher in western as compared with eastern Germany. Among women in eastern Germany, income did not influence the risk of poor health. One reason for the differences in income inequality between the east and the west of the country are the low numbers in the eastern part which lead to only one significant association between low income and impaired daily activities. Another explanation for the more pronounced income inequalities in western Germany is provided by the fact that the data are from the beginning of the 1990s. A few years after the reunification, however, a more equal income distribution could be observed in former East Germany.

Table 14: Poverty and morbidity in western and eastern Germany

	Odds Ratio[1] Household net income[2]	
	High [3]	Low (poverty)[4]
% in Western German sample: Men	28.5	15.9
Women	22.1	19.3
% in Eastern German sample: Men	16.1	11.6
Women	10.4	14.8
Western Germany: men		
Poor self-reported health[5]	1.00	2.16***
Impediment to performing daily activities[6]	1.00	3.23***
Western Germany: Women	1.00	1.87***
Poor self-reported health[5]	1.00	1.83*
Impediment to performing daily activities[6]		
Eastern Germany: men		
Poor self-reported health[5]	1.00	1.56
Impediment to performing daily activities[6]	1.00	2.35*
Eastern Germany: Women	1.00	1.86
Poor self-reported health[5]	1.00	1.08
Impediment to performing daily activities[6]		

*) $p<0.05$; **: $p<0.01$; ***: $p<0.001$.

1) adjusted for age.

2) Per capita, weighted for number and age of persons in household.

3) > 140% of the average income (reference group).

4) < 62.5% of the average income.

5) Recent self-reported health: less well-off or poor .

6) Serious impediment to performing daily activities due to poor health.

Sample: 4,958 (West); 2,186 (East) persons (25-69 years, German nationality).

Data basis: survey 1990/92 (GCP Study, health survey East).

Source: Helmert et al. 1997. Database: GCP.

A more recent investigation based on the representative data of the microcensus showed associations between all-cause morbidity and occupational status (Hein 1996). As can be seen from table 15, crude morbidity rates are highest among blue-collar workers aged 40 to 64 years. The rate ratio is 1.79 in comparison with the self-employed in this age group, and 1.65 in the age group 15 to 39 years. Interestingly, officials have the second highest morbidity rates. Respective rate ratios are 1.42 in both age categories.

Table 15: Occupational position and morbidity

Occupational position	Proportion in the sample (%)		Ill or injured due to an accident (%)	
	15 to 39 years	40 to 64 years	15 to 39 years	40 to 64 years
Trainees	7.6	0.0	7.8	-
Self-employed	6.1	11.9	5.9	7.6
Supporting relatives	0.8	1.6	7.7	7.8
Officials	6.1	7.6	8.4	10.8
White-collar worker	44.2	45.1	8.2	9.6
Blue-collar worker	35.2	33.8	9.7	13.6
	100.0	100.0	8.6	10.7

Sample: 32,407 employed men and women in western and eastern Germany.
Data basis: national survey 1995 (microcensus).
Source: Hein 1996. Database: MC.

In sum, a number of studies that have been conducted largely with data representative for the German population suggest that lower social class membership in Germany is associated with an increased risk of morbidity. Findings compare well with the figures known from other developed countries. Results showing the most markedly social gap in middle age (Helmert 1993, Hein 1996) suggest that working conditions might explain a substantial part of the social gradient. In Germany the proportion of employed people is highest in middle-aged people (30 to 55 years).

B. Socio-economic Status and Mortality

Only limited information is available concerning socio-economic status and mortality. A study with representative data from the SOEP showed differences in life expectancy (at the age of 16) according to education (Klein 1996). The average life expectancy of men with less than 13 years of education was 2.7 years lower in comparison with those who had 13 years of education (table 16). The difference among women was even greater (3.9 years).

Table 16: Education and life expectancy

	Life expectancy at the age of 16 (in years)	
Education	Men	Women
< 12 years	57.0	61.6
≥ 12 years	60.3	65.5

Sample: about 12,000 men and women > 16 years from western Germany .
Data basis: Survey 1984-1993 (Socio-economic Panel).
Source: Klein 1996. Database: SOP.

In a recent prospective cohort study in about 85,000 men and women, social class indicators were associated with increased risk of mortality from all causes of disease (see table 17). Regarding qualifications – an indicator composed of education and training – and occupational position, mortality risk increased with decreasing social status. Concerning relative income – a measure composed of income quintiles – mortality risk steadily increased with declining income over the first 4 quintiles. In the lowest quintile it was as high as in the middle category.

Table 17: Multivariate Cox regression: relative mortality risks for income, qualification, occupational position and gender

	Relative risk	95% confidence intervals
Model 1: Income in percentiles		
Highest 20%*	1.00	
Higher 20%	1.31	1.13, 1.53
Mean 20%	1.78	1.52, 2.08
Lower 20%	2.55	2.18, 2.98
Lowest 20%	1.77	1.48, 2.12
Gender (females) †	0.28	0.25, 0.33
Model 2: Qualifications#		
University degree$	1.00	
Qualification (1)#	2.95	1.71, 5.09
Qualification (2)#	3.21	2.20, 4.71
Qualification (3)#	4.21	2.87, 6.19
Gender (females) †	0.46	0.41, 0.52
Model 3: Occupational position		
Intermediates/executives§	1.00	
Skilled non-manual	1.73	1.28, 2.32
Skilled manual	3.15	2.39, 4.16
Unskilled/ semi-skilled	3.32	2.52, 4.36
Gender (females) †	0.49	0.43, 0.55

* The highest 20% of the income distribution serves as reference category. †Men serve as reference category. § The highest occupational position (intermediates/ executives) serves as reference category. $ The highest qualification (university degree) serves as reference category; #Qualification (1): '13 years of school with or without vocational training'; qualification (2): 'nine or 10 years of school and vocational training'; qualification (3): 'nine or 10 years or less without vocational training'.
Source: Geyer & Peter 2000. Database: HI.

Although no routine data on social inequality in health are available for Germany, findings of existing studies show similar trends in mortality as known from other countries.

5. The Workplace and Health

A. Psychosocial Work Environments

During the past decades the nature of work in socio-economically developed countries has been characterised by remarkable changes (e.g. more information technology, more part-time work and flexible time arrangements, more jobs in the service sector). These developments can also be observed with regard to Germany (see sections 2 to 4). With these changes, occupational mobility and job insecurity increases (Ferrie *et al.* 1999). Germany has been faced with high levels of structural unemployment during recent years. In sum, these developments lead to a shift from traditional physical and chemical hazards to psychosocial work environments, which are becoming more and more important also with regard to health-adverse outcomes (Peter & Siegrist 2000). Thus, epidemiological studies with the aim of defining populations at risk are of growing importance. Nevertheless, the number of studies in this field is limited in Germany and cannot be compared with the number of studies conducted in some other countries like Sweden, the Netherlands, and the United Kingdom. However, a brief summary of available information will be given below.

Contrary to many studies in other countries, German investigations have not used the demand-control or job strain model (Karasek and Theorell 1990) to measure strenuous psychosocial work environments. In Germany, the effort–reward imbalance (ERI) model was developed and tested by Johannes Siegrist and his group (Siegrist 1996). This model assumes that effort at work is spent as part of a socially organised exchange to which society contributes in terms of rewards. Rewards are distributed by three transmitter systems: money, esteem and career opportunities including job security and promotion prospects. According to this model, lack of reciprocity between costs and gains elicits sustained strain reactions in the working person via activation of the autonomic nervous system. In the long run this activation primarily affects the cardiovascular system but probably also immune reactions and the gastrointestinal system.

Meanwhile almost 40 studies have been conducted with this model worldwide including more than 50,000 persons altogether. Seven of these investigations have been carried out in Germany and will be briefly described.

Table 18: Effort–reward imbalance and risk of coronary heart disease: Study overview (German studies)

Author, Year	Sample (% women)	Study design	Outcome	Multi-variate odds ratio	Adjustment
MAPI					
Siegrist *et al.* 1994	416 (0) Blue-collar	Prospec-tive, mean observation period 6.5 years	Incidence of acute, non-fatal myo-cardial infarction	6.1**a)	Age, blood pressure, Body mass index (BMI)
Siegrist *et al.* 1991			Co-manifestation of hyperten-sion and elevated blood lipids	2.7** a)	Cigarette smoking, BMI
Middle-manager study					
Peter *et al.* 1991	179 (0) Middle managers	Cross-sectional	Cigarette smoking	4.3** a)	Age
Peter *et al.* 1997			Hypertension	5.8** a)	Age, BMI
Siegrist *et al.* 1997			Elevated LDL-cholesterol Elevated fibrinogen	3.6* a) 6.7** a)	Cigarette smoking, alcohol con-sumption Cigarette smoking, BMI
Coronary restenosis study					
Joksimovic *et al.* 1999	106 (0) Coronary patients	Prospec-tive, observation period 1 year	Coronary restenosis, angioplasty	2.9* b)	Age, HDL-cholesterol

*p < .05 ** < p .01.*
a) category (3) (simultaneous exposure to high effort and low reward), three-category index.
b) upper tertile of the scale 'over-commitment'.
For details see text.

Three studies have investigated the associations between ERI and risk of cardiovascular disease (table 18). The Marburg Prospective Industrial Worker (MAPI) study was conducted in 416 male, initially healthy blue-collar men aged 20 to 55 years. After 6.5 years the men who were characterised by ERI showed a more than six-fold increased risk of suffering from first acute myocardial infarction (Siegrist & Peter 1994). This finding was adjusted for a number of traditional cardiovascular risk factors. The high odds ratio might be partly explained by the fact that in this study a high-risk population was investigated. ERI was not only associated with myocardial infarction but also with the risk of belonging to a cardiovascular high-risk group with simultaneously elevated blood pressure and blood lipids (Siegrist *et al*. 1991). This latter finding is important with regard to prevention, particularly primary prevention, since it points to the promise of intervention at an early stage of disease development.

In a second study on ERI and cardiovascular risk, male middle-aged middle-mangers were investigated. Again, persons characterised by ERI had an increased risk of belonging to the group of smokers (Peter *et al*. 1991), of hypertensives (Peter & Siegrist 1997), and of those with elevated LDL-cholesterol and elevated fibrinogen values (Siegrist *et al*. 1997). In one prospective clinical study among 106 male coronary patients an increased risk of restenosis after successful angioplasty was observed for those who reported ERI (Joksimovic *et al*. 1999).

Another four studies in Germany investigated associations between ERI and indicators of self-reported health (see table 19). In a cross-sectional study among male and female employees of a public transport company aged 25 to 65 years, differences in the association between ERI and self-reported symptoms were observed according to occupational group (Peter *et al*. 1998). Associations between ERI and all self-reported symptoms under study and the most substantial odds ratios were also observed among unskilled blue-collar workers as compared with skilled workers and white-collar workers. Despite its limitations, this is currently the only study in Germany pointing to the potential explanatory power of work stress with regard to social inequality in health.

In a cross-sectional study conducted by Rothenbacher *et al*. (1998) in 189 white-collar workers, an association between ERI (over-commitment) and gastrointestinal symptoms was observed. Interestingly, this association was independent from an existing helicobacter pylori infection.

A recent cross-sectional study was conducted in male and female bus drivers to investigate associations between ERI and musculoskeletal symptoms and depression. With regard to musculoskeletal symptoms, the odds ratios for ERI ranged from 1.9 to 3.1 (Joksimovic *et al*. 2002). Concerning depression, the respective estimate was 5.9 (Larisch *et al*. 2003).

In a recent study among more than 20,000 nurses from several European countries, associations between ERI and burnout were analysed (Hasselhorn *et al.* 2004). In German nurses the odds ratios were 5.5 (extrinsic model component: upper tertile of the effort-reward-ratio) and 4.7 (intrinsic model component: over-commitment) respectively. Compared with most other countries, higher odds ratios were observed among German nurses.

Table 19: Effort–reward imbalance and physical/psychological symptoms: Study overview (German studies)

Author, Year	Sample (% women)	Study design	Outcome	Multivariate odds ratio§	Adjustment
HHA-Study: Peter *et al.* 1998	1337 (12) Employees of a public transport company	Cross sectional	Physical and psychological symptoms	Unskilled blue-collar: 2.0 – 3.1 a) Skilled blue-collar: 1.7 – 2.6 a) White-collar: 2.9 a)	Gender, subjective health, physically demanding work, physical–chemical hazards
Rothenbacher *et al.* 1998	189 (75) White-collar	Cross-sectional	Gastro-intestinal symptoms	3.2 b)	Age, gender, cigarette smoking, education, inflammation impeding medication, Helicobacter pylori infection
Study 'Social Reciprocity & Health': Joksimovic *et al.* 2002	316 (15) Employees of a public transport company	Cross-sectional	Musculo-skeletal symptoms	3.1 a) 1.9-2.3 b)	Age, gender, socio-economic status, shift work
Larisch *et al.* 2002			Depression	5.9 a) 5.9 b)	Age, gender, socio-economic status, shift work, job control
Hasselhorn *et al.* 2004	21729 (Germany: 2615)	Cross-sectional	Burnout	5.5 c) 4.7 b)	Age, gender, effort–reward-ratio or over-commitment respectively

§ *p of all odds ratios < .05.*
a) *Effort–reward ratio > 1.*
b) *Upper tertile of the scale 'over-commitment'.*
c) *Upper tertile of the effort–reward ratio.*
For details see text.

In sum, these findings underline the importance of psychosocial work environments for health. Even in populations which are relatively homogeneous in terms of social status (blue-collar workers, middle managers, nurses) the influence of work stress on health is documented. These findings point to the assumption that not only between-class inequality, but also within-class inequality plays an important role regarding health (Marmot 1994), since even in homogenous occupational groups, differences regarding adverse health outcomes related to work stress can be observed. In terms of prevention, high-risk populations can be identified and specific preventive programmes tailored to their needs can be developed.

B. Occupational Status, Psychosocial Work Environment and Health

An important question induced by findings on associations between work stress and health such as those discussed above and currently addressed by international research in this field, is how much of the social inequality in health can be explained by psychosocial work environments. Concerning the potential explanation of social inequalities in health by work stress, it is important to know more about the distribution of work stress indicators across social status positions. Such information is limited for Germany since neither large-scaled epidemiological studies nor official data are currently available. However, findings from three smaller studies give some hints regarding the association of work stress in terms of effort–reward imbalance with occupational class in Germany (see table 20). As known from other countries, the prevalence of work stress increases with decreasing occupational position. It has to be kept in mind that these findings need to be interpreted carefully with regard to generalisability, since they are based on studies conducted in specific occupational groups or in single companies.

**Table 20: Prevalence (%) of effort–reward imbalance
by occupational group**

Occupational Group	Men	Women
Blue-collar[1]		
Unskilled	59.6	48.4
Skilled	37.2	57.7
White-collar[1]	34.2	27.1
White-collar[2]	19.7	
Intermediate positions[3]	12.9	xx

1) Based on Peter et al. 1998, n=1337. 2) Based on Rothenbacher et al. 1998, n=189, no separate figures for men and women available. 3) Based on Siegrist et al. 1997, n=170, men only (own calculations).

The next question arising in view of these findings is how much of the association between occupational class and health-adverse outcomes is due to stressful psychosocial work environments. Findings from the study in public transport workers described above indicate that the part of social inequality in health explained by ERI and by physical/chemical hazards is substantial (see table 21). As can be seen, being an unskilled worker (e.g. a bus driver) is associated with a significantly increased risk of poor health as compared with white-collar workers after adjustment for age and gender (model I: odds ratio 2.2). Additional adjustment for ERI (model II) weakens the effect of occupational class substantially: the odds ratio for unskilled workers decreases from 2.2 to 1.4 and is no longer significant, whereas ERI becomes the strongest predictor in the model (OR 4.0, 95% CI 2.9, 5.4). Adjustment for physical and chemical hazards (model III) decreases the odds ratios for occupational group to 1.4, whereas hazards are significant (OR 4.3, 95% CI 2.9, 6.7). Full adjustment for all factors (model IV, i.e. physical/chemical hazards plus ERI) does not change this picture, although the OR for ERI decreases to 3.6 (95% CI 2.5, 5.2) and the one for physical and chemical hazards is diminished to 2.9 (95% CI 1.9, 4.6).

Table 21: Stepwise logistic regression analysis: self-reported symptoms[5] by occupational group, effort–reward imbalance and additional factors[6] (multivariate odds ratios, 95% CI)

Predictors in model	Model I[1]	Model II[2]	Model III[3]	Model IV[4]
Occupational group				
Blue-collar	2.2 (1.4, 3.5)	1.6 (1.0, 2.4)	1.4 (0.8, 2.3)	1.1 (0.6, 1.8)
Unskilled	1.5 (0.9, 2.4)	1.2 (0.8, 1.8)	1.4 (0.8, 2.2)	1.2 (0.8, 2.1)
Skilled	1.0	1.0	1.0	1.0
White-collar (ref.)				
Effort–reward imbalance	x	4.0 (2.9, 5.4)	x	3.6 (2.5, 5.2)
Physical/chemical hazards	x	x	4.3 (2.9, 6.7)	2.9 (1.9, 4.6)

1) *Occupational group adjusted for age and gender.*
2) *Additionally adjusted for ERI.*
3) *Additionally adjusted for physical/chemical hazards.*
4) *Additionally adjusted for ERI and physical/chemical hazards.*
5) *Musculoskeletal, gastrointestinal, fatigue and sleep disturbances, common cold, nausea and dizziness.*
6) *For study population and methods, see Peter et al. 1998, own calculations.*

Table 22 a: Stepwise logistic regression analysis: self-reported musculoskeletal symptoms by occupational group, occupational efforts and resources, physical and chemical hazards[5] (multivariate odds ratios, 95% CI)

Men (n=13771)

Predictors in model	Model I[1]	Model II[2]	Model III[3]	Model IV[4]
Occupational group:				
Unskilled blue-collar	4.7 (3.9, 5.6)	5.3 (4.5, 6.4)	2.2 (1.9, 2.6)	2.7 (2.2, 3.2)
Skilled blue-collar	4.7 (4.0, 5.4)	5.1 (4.4, 6.0)	2.1 (1.8, 2.5)	2.4 (2.1, 2.9)
Low level white-collar	3.3 (2.5, 4.4)	3.3 (2.5, 4.3)	1.7 (1.3, 2.3)	1.8 (1.3, 2.4)
Intermediate white-collar	2.1 (1.7, 2.5)	2.5 (2.0, 3.0)	1.5 (1.3, 1.8)	1.8 (1.5, 2.3)
High level white-collar	1.2 (0.9, 1.4)	1.3 (1.0, 1.6)	1.1 (0.9, 1.3)	1.2 (1.0, 1.5)
Professionals (ref.)	1.0	1.0	1.0	1.0
High efforts	x	1.9 (1.8, 2.1)	x	1.8 (1.6, 2.0)
Poor resources	x	1.8 (1.6, 2.0)	x	1.7 (1.5, 1.9)
Physical/chemical hazards	x	x	4.4 (3.8, 5.1)	3.9 (3.4, 4.6)

1) Occupational group adjusted for age, self-employed not included.
2) Model I additionally adjusted for occupational efforts and resources.
3) Model I additionally adjusted for physical/chemical hazards.
4) Fully adjusted for occupational efforts and resources, physical/chemical hazards.
5) For study population and methods, see BIB/IAB 2001, own calculations.

In another study no explanatory contribution of work stress to social inequality in health has been observed. Analysis was based on data from about 34,000 men and women employed in 1998/99. This group represents a 0.1% sample of the working population who were 15 years or older and employed at least 10 hours per week (see BIBB/IAB 2001). Tables 22 a + b displays associations between occupational group, work stress indicators (efforts, e.g. time pressure, disturbances, responsibility increase in workload; resources, e.g. job insecurity, promotion prospects, social network, changes in the work organisation, income), physical and chemical hazards, and self-reported musculoskeletal symptoms. As can be seen, there is a social gradient regarding reports of musculoskeletal symptoms in model I among both men and women. These figures do not substantially change when additionally adjusted for occupational efforts and resources (model II). When additional physical and chemical hazards are introduced in model III the odds ratios of occupational groups decrease considerably. Full adjustment in model IV does not reveal any further change in the effects of occupational group. The estimations of both work stress indicators and of physical and chemical hazards are quite stable as compared with models II and III. These findings indicate that a substantial part of the observed association between occupational group and musculoskeletal symptoms is explained by physical and chemical hazards. Independently from the occupational group and from physical/chemical hazards, work stress is associated with the outcome. These findings did not change when additional information on part-time/full-time employment was taken into account (results not displayed in detail).

Table 22 b: Stepwise logistic regression analysis: self-reported musculoskeletal symptoms by occupational group, occupational efforts and resources, physical and chemical hazards[5] (multivariate odds ratios, 95% CI)

Women (n=10,640)

Predictors in model	Model I[1]	Model II[2]	Model III[3]	Model IV[4]
Occupational group:				
Unskilled blue-collar	2.7 (2.2, 3.2)	3.0 (2.4, 3.6)	1.6 (1.3, 1.9)	1.8 (1.4, 2.1)
Skilled blue-collar	2.9 (2.2, 3.7)	3.1 (2.4, 4.0)	2.0 (1.6, 2.6)	2.1 (1.6, 2.7)
Low level white-collar	1.4 (0.4, 4.9)	1.5 (0.4, 5.3)	1.6 (0.6, 4.2)	1.0 (0.3, 3.6)
Intermediate white-collar	1.4 (1.2, 1.6)	1.6 (1.4, 1.9)	1.3 (1.1, 1.5)	1.5 (1.2, 1.7)
High level white-collar	1.0 (0.8, 1.2)	1.0 (0.9, 1.2)	1.0 (0.9, 1.2)	1.1 (1.0, 1.3)
Professionals (ref.)	1.0	1.0	1.0	1.0
High efforts	x	2.0 (1.8, 2.3)	x	1.9 (1.7, 2.2)
Poor resources	x	1.9 (1.7, 2.1)	x	1.7 (1.5, 1.9)
Physical/chemical hazards	x	x	4.0 (3.6, 4.4)	3.8 (3.4, 4.3)

1) Occupational group adjusted for age, self-employed not included.
2) Model I additionally adjusted for occupational efforts and resources.
3) Model I additionally adjusted for physical/chemical hazards.
4) Fully adjusted for occupational efforts and resources, physical/chemical hazards.
5) For study population and methods, see BIBB/IAB 2001, own calculations.

In sum, these first preliminary findings suggest that there is mixed evidence for the explanatory role of work stress with regard to social inequality in health in Germany. Yet, these results may depend on the type of disease/symptoms under study and may change when other diseases or symptoms are investigated. However, the observed associations underline the importance of work stress for human health.

C. Accidents at Work

Despite the basic changes in the nature of work described above, accidents still play an important role in today's jobs. Unfortunately there are no official statistics that allow us to stratify the incidence of accidents by type of occupation.

Table 23 shows the incidence of work accidents in relation to the economically active population between 1991 and 2000, the most recent information available. As can be seen, the incidence of reported accidents at work with a minimum of four days of sick leave has decreased by more than 1% since 1991. This development was mainly attributed to improved safety at work and to the changing nature of work, i.e. a decreasing number of people working in dangerous jobs characterised by physical and chemical hazards, and by physical workload.

Table 23: Accidents at work with > 3 days of sick leave in relation to the economically active (%), absolute numbers in brackets)

	1991	1996	2000
Accidents at work	5.7 (2,016,000)	4.9 (1,658,000)	4.5 (1,514,000)
Economically active persons[1]	100 35,521,000	100 33,813,000	100 33,656,000

All persons employed with work contracts or self-employed, part-time and full-time, employment main source of income.
Source: Statistical Yearbook 1993, 1997, 2002 (own calculations).

Since 1960 the incidence of lethal occupational accidents has been constantly decreasing (Bundesregierung 2002). Starting from a peak of about 5,500 deaths at the beginning of the 1960s and another peak with about 4,600 deaths 10 years later, the incidence was 1,107 deaths in 2001. Another peak could be observed around 1992 (about 1,900 deaths, compared with 1,500 in 1990 and 1995). A part of this increase might be attributable to the reunification and the inclusion of East German data. In sum, these findings underline the beneficial effects that are derived from developments in occupational medicine and safety policies.

6. Trade Unions – Unionisation Rates and Changes over Time

Keeping the associations between social class, work stress and health in mind, strong trade unions could help to reduce related health risks. Yet, trends in Germany concerning numbers of union members are talking in different tongues (see table 24).

Numbers concerning the unionisation rates in Germany are usually derived from information on the German Trade Union, the umbrella organisation covering most German unions. Unions like the German Officials' Union with more than 1,200,000 members, or the Christian German Union with 300,000 members in 2000 are not organised under this umbrella. Accordingly, only those officials who are organised in other unions are listed as members of the German Trade Union, except for those who have dual membership. The latter numbers are not listed in the official statistics. Therefore the overall unionisation rate might be underestimated.

Table 24: Proportion of unionisation (German Trade Union)
in relation to the economically active population[1]
(percentages[2], numbers in brackets)

	1991	1996	1998[3]
Totally	31.5 (11,800,402)	24.9 (8,972,172)	22.6 (8,310,783)
Men	36.2 (7,910,251)	30.1 (6,227,686)	28.0 (5,776,720)
Women	25.0 (3,890,151)	18.0 (2,744,486)	15.7 (2,534,063)
Blue-collar	48.1 (7,005,697)	42.0 (5,449,907)	41.4 (4,960,852)
White-collar	16.6 (2,790,159)	15.3 (2,554,633)	13.2 (2,431,727)
Officials	32.2 (809,549)	26.9 (662,901)	27.5 (622,765)

1) All persons employed with work contracts or self-employed, part-time and full-time, numbers are given in table 2.
2) Percentage of union members in relation to the occupational groups in table 2. Accordingly percentages do not add up to 100.
3) Most recent information available.
Source: Statistical Yearbook 1992, 1997, 2001, own calculations.

Nevertheless, if the unionisation rate within a country is an indicator for the balance of economic power in the country, this balance has changed in Germany since 1991. The overall unionisation rate decreased by nearly 9% between 1991 and 1998, the year with the latest available information. The fact that little more than one fifth of the workforce are union members is low by European comparison. Men have higher unionisation rates compared with women, and the decrease in unionisation between 1991 and 1998 is more pronounced among women. With regard to occupational group, blue-collar workers have the highest proportion of union members followed by officials and white-collar workers. Whereas the unionisation rate of white- and blue-collar workers has constantly decreased during recent years, a slight increase can be observed among officials in 1998.

7. Ongoing Research on Social Inequality in Health

A prospective study on biological, behavioural, and psychosocial determinants of cardiovascular diseases – the so-called Heinz Nixdorf RECALL (Risk factors, evaluation of coronary calcium, and lifestyle) study – is being conducted in Northrhine-Westfalia (Schmermund *et al.* 2002). Currently, the baseline screening in more than 4000 initially healthy men and women aged 45 to 75 years is approaching completion. This population is representative for the population living in this area. After 5 years a second screening is planned, focusing particularly on biological risk factors and markers of myocardial infarction, and on incidence rates regarding this disease including sudden cardiac death.

8. National Goals and Strategies to Reduce Social Inequality in Health

In Germany a gap between available data and the importance of social inequality in health can be observed. Whereas social inequality in health is as pronounced as it is in other developed countries, the available data are comparably limited. For two reasons it is not worthwhile justifying the restricted German data situation by hinting at the availability of information from other countries that could be applied to the German situation. Firstly, huge differences in social inequality regarding health can be observed between countries, even if they are at similar levels of socio-economic development (Kunst *et al.* 1998, Marmot 1994). Reasons for these differences are manifold, including differences in political activities per country to reduce social inequality. Secondly, findings from many countries show that social inequality within one country might change over time (Mackenbach & Bakker 2002). Therefore it is not sufficient to measure social inequality once; continuous registration of information is needed. Nevertheless, only few official activities to improve the German data situation with regard to social inequality in health are currently under way. For instance, the Ministry for Education and Family Affairs has offered two grants for research on social inequality in health during the past 4 years. Although these grants were relatively small compared with funding in other research areas, and were not primarily aimed at improving the official data situation, this is a step in the right direction. However, there are some data sources that could be used. For instance, although statutory health insurance data are one of the few sources in Germany containing all information required for reporting on social inequality, and although it is allowed by law to make use of this information for scientific purposes or for official reporting, these data have not often been used up to now. This is even more surprising since parts of the official health reporting are based on a 0.82% sample of members of the statutory health insurance in Germany (Statistisches Bundesamt 1999).

During recent years no official statements by politicians have been made addressing social inequalities in health and activities to reduce the social gap. Moreover, social inequality in terms of poverty has been ignored in official governmental statements (Mielck 2000). Since the PISA study – an investigation initialised among OECD members to evaluate the quality of national educational systems – it cannot be ignored that in Germany access to education depends more on parental social status than is the case in other countries (PISA 2003). However, this situation is counterbalanced by an increasing awareness of social inequality in science, documented by a huge number of publications and conferences, although the data situation is not favourable in Germany (Mielck 2000). The collection and official availability of data is seen as one of the most important challenges for German policy and science in the 21st century (Bardehle 2001).

9. Conclusions

In Germany social inequality in health is a problem that is as impor-tant as in other socio-economically developed countries. Although not many official efforts have been made to collect information during recent years, some data from scientific studies and official sources are available to support this statement. Some of this data is rather old and thereby underlines some of the problems in Germany in collecting information on social inequality in health. Examples given in this chapter have even shown increasing social inequality during the past few years, particularly regarding income. If the current political and economic developments in Germany are taken into account, it seems that a widening social gap can be expected in the future. Although currently still on a high standard compared with other European coun-tries (Eurostat 2004), social security (e.g. job security, pensions, health insurance) and egalitarian welfare policy has already started to be reduced. The most recent reforms contain increasing costs for members of the statutory health insurance system, decreasing levels of pensions combined with the necessity of private precautions, less strict job secu-rity regulations, less money for the unemployed, and financial sanctions for people on social welfare among others. These changes might in-crease the economic and material gap in Germany. Yet, a comparison between different European countries concerning the possible impact of welfare policy on social inequality could not find that the slight differences that were observed between countries in terms of social-status-related mortality were directly attributable to differences in welfare policy between these countries (Kunst *et al.* 1998, Mackenbach *et al.* 1997). The authors argued that social security and welfare policy may influence all social groups and should therefore have an impact on nationwide morbidity and mortality rates rather than on social inequality in health. Yet, it was also concluded that a worsening situation as regards economic and material inequality must be compensated by improvements in other areas (e.g. education, working conditions) if an influence on social inequality in health is to be prevented (Mackenbach *et al.* 1997). Given the cuts in money for education and science during recent years and the bad situation in education reported by PISA (2003), this is not the case in Germany. Therefore, it is likely that the situation in Germany will worsen during the next few years due to an increasing economic and material gap.

Concerning the possible impact of working conditions on social inequality in health, the picture might be clearer. Due to an increasing proportion of part-time work, as well as contracts limited in time, and job insecurity for a broader section of the working force, fragmented occupational careers tend to become more likely. In addition, occupational demands are changing more and more, from traditional physical and chemical hazards to psychologically demanding work, mainly due to increasing numbers of jobs in the service sector and to the diffusion of information technology into more and more jobs. These developments influence the character of work and may lead to an increase in work demands and a decrease in occupational rewards that does not affect all occupational groups to the same extent. It has been discussed that socially less well-off groups may suffer more from these developments (Peter 2001, Siegrist & Marmot 2004). It can therefore be expected that the influence of working conditions on social inequality in health is likely to become more important rather than decrease. Due to the described changes in the nature of work, in combination with a developed occupational medicine and job security in Germany, traditional work exposures (e.g. physically demanding work, physical and chemical hazards) may play a less important role in this context.

Despite the already existing social inequality in health in Germany and the not very promising prognosis for the future, enhanced health policy efforts to reduce the burden of poor health among the socially less privileged have not been made up to now.

Accordingly, the most important aims for the future are as follows:

1. Official data on social inequality in health should be established on a regular basis.

2. Given the importance of work with regard to health and the documented relationship between psychosocial work environments and social status, the role of work in social inequality in health needs to be explored more intensively.

3. Political goals aiming at the reduction of social inequality in health need to be formulated.

4. Public health intervention strategies need to be developed and applied to reduce the health burden of socially less privileged groups in different settings (e.g. school, work).

References

BARDEHLE D. 2001. "Sozial-epidemiologische Indikatoren in der Gesundheits- und Sozialstatistik (Socio-epidemiological indicators in health and social statistics)". In: MIELCK A., BLOMFIELD K (eds.) *Sozialepidemiologie – Einführung in die Grundlagen, Ergebnisse und Umsetzungsmöglichkeiten* (Social epidemiology – introduction to basics, findings, and practical consequences). Weinheim: München: Juventa-Verlag,

BIBB-IAB BIBB/IAB. 2001. *Erwerb und Verwertung beruflicher Qualifikationen von Erwerbstätigkeiten,* BIBB/ IAB – Strukturerhebung: 1998/99.

BUNDESREGIERUNG (Federal Government)(ed.). 2002. *Bericht der Bundesregierung über den Stand von Sicherheit und Gesundheit bei der Arbeit 2001* (Report of the Federal Government concerning safety and health at work 2001). Drucksache 15/279 des Deutschen Bundestages (Document 15/279 of the lower house of the German Parliament). Bonn: Bundesanzeiger Verlagsgesellschaft.

EUROSTAT. The social situation in the European Union 2003 (short version). http://europa.eu.int/comm/eurostat/Public/datashop/print-product/EN. 02 April, 2004.

FERRIE J.E., GRIFFITHS J., MARMOT M.G., ZIGLIO E. (eds.). 1999. *Labour market changes and job insecurity: a challenge for social welfare and health promotion.* Copenhagen: WHO Regional Office for Europe.

GCP RESEARCH GROUP. 1988. "German Cardiovascular Prevention Study (GCP): Design and Methods". *Europ Heart J* 9: 1058-66.

GEYER S., PETER, R. 2000. "Income, occupational position, qualification, and health inequalities – competing risks? (Comparing indicators of social status)". *J Epidemiol Community Health* 54: 299-305.

HANEFELD U. 1987. *Das Sozio-ökonomische Panel. Grundlagen und Konzeption* (The socioeconiomic panel. Basis and conception). Frankfurt a.M./New York: Campus.

HASSELHORN H.M., NÜBLING M. 2004. "Arbeitsbedingte psychische Erschöpfung bei Erwerbstätigen in Deutschland (Work related mental health among employees in Germany)". *Arbeitsmed Sozialmed Umweltmed* 39: 568-76.

HASSELHORN H.M., TACKENBERG P., PETER R. and THE NEXT STUDY GROUP. 2004. "Effort–reward imbalance among nurses in stable countries and in countries in transition". *Int J Occup Environ Health* 10: 401-8.

HEIN B. 1996. "Fragen zur Gesundheit. Ergebnisse des Mikrozensus 1995 (Questions concerning health. Findings of the 1995 Microcensus)". *Wirtschaft und Statistik* 10: 624-32.

HELMERT U., MASCHEWSKY-SCHNEIDER U., MIELCK A., GREISER E. 1993. "Soziale Ungleichheit bei Herzinfarkt und Schlaganfall in West-Deutschland (Social inequalities for myocardial infarction and stroke in West Germany)". *Soz Präventivmed* 38: 123-132.

HELMERT U. 1994. "Sozialschichtspezifische Unterschiede in der selbst wahrgenommenen Morbidität und bei ausgewählten gesundheitsbezogenen Indikatoren in West-Deutschland (Social inequality in self-reported morbidity and in selected indicators of self-reported health in Western Germany)". In: MIELCK A (ed.). *Krankheit und soziale Ungleichheit. Ergebnisse der sozialepidemiologischen Forschung in Deutschland* (Social inequality in illness. Findings of social epidemiological research in Germany). Leske & Budrich: Opladen.

HELMERT U., SHEA S., MASCHWESKY-SCHNEIDER U. 1995. "Social class and cardiovascular disease risk factor changes in West Germany 1984-1991". *Eur J Publ Health* 5: 103-8.

HELMERT U. 1996. "Kardiovaskuläre Risikofaktoren und Beruf: Resultate der Gesundheitssurveys der Deutschen Herz-Kreislauf-Präventionsstudie Cardiovascular risk factors and occupation: Findings of the health survey of the German heart and circulation disease prevention study)". *Soz Präventivmed*: 41: 165-177.

HELMERT U., MIELCK A., SHEA S. 1997. "Poverty, health, and nutrition in Germany", *Rev Environ Health* 12: 159-70.

INTERNATIONAL LABOUR OFFICE (ILO). 1990. *ISCO-88 International Classification of Occupations*. Geneva: ILO.

JOKSIMOVIC L., SIEGRIST, J., MEYER-HAMMER M., PETER R., KLIMEK W., HEINTZEN M. 1999. "Psychosocial factors and restenosis after PTCA: the role of work-related overcommitment". *Int J Behav Med* 6: 356-69.

JOKSIMOVIC L., STARKE D V.D., KNESEBECK O., SIEGRIST J. 2002. "Perceived work stress, overcommitment, and self-reported musculoskeletal pain: a cross-sectional investigation". *Int J Behav Med* 9: 122-138.

KARASEK RA., THEORELL T., 1990. *Healthy Work: Stress, Productivity, and the Reconstruction of Working Life*. New York: Basic Books.

KLEIN T. 1996. "Mortalität in Deutschland: aktuelle Entwicklungen und soziale Unterschiede (Mortality in Germany: recent trends and social differences)". In: ZAPF W., SCHUPP J., HABICH R. (eds.) *Lebenslagen im Wandel. Sozialberichterstattung im Längsschnitt* (Changing social position. Longitudinal Reports on social changes). New York/Frankfurt a. M.: Campus.

KRONES T. 2001. "Nationalität, Migration und Gesundheitszustand (Nationality, migration, and health)", in: MIELCK A., BLOMFIELD K (eds.) *Sozialepidemiologie – Einführung in die Grundlagen, Ergebnisse und Umsetzungsmöglichkeiten* (Social epidemiology – introduction to basics, findings, and possibilities for realization. Weinheim, München: Juventa-Verlag.

KUNST A.E., GROENHOF F., MACKENBACH J.P. and THE EU WORKING GROUP ON SOCIOECONOMIC INEQUALITIES IN HEALTH. 1998. "Mortality by occupational class among men 30-64 years in 11 European countries". *Soc Sci Med* 46: 1459-76.

LARISCH M., JOKSIMOVIC J., KNESEBECK O.V.D., STARKE D., SIEGRIST J. 2003. "Berufliche Gratifikationskrisen und depressive Symptome: Eine Querschnittsstudie bei Erwerbstätigen im mittleren Erwachsenenalter". *Psychotherapie, Psychosomatik, Medizinische Psychologie* 53: 223-28.

LECHNER I., MIELCK A. 1998. "Die Verkleinerung des ‚Healthy Migrant-Effects': Entwicklung der Morbidität von ausländischen und deutschen Befragten im sozio-ökonomischen Panel 1984-1992 (Reduction of the healthy migrant effect: Trends in morbidity among foreign and German respondents in the socio-economic panel 1984-1992)". *Gesundheitswesen* 60: 715-20.

MACKENBACH JP., KUNST A.E., CAVELAARS E.J.M., GROENHOF F., GEURTS J.J.M. and THE EU WORKING GROUP ON SOCIOECONOMIC INEQUALITIES IN HEALTH. 1997. "Socioeconomic inequalities in morbidity and mortality in Western Europe". *The Lancet* 349: 1655-59.

MACKENBACH J., BAKKER M. (eds.). 2002. *Reducing inequalities in health: a European perspective*. London and New York: Routledge.

MARMOT M.G. 1994. "Social differentials in health within and between populations". *Daedalus* 123: 197-216.

MIELCK A., *Soziale Ungleichheit und Gesundheit* (Social inequality in health). 2000. Bern, Göttingen, Toronto, Seattle: Huber.

PETER R., SIEGRIST J., STORK J., MANN H., LABROT B. 1991. "Zigarettenrauchen und psychosoziale Arbeitsbelastungen bei Beschäftigten des mittleren Managements (Cigarette smoking and psychosocial work environment in middle managers)". *Soz Präventivmed* 36: 315-21.

PETER R., SIEGRIST J. 1997. "Chronic work stress, sickness absence, and hypertension in middle-managers – general or specific sociological explanations?". *Soc Sci Med* 45: 1111-20.

PETER R., GEIßLER H., SIEGRIST J. 1998. "Associations of effort–reward imbalance at work and reported symptoms in different groups of male and female public transport workers". *Stress Medicine* 14: 175-82.

PETER R., SIEGRIST J. 2000. "Psychosocial work environment and the risk of coronary heart disease". *Int Arch Occup Environ Health* 73 (Suppl 1): S41-S45.

PETER R. 2001. "Berufsstatus und Gesundheit (Occupational position and health)". In: MIELCK, A., BLOMFIELD, K. (Hrsg.) *Sozialepidemiologie – Einführung in die Grundlagen, Ergebnisse und Umsetzungsmöglichkeiten* (So-

cial epidemiology – introduction to the basics, results, and practical consequences). Weinheim, München: Juventa-Verlag.

PETER R., YONG M., GEYER S. 2003. "Schul- und Berufsausbildung, beruflicher
Status und ischämische Herzkrankheiten- eine prospektive Studie mit Daten
einer gesetzlichen Krankenversicherung in Deutschland (Education and
training, occupational position, and ischaemic heart disease – a prospective
study with data from a statutory health insurance company in Germany)".
Soz Präventivmed 48: 44-54.

PISA 2003: http://www.pisa.oecd.org.

RAZUM O., GEIGER I. 2003. "Migranten (Migrants)". In: SCHWARTZ F.W.,
BADURA B., BUSSE R., LEIDL R., RASPE H., SIEGRIST J., WALTER U. (eds.)
Das Public Health Buch (The Public Health Book). Second Edition. Munich:
Jena: Urban & Fischer: 686-94.

ROTHENBACHER D., PETER R., BODE G., ADLER G., BRENNER H. 1998. "Dyspep-
sia in relation to Helicobacter pylori infection and psychosocial work stress
in white collar employees". *Am J Gastroenterology* 93: 1443-49.

SCHMERMUND A., MÖHLENKAMP S., STANG A., GRÖNEMEYER D., SEIBEL R.,
HIRCHE H., MANN K., SIFFERT W., LAUTERBACH K., SIEGRIST J.,
JÖCKEL K.H., ERBEL R. FOR THE HEINZ NIXDORF RECALL STUDY INVESTI-
GATIVE GROUP. 2002. "Assessment of clinically silent atherosclerotic disease
and novel risk factors for predicting myocardial infarction and cardiac death
in healthy middle-aged subjects: Rationale and design of the Heinz Nixdorf
RECALL Study". *Am Heart J* 144: 212-18.

SIEGRIST J., PETER R. 1994. "Job stressors and coping characteristics in work-
related disease: issues of validity". *Work & Stress* 8: 130-40.

SIEGRIST J., PETER R., GEORG W., CREMER P., SEIDEL D. 1991. "Psychosocial
and biobehavioral characteristics of hypertensive men with elevated atherogenic lipids". *Atherosclerosis* 86: 211-218.

SIEGRIST J. 1996. "Adverse health effects of high-effort/low-reward conditions".
J Occup Health Psychol 1: 27-41.

SIEGRIST J., PETER R., CREMER P., SEIDEL D. 1997. "Chronic work stress is
associated with atherogenic lipids and elevated fibrinogen in middle-aged
men". *J Internal Med* 242: 149-56.

SIEGRIST J., MARMOT M. 2004. "Health inequalities and the psychosocial
environment – two scientific challenges". *Soc Sci Med* 58: 1463-73.

STATISTISCHES BUNDESAMT (Federal Bureau of Statistics), *Mikrozensus.* Zweig-
stelle Bonn; Gruppe VIIIC-Mikrozensus (Microcensus. Office Bonn; Group
VIIIC-Microcensus). Graurheindorferstr 198: DE-53117. Bonn: Germany.

STATISTISCHES BUNDESAMT (Federal Bureau of Statistics) (ed.). 1992. *Statistisches Jahrbuch 1992 für die Bundesrepublik Deutschland* (Statistical Yearbook for Germany 1992). Stuttgart: Metzler-Poeschel.

STATISTISCHES BUNDESAMT (Federal Bureau of Statistics) (ed.). 1993. *Statistisches Jahrbuch 1993 für die Bundesrepublik Deutschland* (Statistical Yearbook for Germany 1993). Stuttgart: Metzler-Poeschel.

STATISTISCHES BUNDESAMT (Federal Bureau of Statistics) (ed.). 1996. *Statistisches Jahrbuch 1996 für die Bundesrepublik Deutschland* (Statistical Yearbook for Germany 1996). Stuttgart: Metzler-Poesche.l

STATISTISCHES BUNDESAMT (Federal Bureau of Statistics) (ed.). 1997. *Statistisches Jahrbuch 1997 für die Bundesrepublik Deutschland* (Statistical Yearbook for Germany 1997). Stuttgart: Metzler-Poeschel.

STATISTISCHES BUNDESAMT (Federal Bureau of Statistics) (ed.). 2001. *Statistisches Jahrbuch 2001 für die Bundesrepublik Deutschland* (Statistical Yearbook for Germany 2001). Stuttgart: Metzler-Poeschel.

STATISTISCHES BUNDESAMT (Federal Bureau of Statistics) (ed.). 2002. *Statistisches Jahrbuch 2002 für die Bundesrepublik Deutschland* (Statistical Yearbook for Germany 2002). Stuttgart: Metzler-Poeschel.

STATISTISCHES BUNDESAMT (Federal Bureau of Statistics) (ed.). 2003. *Statistisches Jahrbuch 2003 für die Bundesrepublik Deutschland* (Statistical Yearbook for Germany 2003). Stuttgart: Metzler-Poeschel.

STATISTISCHES BUNDESAMT (Federal Bureau of Statistics) (ed.). 1999. *Versichertenstichprobe aus der gesetzlichen Krankenversicherung – Kurzfassung* (Sample of the Staturory Health Insurance – short version). Wiesbaden.

The Netherlands

Irene HOUTMAN & Marije EVERS

Introduction

In this chapter we will give an impression of the Dutch situation and development concerning socio-economic status (SES), working conditions and health. Recently a large programme on 'Socio-economic status and health' has been concluded in the Netherlands; however, only 3 out of 25 studies included working life. It seems typical that this combined look at SES and work in relation to health is not so much elaborated on, since in many areas the approach to public health and occupational health appears to be a separate one (see appendix 1 for a more elaborate discussion on the research on social inequalities in health in the Netherlands). In this chapter we will more specifically describe the socio-economic status according to several labour market characteristics, working conditions and health outcomes, and consequently examine to what extent socio-economic status, working conditions and several other relevant labour market characteristics are related to one another and how they contribute to health.

In this present chapter we will first focus on the economic developments over the past 20 years. The national trends in economics, unemployment and other forms of dropout from the labour market, such as sickness absenteeism and disability, are an important background for interpreting the trends in the salary, education, working conditions and health of the Dutch workforce. The majority of data and analyses presented in this chapter will be taken from the national Living Conditions Survey, which includes information on work, socio-economic class and also on health. This source provides the 'core data' which will be described in more detail in the method section.

A paragraph on demographics will provide information about demographic aspects for men and women from the various socio-economic groups in relation to work and health. Finally, the role of socio-economic status and working conditions as explanatory factors for inequalities in determining health will be examined. When discussing these findings, we will elaborate on the emanating issues with respect to social groups, and the role of the Government, social partners and sector organisations with respect to these issues.

1. Economic Development and Social Security

The Gross Domestic Product in the Netherlands shows a net increase every year, and there was an increase from 160,721 GDP in 1980 to 445,160 GDP in 2002 (www.cbs.nl). The growth was, however, not so continuous. Employment and unemployment figures indicate that in the early 1980s (1983-1984) as well as in the early 1990s (1993-1994) there was an increase in unemployment which followed a decrease or stagnation of economic growth. After a period of continuous economic growth and almost no unemployment, the economy worsened again in 2001. Since 2002 the Netherlands finds itself in an economic recession, which appears to be turning to the better in 2004 (http://www.cbs.nl/en/publications/articles/webmagazine/2004/1532k.htm). The changes in unemployment rates co-occur with changes in disability rates (and absence rates), but go in a contrary direction. The pattern appears to be that an increasing unemployment rate is associated with decreasing disability and sickness absence figures and vice versa.

Absenteeism and disability benefits in the Netherlands in the period covered are relatively high. Since 1998 more than 100,000 workers have already been diagnosed as being disabled for work each year. It was predicted that a total number of a million disabled workers would be reached in 2003, resulting in one disabled employee for every seven working persons. This simply did not happen, since a dramatic reduction started in 2002, and progressed during 2003 and 2004. This can be related to the fact that since 2002 there has been a new economic recession at hand in the Netherlands.

The social insurance system in the Netherlands has witnessed continuous change in the past decades (see De Haan & Verboon 2002, Return 1999, Brenninkmeijer *et al.* 2003). Initially, the protective function of the system was of central concern. The system offered insurance against loss of income, with a guaranteed minimum income for everyone. In general, the social insurance system is biased towards workers with a low income. Because of the way access to disability benefits is regulated, low-income workers have less opportunity to receive a disability payment, since their loss of income (relative to being unemployed) may be too small to qualify for disability benefits.

The social insurance system has become an important political issue in the Netherlands, particularly since the beginning of the last decade (the 1990s), when the economic situation deteriorated, as well as during the period of economic growth that followed. The measures which were meant to restructure the disability system aimed to lower absence rates and duration, and consequently the inflow into the disability benefit system (for a description of these measures see appendix 2). However, they were generally found to be short term and only partially effective. At present even more drastic changes in the social security legislation are forthcoming. The general view is that the Dutch legislative system has been too lenient towards both employers and employees.

Most measures were quite general and did not affect one particular group within the population, except the change in the disability criterion in 1993. This measure resulted in a reduced inflow into the disability benefit system of employees who were diagnosed as being disabled for work due to musculoskeletal disorders. Employees with musculoskeletal disorders often work in low-paid blue-collar jobs. It is particularly this group that since then has had less access to the disability benefits, and has been more eligible for lower unemployment benefits or the much lower welfare benefits.

2. Core Data

The data files that were used to furnish this chapter were the Central Bureau of Statistics' (CBS) data from the 'Living Conditions Survey' (LSO, DLO, and POLS) from the years 1980, 1983, 1991, 1992 and 2000. This survey has been the representative source for national information on SES, work and (self-reported) health. Throughout the years the Living Conditions Survey has not only changed its (Dutch) name, but has also changed items, and changed the order of items as well as answering categories. For example, in 2000 as opposed to previous years there was no question about level of income anymore, whereas the section of items on working conditions that started in 1977 with 11 questions had been considerably extended in 2000. This makes comparison over the years difficult. Nevertheless, the Living Conditions Survey contains valuable information as regards the aim of this chapter. Data for this chapter were therefore taken from several sources such as the CBS microdata base of the Living Conditions Survey, as well as the web page of the CBS (Statline: www.cbs.nl), which provides information free of charge on several topics from other data sources they collect, but also sources from other data providers such as the Social Security Administration (UWV).

A. Labour Force

The Central Bureau of Statistics' definition of labour force is people who work at least 12 hours per week on an annual basis. For each table it is specified whether the labour force is defined as all people between

14 and 64 years old or according to the above definition. Using the CBS definition many workers with short or seasonal contracts are lost. These are often women, and workers in specific sectors where many people do seasonal work or work with short, temporary contracts, such as in the hotels & restaurant sector and agriculture.

B. Health Measures

The Living Conditions Surveys only provide subjective information about health, such as the prevalence of chronic illnesses. Unfortunately the questions about these illnesses were not the same throughout the years. Therefore the sum of the psychosomatic health items that return every year (VOEG) was chosen as a dependent variable. The short version of the VOEG is a 13-item scale on psychosomatic health. The items can be answered with yes or no.

Another health measure is the answer to the question about overall state of health. The answer could range from bad to very good.

C. Socio-economic Status

Within the Living Conditions Surveys the concept of social group is defined as a combination of education, occupation and income level. On the one hand a distinction is made between white- versus blue-collar workers and self-employed. Within the white-collar workers, 'higher', 'intermediate' and 'lower' employees are identified. The blue-collar workers consist of labourers, farmers and fishermen (the latter group is extremely small). Although labourers and farmers are rather distinct groups, they cannot be separately identified for all years. For this reason we present them as one group in this chapter.

D. Working Conditions

Initially the survey used 11 items to question workers about their working conditions. These questions could be brought back to three concepts: working at a high work pace (1 question), skill and intellectual discretion (4 questions related to self-employment in one's job; Cronbach alpha ≥ 0.55), and the physical environment (4 questions related to physically heavy work, working in noise, and working in a dirty, smelly environment; Cronbach alpha ≥ 0.63).

E. Analyses

The analyses used to gain a better understanding of the relation between socio-economic status and health were cross-tabulations and stepwise multivariate logistic regression analysis. The regression analyses were stepwise (forced entry of predictor sets) to test to what extent working conditions changed the relation that was found initially for SES and health.

3. Demographics of the Dutch Population

A. *Labour Force Participation and Gender*

Participation in the labour market was assessed using the 'Living Conditions Survey' by asking people what their daily occupation was (work, student, pensioner, etc.) or directly whether they participated in the labour force.

Table 1: Men at work, part-time, full-time, employed, self-employed and inactive from 1980 to 2000. Percentages are based on total number of men aged 15-64 years (CBS, Living Conditions Survey)

	Aged 15-64	Working ≥ 12 h[1]	Employees		Self-employed		Inactive[4]					Total[5]
			Part-time[2]	Full-time[3]	Part-time	Full-time	Unemployed	Disabled	Student	House husband	Early retired	
1980-1983												
N	2,985	2,332	111	1,925	10	233	146	180	162	17	52	2,836
%		78.1	3.7	64.5	0.3	7.8	4.9	6.0	5.4	0.6	1.7	95.0
1991												
N	2,075	1,299	123	1,163	No data	No data	42	137	188	33	90	1,776
%		62.6	5.9	56.1			2.0	6.6	9.1	1.6	4.3	85.6
2000												
N	3,433	2,705	276	2,130	29	253	95	144	280	26	129	3,362
%		78.8	8.0	62.0	0.8	7.4	2.8	4.2	8.2	0.8	3.8	97.9

[1] *In 1980-1983 the cut-off lies at 15 hours per week instead of 12.*
[2] *Part-time: more than 12 hours a week and less than 35 hours a week.*
[3] *Full-time: 35 hours a week or more.*
[4] *Inactive: working less than 11 hours a week, based on self-report.*
[5] *Total does not add up to 100% due to missing data.*

Tables 1 and 2 indicate that the participation in the Dutch labour force is much higher for men as compared with women. This gender difference has become somewhat smaller over the last 20 years, but is still very present. For men, the labour force participation slightly decreased from about 78% in 1980/1983 to about 63% in 1991, and increased again in 2000 to about 79% (table 1). Women showed a continuous growth in labour force participation. Their participation increased from about 30% in 1980/1983 to about 54% in 2000 (table 2).

When women participate in the labour force, an increasingly large proportion of them work part-time, whereas only a small proportion of men work part-time.

Table 2: Women at work, part-time, full-time, employed, self-employed and inactive from 1980 to 2000. Percentages are based on total number of women aged 15-64 years (CBS, Living Conditions Survey)

	Aged 15-64	Working $>12\ h^1$	Employees Part-time[2]	Full-time[3]	Self-employed Part-time	Full-time	Inactive[4] Unemployed	Disabled	Student	Housewife	Early retired	Total[5]
1980-1983												
N	2,829	862	329	455	17	23	49	56	126	1,541	11	2,607
%		30.5	11.6	16.1	0.6	0.8	1.7	2.0	4.5	54.5	0.4	92.2
1991												
N	2,623	931	477	447	No data	No data	14	67	191	1,177	15	2,388
%		35.5	18.2	17.0			0.5	2.6	7.3	44.9	0.6	91.0
2000												
N	3,365	1,812	1,063	602	57	50	148	135	307	642	214	3,217
%		53.9	31.6	17.9	1.7	1.5	4.4	4.0	9.1	19.1	6.4	95.6

[1] *In 1980-1983 the cut-off lies at 15 hours per week instead of 12.*
[2] *Part-time: more than 12 hours a week and less than 35 hours a week.*
[3] *Full-time: 35 hours a week or more.*
[4] *Inactive: working less than 11 hours a week, based on self-report.*
[5] *Total does not add up to 100% due to missing data.*

B. Age and Gender

The population of male workers is growing older. In 1980-1983 the male worker had a mean age of 37.5 years, while in 1991-1992 and in 2000 the mean age had increased to 38.7 and 38.6 years respectively. For women the same trend can be seen: the female worker in 1991-1992 is older than in 1981-1983 (37.1 as opposed to 33.3 years) and in 2000 the mean age seems to be levelling off at 36.9. Thus the whole Dutch labour force is ageing. Figure 1 provides a graphical presentation of the present development of age within the workforce.

Figure 1: The age distribution of the labour force in the Netherlands (CBS, Statline)

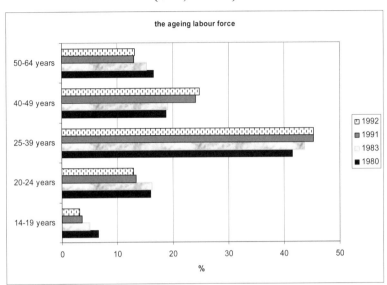

C. Gender and Social Group

Table 3 indicates that both men and women showed a considerable shift towards 'higher' socio-economic categories, although men were still about twice as much represented in the social group of higher employees as compared with women in the year 2000. In comparison with men, women are less likely to be self-employed or to work as labourers or farmers. The percentage of self-employed people has decreased over the last 20 years for both men and women.

**Table 3: Social group by gender across the period of 1980 to 2000.
Between brackets the actual sample sizes are shown
(CBS, Living Conditions Survey)**

	1980-1983	*1991-1992*	*2000*
Men			
Higher employees	13.9 (n=166)	15.3 (n=485)	18.7 (n=493)
Intermediate employees	21.8 (n=261)	31.9 (n=1,012)	26.4 (n=697)
Lower employees	13.5 (n=161)	13.4 (n=424)	11.7 (n=309)
Self-employed	10.3 (n=123)	8.6 (n=272)	5.2 (n=136)
Labourers	40.5 (n=484)	30.8 (n=976)	38.1 (n=1,005)
	100%	100%	100%
Women			
Higher employees	6.9 (n=28)	5.2 (n=126)	10.0 (n=180)
Intermediate employees	20.3 (n=82)	25.7 (n=619)	31.3 (n=563)
Lower employees	41.4 (n=167)	35.4 (n=854)	36.1 (n=649)
Self-employed	8.7 (n=35)	4.1 (n=98)	3.3 (n=59)
Labourers	22.6 (n=91)	29.7 (n=716)	19.4 (n=349)
	100%	100%	100%

Source: data file (POLS).

D. Adult Population outside Employment

Groups outside employment are students, housewives/men, pensioners, the unemployed and the disabled. Percentages are represented in table 4. Table 4 indicates that students amount to almost 10% when the total number is taken as a percentage of the labour force in 2000, with equal participation of men and women. The participation of female and male students has increased over the last two decades. The majority of the women outside the labour force are housewives, whereas only few men appear to take a role as 'househusbands'. Parallel to the increase in labour force participation of women, the percentage of housewives declined markedly from 58% in 1980-1983, to 43% in 1991-1992 and 22% in 2000. The other groups contribute cent to the workforce.

Table 4: Men and women who are students, housewives/men, early retired, disabled, as a percentage of the labour force (15-64 years) throughout 1980-2000. All variables are based on self-report. Actual sample sizes are shown within brackets (CBS, Living Conditions Survey)

Men	Students		Housewives/ men		Early retired		Disabled		Unemployed		Male labour force[1]
	%	N	%	N	%	N	%	N	%	N	
1980-1983	6▼	168	1▼	18	2▼	54	6	177	5▲	148	2,974
1991-1992	10▲	440	2▲	84	5▲	229	6	249	3▼	109	4,298
2000	8	288	1	35	5▲	171	4	147	2	85	3,433

Women	Students		Housewives/ men		Early retired		Disabled		Unemployed		Female labour force[1]
	%	N	%	N	%	N	%	N	%	N	
1980-1983	5▼	127	58▲	1,618	0▼	13	2▼	42	2	49	2,775
1991-1992	8	421	43▲	2,308	1▼	44	2▼	87	1▼	70	5,335
2000	9▲	307	22▼	725	7▲	240	4▲	130	4	143	3,365

[1] *Number of people (men/women) between 15 and 64 years in the surveys.*
▲*Higher percentage in this cell in comparison with the same cell in other years. p<.05.*
▼*Lower percentage in this cell in comparison with the same cell in other years. p<.05.*

Increasingly men and women take early retirement. In 1980-1983 only 2% of the male workforce took early retirement[1]. In the following

---

[1]   Early retirement schemes were introduced in the seventies as an experiment to tackle the problems of youth unemployment, by making it more attractive for older people to leave the labour market. There are several schemes that can be used for early retirement. These schemes are referred to as VUT (Vervroegde UitTreding = Early Retirement). Early retirement schemes are arranged through collective bargaining and established in collective agreements. The schemes are financed from contributions paid by both employees and employers.
Because early retirement gained popularity and was considered to be a social right, employment rates among older people remained low. In a European context, in 1995 the Netherlands in 1995 showed extremely low figures for employment of people between 55 and 64 years old, only to be surpassed by Belgium and Luxembourg (http://www.ouderenenarbeid.nl/). It is generally acknowledged that participation of the elderly in to the workforce has to be increased significantly in view of the significant ageing of the Dutch population, due to the rising life expectancy, the relative

years, 1991-1992 and 2000, this figure rose to 5%. The increase for women is even steeper. In 1980-1983 the percentage that retired was zero, whereas in 1991-1992 1% retired and in 2000 the figure was 8%. In an attempt to counter the recent economic recession the Government has proposed amendments in the regulations on pre-pension-like arrangements. Since the labour force is ageing, more and more people will want to make use of these arrangements, while there will be fewer employees to pay for this and other social services. The amendments are intended to discourage workers from taking early retirement. If these proposals are accepted and regulations are implemented and enforced, it is expected that in the years to come the prevalence of early-retired people will decrease.

The Dutch government supports the transformation of early retirement (VUT) regulations into flexible and pre-pension schemes. Under pre-pension schemes employees can still stop working before the official retirement age of 65. In contrast to the VUT schemes, pre-pension schemes are financed by capital funding, leaving the financial burden to a greater extent on the individual. An early exit will imply a lower pension benefit. It is clear that those with low income will not be so eager to pay for these pre-pension schemes, which will mean that they will either have to work longer or have lower pensions as compared with those often higher educated and wealthier workers, who can easily afford the pre-pension premiums. At present (2004) the Government and the social partners (employer and employee representatives[2]) have had a

---

large size of post-war cohorts and more recent lower fertility rates. Because this ageing process results in growing claims on socials benefits and facilities it will be impossible to sustain the current pensions and social security system (European Commission 2003). Fortunately, there has been a substantial increase in employment rates among older people have been substantially increasing since 1997. Furthermore, the ageing of the population has is slowed down by a relatively strong growth of the non-western national's population. The Dutch government is striving for an employment rate of 50% in 2020 for people between 55 and 64 years of age.

[2] According to Central Bureau of Statistics data the rate of unionisation fluctuated from 27 to 37%. Unfortunately the data are not subdivided for the different branches. In the Netherlands the unions play a less important role than in more Nordic countries such as Norway, Sweden, Denmark and Finland. Higher educated non-manual workers are hardly ever union members.

A fairly direct way unions can influence the working conditions is by maintaining close contact with the works council. Works council members get information and trainings in return. Other ways of influencing working conditions are the collective labour agreements and nationwide nation wide campaigns that aspire to influence the public opinion and politics.

Just like in Norway, the unions accepted moderate wage increases in exchange for low inflation and better chances for full employment. However, there are no objective figures about how and to what which extent trade unions positively affect health

fierce dispute about these pre-pension schemes and have even stopped talking to one another. Until recently there was a good social dialogue. However, this dispute, together with the dispute on the adaptation of the disability benefit system (see previous paragraph) puts the mutual relations on edge.

E. *Unemployment*[3]

In 1980-1983, 5% of the male labour force were reported to be unemployed. In 1991-1992 the unemployment rate for men decreased to 2% and rose slightly in 2000 to 3%. According to the CBS, the current unemployment rates for both men and women have been rising recently, after the onset of the economic recession. Unemployment figures in the Netherlands are, however, still amongst the lowest in Europe. On the other hand, disability figures in the Netherlands are amongst the highest in Europe.

F. *Sickness Absence*

In 1991-1992 and 2000 the employees were asked whether they had been absent from work due to illness in the past two months[4]. In 1991-

---

by regulating working conditions. Social inequality has always been a concern to unions. Nevertheless there is no union policy specific to social inequalities in health.

[3] In the Netherlands the most frequent unemployment benefits are WW benefits and welfare. WW can only be claimed by ex-employees, whereas welfare can also be claimed by unemployed people who have not worked before, or do not meet the WW criteria. The WW benefits comprise 70% of the last salary with a maximum of €2.335,- per month. Roughly the criteria are:
Having worked as an employee at least 26 of the 39 weeks preceding the first unemployment day.
Having worked as an employee four out of five years preceding the year the unemployment started and having received salary for at least 52 days a year.
The duration of the WW benefits depends on previous employment and ranges from 6 months to 5 years. Recently the government has decided to make it more difficult to meet the entry criteria and to restrict the duration of the benefit to 1.5 or 2 years.

When no salary, benefit, or other income is available, the unemployed can claim social security. For single people social security is 50% of the minimum wages. In order to stimulate people to resume work there is a job-search requirement.

[4] Cited from Brenninkmeijer, de Groot, Raes and Houtman, 2003:
According to the Sickness Benefits Act employed persons who are absent from work because they are ill, are entitled to receive at least 70% of their wages, but no less than the minimum wages for a period of 52 weeks. Employers are exempted from paying wages if employees have deliberately caused their illness, if they hinder their recovery, or if they do not accept an adjusted job in their own or in another organisation. However, if employers put insufficient effort in job retention for an employee who is absent due to sickness, they can receive a financial penalty.

In most collective labour agreements (CAO's), it is agreed that the employers supplement the benefit up to 100% of the employed person's wages. Employers are allowed

1992 and in 2000 the male higher employees/workers and – even more so – the male self-employed reported *less* often than the other groups that they had been absent from work. In 1991-1992 and in 2000 the male farmers/labourers *most* often reported that they had been absent from work. Apart from the low absence figures for self-employed females, the *absence* of socio-economic differences in sickness absence figures for women, particularly in 2000, is striking (table 5).

These data thus suggest that particularly male farmers/labourers more often report absent than other socio-economic groups. Self-employed people in general, as well as the male higher employees/workers, are most *un*likely to report sickness absences.

Table 5: Sickness absence percentage by SES for men and women
in 2000 (%) (CBS, Living Conditions Survey)

	Higher employees	Intermediate employees	Lower employees	Self-employed	Labourers	Total
Men	14.5	21.9	19.8	9.5	26.6	21.5
Women	27.3	26.7	26.6	8.5	24.1	25.6

G. The Disabled

Throughout the years, 6% of the male workforce claimed disability benefits. Although the percentage remained rather stable, the absolute numbers steadily increased. For women the percentage rose from 2 to 5%. Data from the Social Security Administration (UWV) show that the total number of employees claiming benefits rose to almost one million. Since 2003 this figure has been declining. The 'Gatekeeper Improvement' law, which is aimed at stimulating work resumption during the first year of sickness absence, may possibly have contributed to this.

In appendix 2 several policies are described that have been implemented over the last ten years in order to increase labour participation of older people and people who are not working because of sickness or disablement, as well as on the availability of occupational health care services. These occupational health care services have a major task in supporting organisations in combating dropout of employees.

---

to wait two days before they start paying the benefit. In that case it has to be explicitly stated in the collective agreement. The latter is hardly ever the case. Employees who are absent from work due to sickness, but are not entitled to continued payment by the employer (e.g. temporary workers, trainees, employees on trial contracts etc.), receive sickness absence benefits from the Social Security Administration (UWV).

H. Social Group, Income and Gender

Since 2000 no data are available in the Living Conditions Survey on income in combination with SES, work and health, and figures are thus only compared for 1980-1983 and 1991-1992. Table 6 shows the relation between social group, income and gender over that time period. In general it can be stated that the higher the socio-economic status, the higher the wages. Labourers have the lowest average income. Self-employed men have an average income that is comparable with 'intermediate employees'. Self-employed women, on the other hand, have an average income that is more comparable with that of labourers. One should however consider that the group of self-employed men is very heterogeneous, and ranges from highly paid specialists and lawyers to self-employed drivers or lower-educated self-employed workers in building and construction or industry. The male self-employed population may even be more heterogeneous in comparison with the female self-employed population.

Table 6: Mean annual net income in euros for different socio-economic groups by period (age 15-64 years; CBS, Living Conditions Survey)

Income from work	Higher employees	Intermediate employees	Lower employees	Self-employed	Labourers
Men					
(N)	166	258	161	123	485
1980-1983	18,902	13,833	10,858	11,598	9,721
(N)	485	1,012	424	272	976
1991	22,900	17,492	14,927	16,601	12,754
Women					
(N)	27	82	167	35	91
1980-1983	10,518	8,970	7,197	7,788	6,553
(N)	126	619	854	98	716
1991	18,386	12,073	10,562	9,572	8,830
Gender pay gap (income of women/men)					
1980-1983	55%	65%	66%	67%	67%
1991	80%	69%	71%	58%	69%

Women's pay is lower than men's. Since women more often work part-time than men do, we should, however, compare full-time working women with full-time working men to properly consider the (change in the) gender pay gap (see table 7). Even when only full-time working men and women are considered, a gender pay gap appears to exist. We should, however, consider that the remaining variation in jobs within socio-economic groups, with men occupying higher-paid jobs within the same socio-economic groups, may be a possible explanation. The next section about sectors suggests some indications on this issue.

Over the period of 1980-1983 to 1991 the gender pay gap appears to have been narrowing somewhat. The relative socio-economic differences in the gender pay gap also appear to have been reduced over this period. In 1991, however, women still earned about 80% of that of men in a comparable socio-economic group. A fairly recent paper on gender pay equity in Europe acknowledges a further narrowing gender pay gap in the Netherlands. (www.eiro.eurofound.eu.int/2002/01/study/tn0201101s.html).

Table 7: Mean and standard deviations (in brackets) of annual net income in euros for full-time working men and women aged 15-64 years (CBS, Living Conditions Survey)

Full-timers	Higher employees	Intermediate employees	Lower employees	Self-employed	Labourers
Men					
1980-1983	19,654 (8,397)	14,177 (4,999)	11,226 (3,584)	12,291 (5,867)	9,904 (3,510)
(N)	140	223	143	104	435
Hours/ week	40-45	45-50	40-44	>55	40-44
1991	22,034 (8,807)	17,080 (5,971)	14,637 (4,014)		12,781 (3,329)
(N)	193	398	171	N<10	390
Hours/ week	41	40	39		39
Women					
1980-1983	11,821 (3,678)	10,176 (3,577)	7,408 (1,654)	9,033 (3,593)	7,287 (1,752)
(N)	12	40	120	18	47
Hours/ week	45-50	40-45	40-45	50-55	45-50
1991	16,914 (5,245)	13,670 (3,778)	11,567 (2,937)		10,490 (2,640)
(N)	32	122	194	N<10	95
Hours/ week	39	39	39		39
Gender pay gap (income of women/ men)					
1980-1983	60%	72%	66%	73%	74%
1991	77%	80%	79%	-	82%

I. Sector and Occupation

Social group is often associated with the sector in which one works. In this paragraph we will present some of the recent trends (1990-2000) in the number of people working in a specific (blue- or white-collar) sector. Because of the strong gender segregation we will distinguish between men and women here too. The gender segregation is strongly present, as can be seen from table 8. Men but hardly any women work in sectors such as agriculture and construction, and many more men than women work in industry and transportation. When women work in these sectors they often perform quite different professional activities as compared with men. In agriculture, women are often the family partner in the business, who does not receive a salary for the work she does. Women tend to work in retail, wholesale and the hotel sector, as well as in profit and non-profit (other) services.

Table 8: Sector by sex in 1991-1992 and 2000 (%)
(CBS, Living Conditions Survey)

Sector	*1991-1992*	*2000*	*1991-1992*	*2000*
	Men	Men	Women	Women
Agriculture and fishing	5.6	4.2	1.9	1.9
Mining and quarrying	0.2	0.1	0.0	0.0
Industry	21.5	20.0	10.1	7.5
Utility companies	1.0	0.0	0.3	0.0
Construction	8.9	12.1	1.1	1.3
Wholesale, retail and hotels	16.6	16.3	18.8	20.0
Transport, storage and communications	6.5	7.2	3.6	3.8
Financial intermediation: banking and insurance	13.1	14.2	10.5	13.1
Other services	26.6	25.8	53.7	52.4
Total	100	100	100	100

Table 8 shows that there has been a reduction in employment in agriculture and utilities, but a rise in employment in the construction sector, as far as male employment is concerned. When we look at female employment we can see a reduction in industry and in utilities as well, but a rise in financial services (banks and insurance).

4. Working Conditions and Social Group

A. Physical Demands at Work: Noisy, Dirty, Smelly, Dangerous, Physically Heavy Work.

Houtman, Andries and Hupkens (2004) report in their 'Trends in Work and Employment 2004' that the prevalence of physical and chemical risks at work appears to be decreasing in general (as much of it as can be measured by questionnaire). Dirty work slightly decreased between 1990 and 2002 to 17% being exposed. The prevalence of a bad smell at work was quite stable in the years 1990-1993, started to decrease in the period of 1994-1997 and then stabilised at 8% until 2000. In 2002 it showed a further decrease to 7%. The percentage of people performing dangerous work remained quite stable over time until 2002 at about 5%. The prevalence of doing physically heavy work decreased slightly until it reached the level where 19% of workers were exposed in 2002.

Table 9: Physical working conditions for men and women in 2000 (CBS, Living Conditions Survey)

	Higher employees	Intermediate employees	Lower employees	Self-employed	Labourers
Scale physical working conditions (10= max. score. neg.)	Mean (Sd)	Mean (Sd)	Mean (Sd)	Mean (Sd)	Mean (Sd)
Men	0.86	1.22	1.32	2.65 ▲	4.21 ▲
	(1.82)	(2.07)	(1.79)	(2.58)	(.07)
Women	0.50	1.11 ▲	1.29 ▲	1.39 ▲	2.56 ▲
	(.92)	(1.67)	(1.83)	(1.79)	(2.15)
Total	0.76	1.17 ▲	1.30 ▲	2.24 ▲	3.77 ▲
	(1.63)	(1.90)	(1.82)	(2.42)	(2.71)

For each year the higher employees are taken as the reference group.
▲ indicates that the score is higher than the score in the reference group.
p<.05.

For the time period of 1980-1983 and the year 2000 these working conditions were related to social group. The working conditions noise, dirty, smelly, dangerous and physically heavy work constituted a physical working conditions scale. The data for 1980-1983 and 1991-1992 cannot easily be compared with those from 2000, since the answering categories for most items on working conditions changed in 1994. The pattern by gender and SES are, however, very comparable over the years. Table 9 shows that men consistently reported that they were more exposed to physical working conditions than women. There was also a main effect of socio-economic group consistently indicating higher physical load for labourers and the self-employed. Next to main effects of gender and socio-economic group, an interaction of gender and socio-economic group also appeared to be significant, indicating a highly prevalent physical load particularly in male labourers and the self-employed[5], whereas there were no (large[6]) gender differences in the other socio-economic groups.

---

[5]   Significant for women only in 2000.

[6]   In 1980-1983 there were no differences in physical load for either male and female employees. In 2000, however, the female higher employees reported less physical

B. *Psychosocial Risks at Work: Demands,*
Reward and Skill & Intellectual Discretion

The demand to work at a very high pace has been increasing since 1977, i.e. since the Living Conditions Survey started, and the increase was 1.5% on a yearly basis until 1997. From 1997 onwards the high work pace of the Dutch workforce appears to have stabilised (Houtman, Otten &Venema 2001) and even appears to be dropping (Houtman, Andries & Hupkens 2004). At the European level the Dutch were leading on work pace until the second survey of the European Foundation for the Improvement of Living and Working Conditions (EFILWC, 1995/96), and they were still in a high position at the third survey set out by the EFILWC (2000, Paoli and Merllié 2001).

Figure 2: High work pace by SES in men and women in 2000
(CBS; Living Conditions Survey)

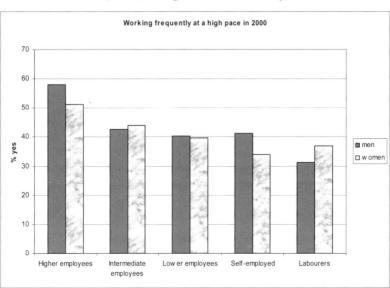

When considering perceived high work pace by social group, we can see that the lower the SES, the lower the work pace in men and women (figure 2). The change of answering categories and changed order of questions appeared to have had a tremendous effect on the prevalence of

---

load than all other socio-economic groups. Apart from labourers and the self-employed, however, the gender differences within socio-economic groups were non-significant.

a high work pace in 1994. Therefore we only present the most recent 2000 figures on work pace here. The SES pattern in work pace was, however, comparable in the earlier years.

Since 1996 we have some information on autonomy in work as perceived by workers in the Netherlands. The information on decision authority in the work situation has been available since 1994.

Trend information on immaterial reward as related to personal development (skill and intellectual discretion) as well as material reward, i.e. pay, can go back to the start of the Living Conditions Survey in the 1970s. In 1990-2000 an almost stable percentage of about 34% of the workers reported poor opportunities for promotion.

Figures 3 and 4 show the scores on skill and intellectual discretion for men and women belonging to the various social groups for the period covering 1980 to 2000. Again, we have to point out that the scores between 1992 and 2000 are not comparable in an absolute way, although the changes in the questionnaire in 1994 did not appear to have a very great effect on the answers to these particular questions. Only the average scores among social groups will be discussed.

Women consistently reported more unfavourable skill and intellectual discretion as compared with males. As far as social group is concerned, the lower the SES of the social group, the more problematic the skill and intellectual discretion. Labourers and farmers report that they have the most unfavourable skill and intellectual discretion. In general, we can see a somewhat negative development of skill and intellectual discretion for almost all socio-economic groups over time (1980 to 1992), except for higher employees (stable situation) and the self-employed men (less unfavourable skill discretion).

Figure 3: Unfavourable skill discretion by SES in men across 1980-2000 (CBS, Living Conditions Survey)

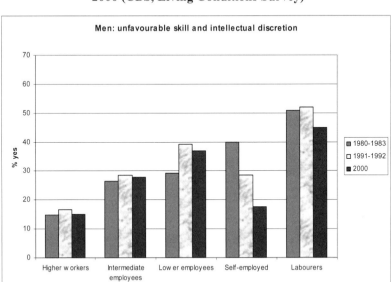

Figure 4: Skill discretion by SES in women across 1980-2000 (CBS, Living Conditions Survey)

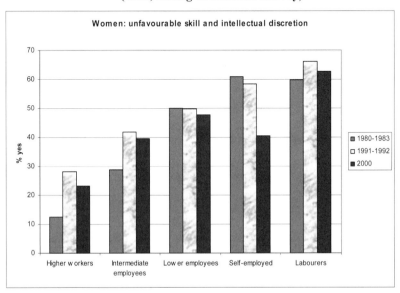

5. Health and Health Behaviour and Social Group

Within the general working population no significant changes in psychosomatic health (VOEG) and general health were shown over the period of 1980-2000. One of the interpretations of this in combination with the increasing inflow of workers into the disability benefit system is that there has been a health-based selection out of the Dutch work-force over the last few decades. Nor do we see more specific cases of ill health, such as burnout, in the working population, despite an ever-increasing number of people diagnosed as being disabled for work due to mental health problems (Houtman *et al.* 2004).

Figure 5: Less then good self-reported health by SES in men 1980-2000 (CBS, Living Conditions Survey)

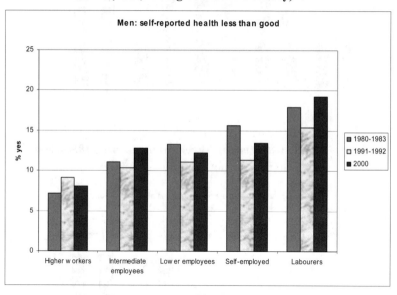

Figure 6: Less then good self-reported health by SES in women 1980-2000 (CBS, Living Conditions Survey)

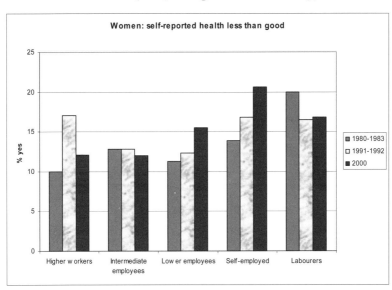

In figures 5 and 6 self-reported general health is presented by gender and social group. The percentage of men and women who report that their self-reported health is less than good is quite low: on average 14.5% in 2000. Men and women do not appear to differ much, but particularly for the men, the differences by social group are strong and consistent. The lowest percentages of less than good health are reported by the higher employees, whereas the highest percentages are reported for the labourers and farmers. For the women, self-reported health was not so distinctly different for the social groups. The self-reported poor health of higher employees appeared to rise in 1991-1992 and dropped to the level of the beginning of the 1980s again in 2000. Whereas an average percentage of self-employed men reported their health to be less than good over the years this percentage is rising in the self-employed women.

A somewhat comparable picture is observed for self-reported psychosomatic health (see figures 7 and 8). However, women consistently report more psychosomatic health problems than men. Some pronounced differences in psychosomatic health are found by social group, but in the women, social group differences diminished over the period of 20 years. In the 1980s, self-employed females and labourers reported high psychosomatic complaints. The prevalence of high complaints for all groups was found to rather similar since 1991-1992.

Figure 7: Psychosomatic complaints by SES in men 1980-2000 (CBS, Living Conditions Survey)

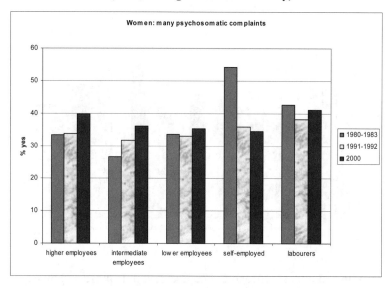

Figure 8: Psychosomatic complaints by SES in women 1980-2000 (CBS, Living Conditions Survey)

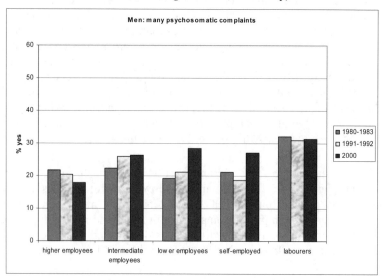

For the men, particularly labourers and farmers are high on psycho-somatic complaints, whereas higher employees report relatively few psychosomatic complaints. The difference in psychosomatic complaints between the male higher employees and the other groups is increasing over time, because the male labourers remain high in psychosomatic complaints, whereas the male intermediate and lower employees, as well as self-employed males show an increase in psychosomatic com-plaints over the 20-year period. The male higher employees, on the other hand, remain rather low on psychosomatic complaints.

Next to self-reported general and psychosomatic health the Living Conditions Survey provided information on heart attacks and back injuries, as well as on some health behaviours such as alcohol abuse and smoking. It should, however, be noted that differences in prevalence of heart attack, back injury and alcohol abuse among the different social groups should be interpreted with caution due to small numbers.

Figures 9 and 10 show the prevalence of having had self-reported back injuries in the last year. We see quite different trends for the genders and for the social groups. In general the level of self-reported back problems is higher for women as compared to men. For both higher employee men and women we see an initial increase in back problems followed by a reduction. For women intermediate and lower employees and for labourers in both genders there is some rise in self-reported back injury 1980-2000. In 2000 most back problems are re-ported for self-employed women and for labourers and farmers among men.

In the above trends an implicit different gender ranking has been de-scribed, particularly as related to the self-employed and labour-ers/farmers. Whereas self-reported back pain does not appear to be highly prevalent in self-employed men, particularly in 2000 it has become a big problem in the (small group of) self-employed women.

Figure 9: Back injuries by SES in men 1980-2000
(CBS, Living Conditions Survey)

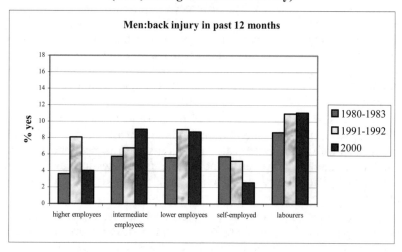

Figure 10: Back injuries by SES in women 1980-2000
(CBS, Living Conditions Survey)

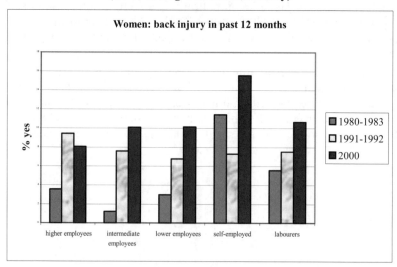

**Figure 11: Alcohol abuse by SES in men 1980-2000
(CBS, Living Conditions Survey)**

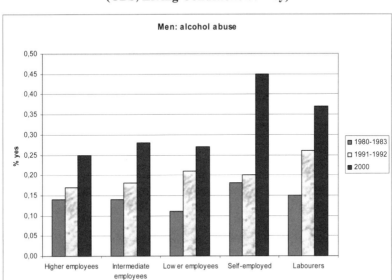

**Figure 12: Alcohol abuse by SES in women 1980-2000
(CBS, Living Conditions Survey)**

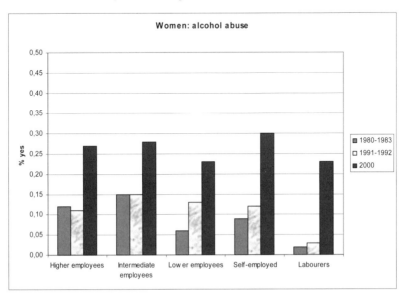

According to the Ministry of Health, alcohol consumption is safe when women drink maximally two glasses a day five days a week. Men can drink up to three glasses a day, five days a week. Alcohol consumption has not been reported in the same way over the years, and items have varied from estimated number of glasses a day, a week, per weekend, and on weekdays. Therefore every year the items on alcohol consumption were converted to estimated number of glasses a week. Based on the guidelines of the Ministry, *alcohol abuse* was defined as drinking more than 10 glasses a week for women, and more than 15 glasses a week for men. Figures 11 and 12 show the percentages of men and women in the different social groups with alcohol abuse. Alcohol abuse increased considerably over the 20-year period and increased most in the period 1990-2000. For women there was no clear relationship between social class and alcohol abuse. For men, a stronger relation emerged, particularly at the end of this 20-year period, indicating more alcohol abuse in the lower social groups, and particularly among the self-employed.

Every year the Living Conditions Survey has included some questions on smoking behaviour. Differences on what questions were asked occurred from year to year. Therefore only smoking or non-smoking is reported. Figures 13 and 14 show the percentages of male and female smokers by SES groups over the years. In general an increase in cigarette smoking can be seen. In many cases both men and women showed an initial increase in smoking from 1980-1991, with the exception of higher and intermediate female employees who decreased their smoking all along, and the self-employed in both sexes who reduced their smoking behaviour in this period. Since 1991 all groups, except the female self-employed as well as male and female labourers, showed a decrease in smoking. For women, smoking is most prevalent among the self-employed, and labourers. For men, smoking is most prevalent among labourers and farmers.

Figure 13: Smoking by SES in men 1980-2000
(CBS; Living Conditions Survey)

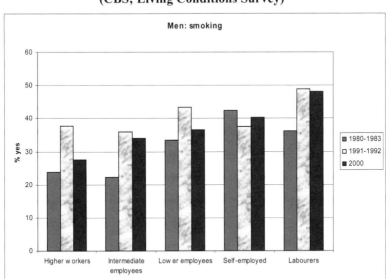

Figure 14: Smoking by SES in women 1980-2000
(CBS, Living Conditions Survey)

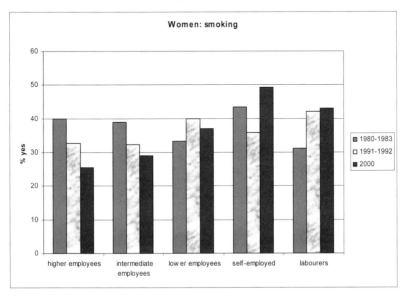

6. Socio-economic Status, Working Conditions and Health Behaviours as Contributing to Health

Thus far we have extensively described social groups by employment characteristics, risk factors at work, health outcomes and health behaviours. In this paragraph we are going to explain the psychosomatic complaints (highest quartile vs. the rest) and self-reported health (good and very good vs. poor and average) by social group, risk factors at work and health behaviours. Stepwise multivariate logistic regression analyses were performed. The social group variable is entered first, working conditions next, and lifestyle variables last. A fixed set of predictors was entered at each step. Because the questions, as well as the answering categories of the questions on working conditions in the Living Conditions Survey were changed in 1994, the information on working conditions cannot be aggregated over the whole period of 20 years. Therefore we only present the results of the data from 2000 here. The analyses were, however, also performed for 1980-1983 and 1991-1992, resulting in a comparable outcome. An overview of the variables used for the logistic regressions in the different years, as well as the results from the analyses for 1980-19983 and 1991-1992 are presented in appendix A to C.

A. Psychosomatic Complaints

Psychosomatic health is explained to a limited extent: about 5% (table 10). As shown above there were no initial SES differences in psychosomatic health among women. Among men the results from the first step indicate that higher employees report psychosomatic complaints least, as compared with all other social groups except the self-employed. When working conditions are entered, the explanatory power of social group is significantly reduced. Only intermediate and lower employees still have more psychosomatic complaints than the higher employees, but the odds ratios are reduced. The working conditions that add to the explanation of psychosomatic complaints are poor skill discretion and high work pace while physical risk factors do not. Lifestyle factors do not contribute to the explanation of psychosomatic health.

Table 10: Logistic regression on psychosomatic health complaints (VOEG) for the year 2000 (n.s. = not significant). See appendix 3 (CBS, Living Conditions Survey)

Predictor		Men (N=1216)		Women (N=656)	
		Odds ratio	p-value	Odds ratio	p-value
Step 1: SES	SES		.010		n.s.
	Higher employees (ref)	1.00		1.00	
	Intermediate employees	1.499	.021	1.194	n.s.
	Lower employees	1.963	.002	1.191	n.s.
	Self-employed	1.461	n.s.	2.254	n.s.
	Labourers	1.739	.001	1.092	n.s.
Step 2: SES	SES		n.s.		n.s.
	Higher employees (ref)	1.00		1.00	
	Intermediate employees	1.451	.041	1.158	n.s.
	Lower employees	1.891	.004	1.073	n.s.
	Self-employed	1.337	n.s.	2.174	n.s.
	Labourers	1.247	n.s.	.779	n.s.
Work	High skill discretion (ref)	1.00		1.00	
	Intermediate skill discretion	1.448	n.s.	1.100	n.s.
	Low skill discretion	2.254	.000	2.082	.001
	High work pace	1.206	.003	1.170	n.s.
	Smell	1.237	n.s.	1.022	n.s.
	Danger	1.077	n.s.	.648	n.s.
	Physically demanding	1.138	n.s.	1.090	n.s.
	Noise	1.419	n.s.	1.571	n.s.
	Dirty work	1.206	n.s.	1.343	n.s.
Step 3: SES	SES		n.s.		n.s.
	Higher employees (ref)	1.00		1.00	
	Intermediate employees	1.437	.047	1.164	n.s.
	Lower employees	1.847	.006	1.066	n.s.
	Self-employed	1.366	n.s.	2.038	n.s.
	Labourers	1.225	n.s.	.772	n.s.
Work	High skill discretion (ref)	1.00		1.00	
	Intermediate skill discretion	1.156	n.s.	1.117	n.s.
	Low skill discretion	2.260	.000	2.100	.001
	High work pace	1.442	.004	1.158	n.s.
	Smell	1.201	n.s.	1.025	n.s.
	Danger	1.237	n.s.	.629	n.s.
	Physically demanding	1.070	n.s.	1.119	n.s.
	Noise	1.133	n.s.	1.564	n.s.
	Dirty work	1.413	n.s.	1.326	n.s.
Lifestyle	Alcohol abuse	.882	n.s.	1.150	n.s.
	Smoking	1.201	n.s.	1.120	n.s.
Cox & Snell's R^2			5.5%		3.6%

The analyses performed for men and women compare well with the overall results. In women, social group differences are completely absent and work pace is not a significant explanatory factor for psychosomatic complaints. The only explanatory factor for psychosomatic complaints in women is low skill discretion.

B. *Self-reported Health*

Among women there were only small initial SES differences in self-reported health and none of the variables entered in logistic regression contributed to their explanation. Among men labourers and farmers most often reported less than good health followed by lower employees (table 11). Social group, however, becomes insignificant when working conditions are taken into account. We can see that this is mainly the result of having poor skill discretion. Again, lifestyle does not contribute to the explanation of social class differences.

Table 11: Logistic regression on self-reported poor health for the year 2000 (n.s. = not significant). See appendix 3 (CBS, Living Conditions Survey)

Predictor		Men (N=1691)		Women (N=863)	
		OR	P	OR	P
Step 1: SES	SES		.000		n.s.
	Higher employees(ref)	1.00		1.00	
	Intermediate employees	1.682	.046	.696	n.s.
	Lower employees	1.819	.049	1.236	n.s.
	Self-employed	1.640	n.s.	.989	n.s.
	Labourers	2.883	.000	.806	n.s.
Step 2: SES	SES		.032		n.s.
	Higher employees(ref)	1.00		1.00	
	Intermediate employees	1.564	n.s.	.687	n.s.
	Lower employees	1.579	n.s.	1.203	n.s.
	Self-employed	1.561	n.s.	.828	n.s.
	Labourers	2.304	.002	.708	n.s.
Work	High skill discretion (ref)	1.00		1.00	
	Intermediate skill discretion	.927	n.s.	.880	n.s.
	Low skill discretion	2.147	.000	1.018	n.s.
	High work pace	1.114	n.s.	.966	n.s.
	Smell	1.500	n.s.	.432	n.s.
	Danger	1.069	n.s.	2.792	n.s.
	Physically demanding	1.149	n.s.	1.222	n.s.
	Noise	.745	n.s.	1.586	n.s.
	Dirty work	1.085	n.s.	1.079	n.s.
Step 3: SES	SES		.016		n.s.
	Higher employees (ref)	1.00		1.00	
	Intermediate employees	1.599	n.s.	.690	n.s.
	Lower employees	1.638	n.s.	1.267	n.s.
	Self-employed	1.648	n.s.	.860	n.s.
	Labourers	2.471	.001	.753	n.s.
Work	High skill discretion (ref)	1.00		1.00	
	Intermediate skill discretion	.912	n.s.	.872	n.s.
	Low skill discretion	2.141	.000	.999	n.s.
	High work pace	1.119	n.s.	.981	n.s.
	Smell	1.487	n.s.	.409	n.s.
	Danger	1.121	n.s.	2.862	n.s.
	Physically demanding	1.157	n.s.	1.212	n.s.
	Noise	.746	n.s.	1.663	n.s.
	Dirty work	1.093	n.s.	1.100	n.s.
Lifestyle	Alcohol abuse	.843	n.s.	1.340	n.s.
	Smoking	.779	n.s.	.753	n.s.
Cox & Snell's R^2			3.5%		1.6%

211

7. Conclusions and Discussion

In the Netherlands, there is no general trend as to an increase or decrease of social groups. We do see, however, that for women there has been a rise in higher and intermediate employees over the last two decades.

Part-time employed women increased as a percentage of the female workforce and part-time employment increased among men too but the increase was much smaller. This may be explained by the fact that in more recent years, women have more often retained their working position when starting a family, but have reduced their number of contractual hours, whereas men in most of these situations have continued to work full-time or reduced their working hours to a limited extent.

A second major labour force trend in the Netherlands is the ageing workforce. This is paralleled by an increase in early retirement. New regulations will probably put a stop to the early retirement regulations of the recent past, in an attempt to keep workers in the labour force. This will be necessary in order to pay for the future old-age pensions. Newly proposed pre-pension arrangements are to be financed by capital funding. The financial burden for this will be more on the individual. This will have negative consequences for those who have a low income. It will probably mainly be the better-paid workers who can afford to pay for this kind of early-retirement arrangements. At present the social dialogue that has always been very good in the Netherlands, has stopped because of these and other Government proposals. It is not only the pre-pension arrangements that will probably be changed, but the disability regulations as well.

Apart from getting an old-age pension, the other 'way out' of the work force is to be diagnosed as being disabled for work. In the Netherlands this means that one has to be long-term absent from work and has to be diagnosed as being disabled for work at the end of the first year of absence (since January 1, 2004 this has changed to after two years of absence). The national data show that labourers have most sickness absence, whereas the self-employed (men and women) as well as the higher employees (men) have least.

Somewhat more than a decade ago, having employees diagnosed as being disabled for work was indeed used as a way out: cheap both for the employer and the employee. For the employee this would mean being unemployed but 'enjoying' a good financial arrangement. For the employer this used to be a way of 'getting rid' of 'less productive workers'. This 'way out' became a heavy issue of social debate in the early 1990s, when many examples were put forward of the arrangement being abused. Due to this initiatives were promoted and implemented for both employers and employees to stimulate work retention and work resumption. As a result of these changes it became more difficult to get into the disability benefit system for those who had been absent from work and probably for those who reported disability due to psychological as well as musculoskeletal disorders, and for blue-collar workers. This trend appears to be strengthened by the receding economy.

As to income, we also see some major differences amongst the different socio-economic groups. Again, labourers earn the lowest income. The most apparent finding here is the gender gap. Even with respect to full-time employment, women earn considerably less than men. It appears that this gender gap is narrowing in the Dutch case but it is still very present in recent data. (www.eiro.eurofound.eu.int/2002/01/study/tn0201101s.html).

The problem of gender and income may be related to the gender segregation in different occupations and sectors. Women tend to work in other occupations and sectors than men do, and are less often likely to work in more senior positions (Kauppinen *et al.* 2003).

Also, men and women report different kinds of health problems. In general women report more health complaints than men do, particularly health complaints that are related to upper-limb disorders and stress-related disorders. Men are more likely to suffer accidents and injuries at work (Kauppinen *et al.* 2003). The gender segregation results in the fact that men and women are exposed to different risks at work, and even when men and women work in the same occupation they do different things, resulting in different exposures. When men and women work in cleaning professions or as gardeners, men often appear to do the heavy work (Messing *et al.* 1994, 1998). Career prospects are more important for male nurses than for female nurses, resulting in extra courses and work at the intensive care unit, in the operating room or as a head nurse. Female nurses work in the wards, nursing patients, which often results in more physical load for female nurses as compared with male nurses (Dassen, Nijhuis & Philipsen 1990). This gender segregation implies that men and women are differently exposed to risk factors at work, as has also been shown in the data presented in this chapter. In general, women often report lower physical risks, but are more often subject to psychosocial risks, particularly relating to autonomy, and skill and intellectual discretion (Kauppinen *et al.* 2003).

Despite the confirmation of the gender segregation as related to the work-related risks in the present study, the socio-economic differences of women in relation to outcome variables were much lower as compared to men. Explanations may be found in the fact that women at work – as a group – more often work part-time and perform their job systematically in less time than men do. Less unfavourable work exposure for females may be the explanation of the findings indicating less social-economic differences.

Social groups report differences in occupational risk factors, but the presence of these risks are highly gender segregated. Labourers and farmers report high physical risks as well as a poor potential to develop skill (and intellectual) discretion. Higher employees, on the other hand, report a high work pace and much room for skill (and intellectual) discretion. Typical (public) service-oriented occupations, however, often with a relatively high percentage of women, score high on work pace but low on decision authority and skills (and intellectual) discretion as well. This compares with the findings of other reports on work and gender (e.g. Houtman *et al*. 2004).

Analyses were performed to explain psychosomatic health complaints and self-reported health by social group, working conditions and health behaviour. The explained variance was very low, particularly for self-reported health, and lifestyle factors did not contribute to the explanation of self-reported or psychosomatic health.

The finding on the low explained variance is a very salient one, and a completely different result than was reported by Schrijvers *et al*. (1998). Although they did not report on the total variance explained, they reported odds ratios for the associations between e.g. hazardous physical conditions and self-reported health (the same question as was used in the present chapter) ranging from 0.7 to 17.6 for different levels of occupational class, indicating much stronger effects, as compared with the effect size presently found. One explanation for the limited effects and low amount of variance explained in the present study is that the present analyses were performed on a representative population sample. These samples are not really the best ones to test causal relationships, since they – by definition – include many respondents with 'average' scores on the independent variables, which do not contribute to the explanation of the causal relationship but instead tend to reduce the power to find causal relations. It is clear that the sample used by Schrijvers *et al*. consisted of a much larger group of blue-collar workers, and their study group was significantly unhealthier as compared to the population presently under study (the present study identified 14.5% as 'less than good' health, whereas in the Schrijvers *et al*. study this was 18.4%).

Despite the much smaller effects reported in this chapter as compared with Schrijvers *et al*. (1998), the conclusion to be drawn was comparable. When working conditions, and particularly skill discretion was entered into the regression, the odds ratio of poor health for the labourers was significantly reduced, or even became insignificant. In the study of Schrijvers *et al*. (1998) the effect of physical working conditions had strong effects as well, together with 'lack of decision latitude' or 'skill discretion'. Again, the problem of the present study may have been that the contrast with physically heavy blue-collar work was not as robust as in the Schrijvers *et al.* study, resulting in less discriminative power for the physical risks. The present study, which included a representative study of workers in the Netherlands, also including many women who do not have such physically demanding jobs, but who do have low decision latitude. The Schrijvers *et al.* study (1998) mostly took its subjects from an area where there is a great deal of industrial, blue-collar labour, but mainly 'male labour' (it was a Catholic area). The effect of the gender segregation may have even strengthened the findings reported by Schrijvers *et al.* (1998).

Final summary of conclusions:

- Low social groups are worst off with respect to working conditions, income and health (particularly blue-collar and male self-employed), and they are also at high risk of becoming (long-term) absent or disabled;

- Future developments regarding old-age pensions and pre-pensions favour the workers with higher incomes. At present it is unclear how the disability benefit system will be changed, and how this will work out for the lower social groups. It should, however, be clear that the lower social groups are worst off when – as expected – future arrangements regarding (pre-)pensions or related benefits and care have to be paid for by capital funding;

- Working conditions, particularly poor skill discretion, explain the variance attributed to SES in self-reported general health and psychosomatic health complaints. The lack of physical load as an eminent predictor of ill health may be explained by the fact that the present study was based on a representative sample of workers in the Netherlands, of whom a large group did not contribute to causal relations at all. Another sample including more blue-collar workers showed that physical load explained a substantial part of social class differences in self-reported health (Schrijvers *et al.* 1998).

References

ARBEIDSINSPECTIE (Labour Inspectorate). 2002a. *Najaarsrapportage CAO afspraken 2002 (Autumn Report CAO-agreements 2002)*. Den Haag: Arbeidsinspectie.

ARBEIDSINSPECTIE (Labour Inspectorate). 2002b. *Jaarverslag 2002 (Annual report 2002)*. Den Haag: Arbeidsinspectie.

BRENNINKMEIJER, V., RAES, A., HOUTMAN, I.L.D. 2003. "Stress Impact project: Report work package 2". *A review and inventory of national social insurance systems and related policies in the Netherlands on sickness and long-term absence*. Hoofddorp: The Netherlands Association of Applied Scientific Research/TNO Work and Employment. http://www.surrey.ac.uk/Psychology/stressimpact/publications/wp2/wp2_ reportNetherland.pdf.

DASSEN, T.W.N., NIJHUIS, F.J.N., PHILIPSEN, H. 1990. Carriereperspectieven bij mannelijke intensive care verpleegkundigen (Career prospects for male intensive care nurses). *Gedrag & Organisatie* 1: 32-47.

DE HAAN, F., VERBOON, F. 2002. Integrated approaches to active welfare and employment policies: The Netherlands. European Foundation for the Improvement of Living and Working Conditions.

EUROPEAN COMMISSION, *EUROPEAN EMPLOYMENT OBSERVATORY REVIEW: Spring 2003*. 2003. Luxembourg: Office for Official Publications of the European Communities.

HUIJSMAN, R., VERGRIJZING (Greying). 1996. *ESB*. 24 februari: 360.

GRÜNDEMANN, R.W.M. & VUUREN, T.D. VAN. 1997. *Preventing absenteeism at the workplace*. Dublin: Loughlinstown: EFILWC.

HOUTMAN, I., ANDRIES, F., HUPKES, C. 2004. "Kerncijfers gezondheid, productiviteit en sociale zekerheid (Core figures on health, productivity and social security". In I.L.D. HOUTMAN, P.G.W. SMULDERS & D.J. KLEIN HESSELINK (eds.). *Trends in arbeid 2004* (Trends in Work and Employment 2004). Hoofddorp: TNO Arbeid: 67-93.

HOUTMAN, I., OTTEN, F., VENEMA, A. 2001. Kerncijfers arbeid, gezondheid en sociale zekerheid (Core figures on work, health and social security). In P.G.W. Smulders, I.L.D. Houtman & D.J. Klein Hesselink (eds.). *Trends in arbeid 2002* (Trend report on Work and Employment 2002). Kluwer: Alphen a/d Rijn: 69-102.

HOUTMAN I., SMULDERS P. 2003. De praktische (ir)relevantie van het Job Demand-Control-model (The practical (ir)relevance of the Job Demand-Control-model). *Gedrag & Organisatie* 5: 258-265.

KARASEK, R., THEORELL, T. 1990. *Healthy work: stress, productivity and the reconstruction of working life*. New York: Basic Books: 381.

KAUPPINEN, K., KUMPULAINEN, R., HOUTMAN, I. & COPSEY, S. 2003. *Gender issues in safety and health at work: A review*. Luxembourg: European Agency for Safety and Health at Work, Luxembourg, Office for Official Publications of the European Communities, http://agency.osha.eu.int/publications/reports/209/en/index.htm.

MESSING, K., CHATIGNY, C., COURVILLE, J. 1998. "Light" and "heavy" work in the housekeeping service of a hospital. *Applied Ergonomics* 29: 451-459.

MESSING, K., DUMAIS, L., COURVILLE, J., SEIFERT, A. & BOUCHER, M. 1994. Evaluation of exposure data from men and women with the same job title. *Journal of Occupational Medicine* 36 (8): 913-918.

PAOLI, P., MERLLI, É. 2001. *Third European survey on working conditions.* Dublin/Loughlinstown: EFILWC.

RETURN. 1999. *Between work and welfare: Improving return to work strategies for long-term absent employees: The Netherlands.* www.wrc-research.ie/return.

SCHRIJVERS, C.T.M., MHEEN, H.D. VAN DE, STRONKS, K. & MACKENBACH, J.P. 1998. Socioeconomic inequalities in health in the working population: the contribution of working conditions. *International Journal of Epidemiology* 27: 1011-1018.

Websites

www.cbs.nl

www.uwv.nl

Appendix 1

1. Research in the Netherlands on Social Inequalities in Health

In **1987** the Ministry of Welfare, Health and Cultural Affairs in the Netherlands initiated a large research project on social inequalities in health. In preparation for the research project a survey was done among researchers who were experts on the topic. The authors (Mackenbach & Stronks 1987) reviewed and summarised 56 studies that were concluded or were still running, in the years 1982-1987. They grouped the aspects of health that emerged in the reviewed studies into three categories: health-influencing factors, health problems and consequences of health problems. Examples of health-influencing factors are smoking, drinking, body weight, but also seeing a doctor when necessary, or working conditions. Health problems can be subdivided into physical and mental health problems. Consequences of health problems are the use of medical facilities and (physical) impairment as a consequence of health problems. In most studies low socio-economic status tended to coincide with factors that negatively influence health. People of lower socio-economic status were more obese or more underweight than others. On the other hand, higher social groups consumed more alcohol. Lifestyle factors and diet were more favourable among higher social groups. Also concerning psychological factors that influence health, such as social support and social deprivation, lower social groups were at a disadvantage. Adequate usage of medical facilities was sometimes related to low socio-economic status and sometimes to high socio-economic status. On average, lower social groups had poorer health than higher social groups. This social inequality in health does not only apply to 'objective' health, e.g. mortality, chronic disease, etc., but also to self-reported health. In contrast, psychosocial problems are more frequent among higher social groups. The relation between socio-economic status and use of medical facilities is equivocal: higher social groups more often visit the dentist, whereas lower social groups consume more drugs only available on prescription. Also lower social groups are more frequently hospitalised, while higher social groups stay in the hospital for a longer period. Regarding impairment, the likelihood of becoming unable to work is higher for people of lower socio-economic status.

In **1997** the research committee presented the second report on inequalities in health. This time the data used came from the Living Conditions Survey (Central Bureau of Statistics) and the Central Bureau of Statistics' statistics on causes of death. The role of socio-economic status for inequalities in health was examined by relating educational level, income and occupational status to health. The risk of poor health diminished gradually as the level of education rose. Highly educated people ran a lower risk of chronic physical diseases, chronic impairments, worse self-reported health, and even death. With regard to differences in psychological disorders, the expected tendency was found for women but not for men. Women with a low level of education were two to four times more likely to develop an anxiety or mood disorder.

A measure which gives insight into the sum of inequalities in health and death is healthy life expectancy. The expected number of years in good health was 11.8 and 11.5 years longer for highly educated men and women respectively, as opposed to men and women with a low educational level. Differences in health by income consistently showed that higher income was associated with better health.

In **2001** the research committee complemented the overview of social inequalities in health in the Netherlands with a review of interventions aimed at reducing social inequalities in health.

Their final report can be found at: http://www.siswo.uva.nl/sznet/Onderzoek_publicaties/Themas/abstractsthemas.asp?id=1435). The committee came to the conclusion that the present social inequalities in the prevalence of morbidity and mortality rates are comparable with those in other north-western European countries. The authors remarked that the mechanisms that underlie social inequalities in health are social causation and social selection. According to social causation, socioeconomic status leads via specific factors to poorer health, but poor health also leads via negative effects on work to lower socio-economic status. Social causation appeared to be the more important mechanism. Three groups of predictors contributed to social inequalities in health: behavioural factors, psychosocial factors and environmental factors. From the interventions that were reviewed, the following appeared to be effective, or were at least considered promising:

- Community-based intervention. Community members have to participate actively in goal-setting and developing activities aimed at reducing social inequality. Effect: still unknown, but seems promising.
- Brushing teeth at school. Children had to brush their teeth once a day at school. After the intervention there were no more differences in teeth-brushing behaviour between children from differ-

ent socio-economic status. Effect: positive in the short term, unknown in the long term.

- Raise duties on tobacco. According to foreign research, raising duties especially affects lower social groups. Effect: promising.
- Improving working conditions among lower occupational groups. Technical, organisational and system measures reduced social inequalities in health. Effect: positive.
- Autonomous teams in work-places. Production teams were made responsible for the whole process. This implied multiple roles for the team. As autonomy increased, the psychosomatic health of the workers improved. Effect: promising, the results were positive.
- Nurse practitioners. Nurse practitioners paid extra attention to asthma patients from lower social groups. Positive effect on medication compliance and satisfaction, fewer visits to the GP and less exacerbation of the disease. The committee's remark was that it is the differentiation in health care in this intervention that had led to positive results. People from lower social groups need more time and explanation from the doctor/nurse.

Appendix 2

1. Policies Aimed at Increasing Labour Force Participation and the Availability of Occupational Health Care Services.

A. *Policies to Increase the Participation of Older Workers in the Workforce*

In 1999 the Labour Inspectorate presented an overview of policies on labour participation of older workers in collective labour agreements. In the collective labour agreements there were no guidelines about age for the recruitment and selection of new employees. Nor were there any age requirements with respect to specific jobs. In accordance with European law, age discrimination is not allowed.

In 7% of the collective labour agreements there are agreements on career counselling specifically for older workers. 32% consists of agreements on examining the ways in which the specific sector could give meaning to older workers' policies. In 14% of the collective labour agreements, guidelines have been put forward concerning the adaptation of tasks for older workers. Usually the minimum age to qualify was 55 years. Some agreements also proposed job change and older workers being a mentor for young workers. In the majority of the collective labour agreements (51%), older workers are given the opportunity to reduce their working hours. This can be an effective strategy to keep older workers working. Fewer working hours, however, may mean less pay and less pension, thus making this option unattractive, particularly for those with low income. Until now pensions have been related to the last earned wages. In contrast, for people with a pension based on their average salary it might be less problematic to cut working hours: they earn less money, but their pension is not as heavily affected. Older workers are not expected to do overtime, irregular duties and shift work.

2. Policies to Improve Occupational Health and to Stimulate Work Resumption

A. Publicly-financed Incentives for Employers to Make Work Environments Healthier

Firms and non-profit organisations that want to carry out projects focused on reducing risks in the work content, work organisation and work environment can apply for financial support. These arrangements regarding risk management have to be concluded upon at sector level, and are to be known as 'Working Conditions Covenants' (*Arboconvenanten*). The risks that are specifically mentioned in this respect concern (1) risks of work stress, (2) risks of Repetitive Strain Injuries (RSI), (3) damaging noise, (4) dust, or (5) solvents. In order to apply for financial support, the project has to be innovative and has to contribute to the prevention or reduction of one of the risks mentioned. The proposed solution has to have long-term effects, and be cost-effective; it must also be possible to generalise the findings to other organisations or sectors.

B. Public Incentives for Employers to Organise Work Resumption

Since 1994, several regulations have been implemented that give the employer the financial burden of paying the salary of employees who are absent from work due to sickness. In 1994, employers had to pay the salary of their employees for the first two or six weeks of sickness absence. Since 1996, they have to do this for the first whole year of sickness absence, and since January 2004 this period has become the first two years of sickness absence. The idea behind this financial incentive is to make the employers feel responsible for their sick employees, and put efforts into their work resumption. What happens in practice is that employers insure themselves against this kind of risk, and make it the 'problem' of the private insurance sector.

Apart from the fact that employers have to pay sickness benefits in the Netherlands, there are also other incentives to stimulate work resumption. In April 2002 the new 'Gatekeeper Improvement' law was implemented. This law comprises regulations in order to stimulate the quick return to work of a sick employee. The employer has to report a sick employee to the organisation's occupational health services. After six weeks of absence the occupational health services advise the employer about the employee's possibilities to recover and resume work. If there is a chance that he/she can go back to work, the employer and the employee have to draw up a plan of action for recovery and rehabilitation, which is based on the advice of the occupational health services.

A case manager supervises the implementation of the plan. After 13 weeks of illness this should also be reported to the Social Security Administration. During the absence, the employer makes a rehabilitation file in which all the agreements and activities focused on recovery and resumption of work are described. In the eighth month the employer and employee write a rehabilitation report together, based on the rehabilitation file. The report summarises the efforts that were made to get the employee back to work. It is only if the efforts of both employer and employee have been found sufficient, that the sickness benefit paid by the employer will be replaced by a public disability benefit. If the efforts of the employer are insufficient, the employer can be forced to pay sickness benefits for up to one more year. On the other hand, there are also rewards for employers. If an employee has become disabled to work and resumes work, the employer receives a one-year reduction on employee insurance. If the disabled person was not a former employee, the reduction is for three years. If a disabled employee is rehabilitated in another organisation, the former employer receives compensation for the expenses incurred for the rehabilitation.

3. The Availability of Occupational Health Care Services

Since 1998 all organisations that have employees must use (buy) services from an 'Occupational Health Care Service' (*arbodienst*). The occupational health care services aim to help employers to outline and implement policies directed at the management of working conditions and absenteeism. Occupational health care services are required to have at least one expert in the area of occupational medicine, work-related hygiene, occupational safety, and industrial and organisational risk management. The employer can choose from a broad spectrum of services, but at least five are compulsory: a risk inventory and evaluation, coaching of ill employees, a voluntary work occupational health check-up for employees, a working conditions consultation, and a medical examination if necessary for the job. Recently the European Court ruled that the Dutch law is to be amended: organisations have to designate an internal prevention worker who will be responsible for the management of occupational risks and for the risk inventory and evaluation. Only if the organisation is unable to do so, is it allowed to call in an occupational health service.

Appendix 3

Table A: Overview of variables used in the logistic regression analyses

Variables	Year	Range	Recode
Psychosomatic health complaints	All	0-11	0-1= no (hardly any) complaints (ref) 2-11= many complaints
Self-reported health	All	1-5	1-3= poor 4-5= good
Skill discretion	All	0-20	0-8= a lot of skill discretion (ref) 9-11= average skill discretion 12-20= little skill discretion
Work pace	1980-1992	1-5	1-3= little (ref) 4-5= a lot
Smell	1980-1992	1-5	1-3= little (ref) 4-5= a lot
Danger	1980-1992	1-5	1-3= little (ref) 4-5= a lot
Physically demanding	1980-1992	1-5	1-3= little (ref) 4-5= a lot
Noise	1980-1992	1-2	1= no (ref) 2= yes
Dirt	1980-1992	1-2	1= no (ref) 2= yes
Work pace	2000	1-3	1-2= no/ yes, sometimes (ref) 3= yes, regularly
Smell	2000	1-3	1-2= no/ yes, sometimes (ref) 3= yes, regularly
Danger	2000	1-3	1-2= no/ yes, sometimes (ref) 3= yes, regularly
Physically demanding	2000	1-3	1-2= no/ yes, sometimes (ref) 3= yes, regularly
Noise	2000	1-3	1-2= no/ yes, sometimes (ref) 3= yes, regularly
Dirt	2000	1-3	1-2= no/ yes, sometimes (ref) 3= yes, regularly
Smoking	All	0-1	0=no (ref) 1=yes
Alcohol abuse	All	0-1	0=no (ref) 1=yes

Table B: Logistic regression on psychosomatic health complaints for the years 1980-1983 – 1991-1992 (n.s. = not significant)

redictor		Total group (N=2141)		Men (N=1317)		Women (N=824)	
		OR	P	OR	P	OR	P
Step 1: SES	Higher employees (ref)	1.00		1.00		1.00	
	Intermediate employees	1.516	.005	1.513	.018	.923	n.s.
	Lower employees	1.545	.007	1.609	.028	.736	n.s.
	Self-employed	1.319	n.s.	.991	n.s.	1.615	n.s.
	Labourers	1.701	.000	1.750	.002	.976	n.s.
Step 2: SES	Higher employees (ref)	1.00		1.00		1.00	
	Intermediate employees	1.397	.027	1.411	n.s.	.873	n.s.
	Lower employees	1.397	.042	1.522	n.s.	.716	n.s.
	Self-employed	1.146	n.s.	.782	n.s.	1.786	n.s.
	Labourers	1.354	n.s.	1.271	n.s.	.897	n.s.
Work	High skill discretion (ref)	1.00		1.00		1.00	
	Intermediate skill discretion	1.273	.026	1.070	n.s.	1.510	.026
	Low skill discretion	1.714	.000	1.608	.002	1.522	.022
	High work pace	1.197	.047	1.132	n.s.	1.382	.030
	Smell	1.061	n.s.	1.077	n.s.	.979	n.s.
	Danger	1.246	n.s.	1.061	n.s.	1.706	.042
	Physically demanding	.854	n.s.	.872	n.s.	.950	n.s.
	Noise	1.246	.047	1.196	n.s.	1.458	n.s.
	Dirty work	1.246	n.s.	1.336	n.s.	1.381	n.s.
Step 3: SES	Higher employees (ref)	1.00		1.00		1.00	
	Intermediate employees	1.396	.028	1.409	n.s.	.856	n.s.
	Lower employees	1.366	n.s.	1.466	n.s.	.690	n.s.
	Self-employed	1.134	n.s.	.767	n.s.	1.796	n.s.
	Labourers	1.343	n.s.	1.229	n.s.	.916	n.s.
Work	High skill discretion (ref)	1.00		1.00		1.00	
	Intermediate skill discretion	1.295	.017	1.091	n.s.	1.537	.021
	Low skill discretion	1.737	.000	1.629	.001	1.520	.023
	High work pace	1.193	n.s.	1.126	n.s.	1.382	.031
	Smell	1.045	n.s.	1.064	n.s.	.947	n.s.
	Danger	1.267	n.s.	1.077	n.s.	1.719	.040
	Physically demanding	.862	n.s.	.878	n.s.	.982	n.s.
	Noise	1.250	.045	1.225	n.s.	1.421	n.s.
	Dirty work	1.081	n.s.	1.294	n.s.	1.365	n.s.
Lifestyle	Alcohol abuse	1.220	n.s.	1.314	n.s.	1.389	n.s.
	Smoking	1.283	.006	1.286	.034	1.307	n.s.
Cox & Snell's R^2			3.1%		3.8%		4.4%

Table C: Logistic regression on self-reported health for the years 1980-1983 – 1991-1992 (n.s. = not significant)

Predictor		Men (N=1321)		Women (N=825)	
		Odds ratio	p-value	Odds ratio	p-value
Step 1: SES	SES		.013		n.s.
	Higher employees(ref)	1.00		1.00	
	Intermediate employees	1.756	n.s.	.650	n.s.
	Lower employees	2.419	.012	.614	n.s.
	Self-employed	1.382	n.s.	.734	n.s.
	Labourers	2.578	.002	.653	n.s.
Step 2: SES	Ses		n.s.		n.s.
	Higher employees(ref)	1.00		1.00	
	Intermediate employees	1.608	n.s.	.612	n.s.
	Lower employees	2.073	.041	.607	n.s.
	Self-employed	1.190	n.s.	.805	n.s.
	Labourers	2.089	.028	.631	n.s.
Work	Skill discretion		.008		n.s.
	High skill discretion (ref)	1.00		1.00	
	Intermediate skill discretion	1.048	n.s.	1.434	n.s.
	Low skill discretion	1.827	.006	1.033	n.s.
	High work pace	.900	n.s.	1.005	n.s.
	Smell	.572	.007	1.177	n.s.
	Danger	1.363	n.s.	1.794	n.s.
	Physically demanding	.889	n.s.	.952	n.s.
	Noise	.897	n.s.	1.329	n.s.
	Dirty work	.827	n.s.	1.627	n.s.
Step 3: SES	SES		n.s.		n.s.
	Higher employees(ref)	1.00		1.00	
	Intermediate employees	1.599	n.s.	.603	n.s.
	Lower employees	2.034	.047	.582	n.s.
	Self-employed	1.176	n.s.	.783	n.s.
	Labourers	2.061	.031	.629	n.s.
Work	Skill discretion		.010		n.s.
	High skill discretion (ref)	1.00		1.00	
	Intermediate skill discretion	1.061	n.s.	1.458	n.s.
	Low skill discretion	1.817	.007	1.029	n.s.
	High work pace	.894	n.s.	.995	n.s.
	Smell	.572	.008	1.152	n.s.
	Danger	1.356	n.s.	1.827	n.s.
	Physically demanding	.890	n.s.	.983	n.s.
	Noise	.906	n.s.	1.296	n.s.
	Dirty work	.810	n.s.	1.598	n.s.
Lifestyle	Alcohol abuse	1.281	n.s.	1.083	n.s.
	Smoking	1.039	n.s.	1.384	n.s.
Cox & Snell's R^2			2.5%		1.5%

Norway

Espen DAHL & Jon Ivar ELSTAD

1. Structural Features of the Norwegian Labour Market

This section describes the structure of the Norwegian labour market and some changes over the last few decades. We focus on the social composition of the adult population, on employment rates and their developments, and on the composition of those outside paid labour. Information is given about early retirement, household work, students, sickness absence, unemployment, and precarious work, i.e. in temporary employment. Furthermore, we describe the industrial transformation during these decades.

A. *Employment Rates, Part-time Work, and Working Hours*

We see from table 1 below that among men, the percentage of the whole population aged 16-74 in some kind of employment dropped during the period 1980-1995 (from 78 to 71%), but has fluctuated since then. Among women, however, the percentage employed has increased steadily, and in the new century two thirds of all women aged 16-74 have had some kind of employment.

Table 1: Employed as percentage of the whole population aged 16-74, during the period 1980-2003

	1980	1985	1990	1995	2000	2003
Men	78.3	76.4	71.8	71.3	75.1	72.9
Women	53.8	57.7	59.4	61.1	66.6	66.3

Source: SSB 2003, table 1, SSB 2005. In this table, all employed, not only those with employment as their main activity, are counted as being employed.

Thus, the transformation of the economy during the last few decades has hardly reduced employment activity in the population. Employment rates are still high for men, and increasing for women. This has meant a feminisation of the workforce: of all employees aged 16-74, women constituted 41% in 1980 and 47% in 2000.

Part-time employment (i.e. less than approx. 35 hours per week) is however continuously more prevalent among women than among men.

While about 10% of all employed men had part-time employment during the entire period 1980-2000, this proportion among women dropped from 53% in 1980 to 43% in 2000 (SSB 2003, table 1). Part-time employment has therefore not become more prevalent during these decades, but rather the contrary.

The number of actual average working hours per week has however decreased somewhat among men (from 41.5 in 1980 to 38.8 in 2000), primarily due to a reduction in the standard number of working hours. Among employed women, average working hours per week increased slightly (29.2 in 1980, 30.6 in 2000), primarily because of fewer part-time jobs (SSB 2003, table 11).

During the period 1980-2000, employment rates were generally rather stable among men and increased among women for practically every age group. A clear exception is the rates among older men. In 1980, more than 70% of men aged 60-66 were employed, dropping to about 55% in the late 1990s (Birkeland 1999).

B. Composition of the Adult Population Outside Employment

When considering *main activity*, about 35% of the whole population aged 16-74 had other types of main activity than employment during the 1980s and 1990s (table 2). Considerable changes in the composition of those outside the ordinary labour market have occurred. The number and proportion of homemakers (practically all housewives) has dropped, while the proportion of students has increased. Even more conspicuous growth is observed among 'pensioners, disabled and sick' (old-age pension, pre-retirement, disability pension): they numbered approximately 300,000 in 1981, but more than 550,000 in 2003.

Table 2: The Norwegian population, men and women together, aged 16-74, grouped according to main activity. %, annual average, 1981, 1995, and 2003

Main activity	1981	1995	2003
Employed	64.3	65.9	63.1
Education	8.2	9.0	11.5
Homemakers	14.7	4.4	3.1
Pension, social security	10.2	15.7	17.2
Others, including unspecified	2.6	5.0	5.1
Total	100.0	100.0	100.0
All persons 16-74	2,909,000	3,140,000	3,257,000

Source: SSB 2002, table 233; SSB 2004, table 234.

The number of early-retired people has grown substantially over the last decades, especially among men. These are predominantly receiving contractual pension, now available from 62 years of age, and the state disability pension. Among the whole population aged 18-67, about 6% were recipients of disability pension in 1980, increasing to 10% in 2001. The consequence has been that over less than a decade, the average retirement age has dropped from 62 years in the early 1990s to slightly less than 60 years of age at present. The official retirement age in Norway is 67. Yet there are huge variations according to occupational group and educational level. Generally, employees who have a higher education and good jobs stay in work longer.

According to the Labour Force Survey (AKU), sickness absence has risen each year from the mid-1990s. In 1994 the percentage reported sick was 2.4, while in 2001, 4% of the economically active were absent because of illness. This development parallels the trend pictured by data coming from other sources, i.e. the Employers Association and the National Insurance Administration. According to these sources, sickness absence dropped from the late 1980s to the mid-1990s and then started to grow. This development was one of the major sources of the concern that led to the 'Inclusive Working Life Agreement' discussed below.

C. Unemployment and Precarious Work

Table 3 shows unemployment rates over the last few decades. A steep increase started in the late 1980s that culminated towards the mid-1990s. From that point it dropped drastically to a level below 60,000 unemployed, equivalent to about 3% of the workforce. Since late 1999, this decline has stopped, and during the most recent years unemployment rates have risen slowly.

Table 3. Unemployed men and women aged 16-74 as percentages of the labour force. Annual average 1980-2003

	1980	1985	1990	1995	2000	2003
Men	1.3	2.2	5.6	5.2	3.6	4.9
Women	2.3	3.1	4.8	4.6	3.2	4.0

Source: SSB 2003, table 22, SSB 2004, table 251. Labour force = sum of the employed and the unemployed (those actively seeking work).

Over the last half of the 1990s, the percentage among the employed who had 'precarious work' in terms of temporary labour contracts, seemed to have slightly decreased, from 12% in 1997 to 9% in 2001 (SSB 2001, table 243, SSB 2002, table 243), in contrast to prevailing hypotheses about the increasing role of flexible employment. Yet in several branches, temporary labour contracts are rather widespread and exist among about 15% of those employed in hotels and restaurants, educational services, and health and social services. It is supposed that precarious work is more widespread among women employees.

D. Composition of Industries

As in many other countries, Norway has gradually transformed over the past few decades away from a society of peasants, farmers and manual workers and towards a society of service providers. Developments since 1980 are indicated in table 4.

Table 4: Distribution of the employed population in industries, 1980 and 2000 (%)

Industry	1980	2000
Agriculture, hunting, forestry, fishing	8.4	4.1
Manufacture, mining, oil, electricity, gas, water supply	22.0	15.0
Construction	7.6	6.5
Wholesale and retail trade, restaurants, hotels	17.1	18.5
Transport, storage, communication	8.9	7.4
Financing, insurance, real estate and business services	5.8	11.3
Public administration, defence	5.2	6.9
Education	7.0	8.1
Health services, social services	13.1	17.7
Other services, unspecified	5.0	4.5
Total %	100.1	100.0
Total number of employed people	1,913,000	2,269,000

Source: SSB 1982, table 82; SSB 2002, table 241.

De-agriculturisation is continuing, as is de-industrialisation. The oil industry, which has expanded considerably since the late 1970s and is extremely important for the Norwegian gross national product, had no more than about 30,000 employees around 2000. Manufacturing and mining are down from 401,100 employees in 1980 to 295,000 in 2000. The decline in primary and secondary industries is more than offset by the growth in several other branches of industry. Private services in bank, insurance etc. are significantly up from 110,000 in 1980 to 256,000 in 2000. Health and social services increased from about 250,000 in 1980 to 402,000 in 2000. Education also shows a growth in absolute terms, from 133,000 to 184,000 in the same period.

The distribution of employment in different industries is clearly gendered. In 2000, women constituted about 25% of the employees in manufacturing etc., but 83% of the employees in health and social services. The proportion of self-employed (not including family workers) declined from approx. 10% in 1980 to 7% in 2000, primarily be-cause of the disappearance of smaller farms.

Norwegian society is more and more based on a post-industrial economy that produces services to meet a diversity of needs. This "new economy" is also clearly gendered; women are predominantly occupied in human and welfare services, often in the public sector, while men hold positions in private businesses, for example in finance and manu-facturing.

2. Changes in Class Composition During Recent Decades

The relative size of socio-economic groups among men and women has changed considerably during the 1980s and 1990s. This is shown in table 5, using data from Statistics Norway's Surveys of Level of Living (1980/1983 pooled and 1995/1998 pooled). The socio-economic groups shown here are the ones that Statistics Norway has used for classifying the employed population during the 1980s and 1990s. In the following we will also sometimes refer to these socio-economic groups as 'social classes' or 'occupational classes'.

Table 5: Distribution of the employed population, aged 20-64, in socio-economic groups (%). Surveys of Level of Living, 1980+1983 (pooled) and 1995+1998 (pooled)

	All		*Men*		*Women*	
	1980-83	1995-98	1980-83	1995-98	1980-83	1995-98
Workers						
– unskilled	21.9	12.7	26.7	17.0	15.2	7.8
– skilled	10.8	10.8	17.0	17.6	1.9	3.0
Salaried employees						
– lower level	16.9	12.7	4.1	3.4	35.1	23.2
– intermediate	27.6	33.7	23.7	28.2	33.2	39.9
– higher	9.7	21.5	13.0	23.1	4.9	19.7
Farmers, fishermen, etc.	5.6	3.1	6.4	4.4	4.4	1.6
Other self-employed	7.6	5.5	9.1	6.1	5.3	4.9
Total %	100.0	100.0	100.0	100.0	100.0	100.0
(Sample N)	(4,357)	(4,279)	(2,559)	(2,270)	(1,798)	(2,009)

Source: Statistics Norway, Surveys of Level of Living (Rommetveit 1997, Ramm 2000), own analyses of data files.

Table 5 indicates the emergence of a predominantly post-industrial society over these two decades. Workers, especially unskilled workers, have been steadily declining. At the same time, the class of salaried employees has expanded, in particular the higher segments. This trend is more pronounced for women than for men. It should be noted that the particularly low percentage of unskilled workers among women occurs because low-ranking staff in health and care services etc. are classified as lower-level salaried employees.

More recent surveys can also be used to show the current distribution of the employed population in social/occupational classes. Unfortunately for the study of time trends, however, in the late 1990s Statistics Norway switched to a Norwegian version of ISCO-88 (COM), making trend comparisons difficult. This new classification also indicates how a large proportion of the current working population are in 'high-status' occupations – see table 6 as regards the distribution in 2003.

Table 6: Distribution in 2003 of the employed population, all ages, main ISCO-88 (COM) categories (%)

Major groups ISCO-88 (COM)	Men	Women
1. Legislators, senior officials, managers	9.9	4.8
2. Professionals	12.0	9.9
3. Technicians and associated professionals	20.5	26.1
4. Clerks	4.9	11.0
5. Service, shop and market sales workers	11.6	34.3
6. Skilled agricultural and fishery workers	4.8	1.7
7. Craft and related trades workers	19.4	1.7
8. Plant and machine operators and assemblers	12.3	2.6
9. Elementary occupations, unspecified	4.7	8.0
Total %	100.0	100.0
Total number of employed population in 2003	1,198,000	1,071,000

Source: SSB 2004, table 243.

3. Social Class and Health among Men and Women

Social and socio-economic inequalities in health in Norway have been demonstrated in quite a large number of studies. Analyses have been made for all age groups, from infants (Arntzen *et al.* 1996) to old age (Dahl and Birkelund 1997); social positions have been indicated in a number of ways (socio-economic group, education, occupation, income, employment status, area of residence grouped according to deprivation, etc.); and health has been measured by overall mortality and cause-specific mortality, as well as by various indicators of disease and illness such as chronic conditions, limitations to activity because of illness, disability pension, self-assessed overall health, mental health problems, etc.

In this section we will concentrate on evidence related to health differences between social classes/socio-economic groups among the adult population. We will focus on four health indicators: overall mortality, cardiovascular mortality, long-standing (chronic) illness, and self-assessed overall health status, and try also to show some trends during recent decades.

A. Social Class Differentials in Overall Mortality

A number of studies have shown clear social class differentials in mortality among the adult population. Mortality differences between occupational classes during the 1970s were for instance demonstrated by analyses performed by Statistics Norway (Borgan and Kristofersen 1986), and by a large study in the capital, Oslo (Holme *et al.* 1980). Norwegian data sets have also been exploited in international comparisons that indicate that during the 1970s and early 1980s Norwegian socio-economic mortality differentials were of more or less the same magnitude as in other countries in North-Western Europe (Kunst 1997), at least in relative terms.

Table 7 reproduces the results from one of these studies (Borgan 1996), as to overall mortality according to socio-economic status among men 30-64 years of age, made by linking census information on occupations to the death registers during the following five-year periods. Clear mortality differences are seen. Those who were economically inactive at the time of the censuses had much higher mortality than those who were employed, and among the employed there are marked differences between the occupational classes. It can be inferred from table 8, first, that overall mortality among men in these age groups increased somewhat during the 1960s, but declined afterwards; and, second, that relative differences seemed to increase even after some possible selection effects were removed (i.e., the figures for the latter part of each decade – 1965-1970, 1975-1980, and 1985-1990 – are to some extent purged for selection effects immediately prior to the observation period, because socio-economic status here refers to a time point five years earlier than the observation period for mortality). A similar study (Dahl and Kjaersgaard 1993) also found that among men, relative mortality differences between the occupational classes increased from the early 1960s to the early 1980s, but they also demonstrated that mortality differences were much less marked among women than men.

Table 7: Age-standardised mortality according to socio-economic status for Norwegian males aged 30-64 years. Five-year periods, 1960-1990

	1960-65	*1965-70*	*1970-75*	*1975-80*	*1980-85*	*1985-90*
All men	100	105	102	100	95	92
All employed men	92	101	84	91	72	78
Workers						
– unskilled	93	106	88	99	80	92
– skilled	102	112	87	97	75	80
Salaried employees						
– lower level	114	107	97	98	89	95
– intermediate	99	104	85	84	67	69
– higher	83	87	65	66	55	53
Farmers etc.	70	79	67	75	64	71
Other self-employed	104	107	91	96	76	79
All not-employed men	240	242	243	220	196	195

Source: Reproduced from Borgan (1996), table 2. Reference category (= 100) is age-standardized mortality among all men aged 30-64 in 1960-1965. Socio-economic status is according to information given at the censuses in 1960, 1970 and 1980, respectively.

Studies of later occupational class mortality differentials have been hampered because the census in 1990, unlike previous censuses, did not register occupation. However, a large study of the population in Oslo has linked mortality during 1990-1994 to census information about occupations in 1980 and found a marked social gradient, which the authors argued was even steeper than comparable mortality differentials in England/Wales (Claussen and Næss 2002). Another recent study which compared educational differences in mortality during 1970-1977, 1980-1987, and 1990-1997, has suggested that the social gradient was indeed steeper in the latter period than in the previous ones, for men as well as for women (Zahl *et al.* 2003).

Several of the above-mentioned studies, as well as other studies, discuss to what extent selection might be (part of) the processes behind the observed occupational differentials. Most of them conclude that selection has probably played only a minor part (Borgan 1996, Dahl 1993a, Dahl 1993b, Dahl and Kjaersgaard 1993). The most recent study (Zahl *et al.* 2003), however, argues that the educational mortality differences seem to be connected to household and marital status effects, suggesting a larger role for selective processes.

B. Social Class Differentials in Cardiovascular Mortality

It can be assumed that socio-economic differences in cardiovascular mortality will be very similar to the pattern for overall mortality because cardiovascular diseases (CVD) constitute such a large proportion of all causes of death. However, this applies primarily for age groups from about 40 years of age and above. The above-mentioned Oslo study during the 1970s and early 1980s found marked socio-economic differences in CVD mortality and CVD risk factors (Holme *et al.* 1980, Holme *et al.* 1982) as also the more recent Oslo study of mortality 1990-1994 has done (Claussen *et al.* 2003). Another large county study (Thürmer 1993) has comparable results. On the national level, Borgan's study, referred to above, shows how the social gradient for CVD mortality for age groups 30-64 to a large extent replicates the pattern found for overall mortality, see table 8.

Table 8: Age-standardised mortality according to socio-economic status for males aged 30-64 years. Cardiovascular diseases. Five-year periods, 1960-1990

	1960-65	1965-70	1970-75	1975-80	1980-85	1985-90
All men	100	111	108	103	96	89
All employed men	92	108	89	94	75	77
Workers						
– unskilled	85	107	88	98	79	89
– skilled	107	126	94	108	79	80
Salaried employees						
– lower level	137	128	105	101	97	96
– intermediate	111	122	97	92	73	69
– higher	92	99	73	71	58	51
Farmers etc.	65	80	66	77	62	69
Other self-employed	116	120	102	97	80	76
All not-employed men	216	225	244	208	182	179

Source: Reproduced from Borgan (1996), table 3. Reference category (= 100) is age-standardised mortality among all men aged 30-64 in 1960-1965. Socio-economic status is according to information given at the censuses in 1960, 1970 and 1980, respectively.

C. Social Class Differentials in Long-standing Illness and Self-assessed Health

The size and trends of social class variations in chronic conditions and self-assessed overall health have been demonstrated in a number of surveys conducted in Norway during the 1970s, 1980s and 1990s. This is exemplified by our own analyses of the Surveys of Level of Living (for chronic conditions, see table 9) and of the Health Surveys (for self-perceived health, see table 10).

Table 9: Average number of reported chronic illnesses (i.e., long-standing medical conditions). Currently employed, socio-economic groups, age 20-64, men and women. Surveys of Level of Living, 1980-1983 (pooled) and 1995-1998 (pooled)

	Men				Women			
Survey year	1980-83		1995-98		1980-83		1995-98	
Age group	20-44	45-64	20-44	45-64	20-44	45-64	20-44	45-64
Workers								
– unskilled	0.53	0.82	0.70	0.89	0.55	0.95	0.84	1.40
– skilled	0.58	0.72	0.75	0.96	-	-	0.82	-
Salaried employees								
– lower level	0.37	-	0.67	-	0.51	0.80	0.74	1.14
– intermediate	0.41	0.68	0.60	0.78	0.45	0.79	0.89	1.03
– higher	0.40	0.64	0.65	0.75	0.49	0.92	0.79	1.22
Farmers, fishermen, etc.	0.34	0.87	0.66	0.98	0.56	1.04	-	-
Other self-employed	0.38	0.63	0.72	0.66	0.52	0.71	0.90	1.38
Average	0.46	0.73	0.67	0.82	0.50	0.85	0.83	1.16
(Sample N)	1620	939	1414	856	1141	657	1268	741

Source: Statistics Norway's Surveys of Level of Living, 1980-83 (pooled) and 1995-98 (pooled), own analyses of data files. Subcategories with fewer than 25 respondents not reported.

On average, workers have more chronic/long-standing conditions than salaried employees, but social differences within the worker groups, and within the salaried employee groups, are small and unsystematic. Male farmers/self-employed often have more chronic diseases than salaried employees. Whether socio-economic differences among men as regards this health indicator have increased from the early 1980s to the late 1990s is hard to determine. It should be noted that the most conspicuous change is the overall *increase* of reported chronic illnesses during this period, in all groups, for which there could be methodological reasons (the questionnaires were somewhat changed), but which is also probably due to more health service attendance and a general 'medicalisation' during these years. The same social pattern is to some extent also present among women; however, socio-economic differences in average number of chronic diseases among women seem smaller and more unsystematic.

Table 10: Percentages reporting overall self-assessed health as 'less than good'. Currently employed, socio-economic groups, age 25-64, men and women. Health Surveys 1985 and 1995

	Men				Women			
Survey year	1985		1995		1985		1995	
Age group	25-44	45-64	25-44	45-64	25-44	45-64	25-44	45-64
Workers								
– unskilled	20	28	7	27	19	29	10	26
– skilled	9	24	11	16	-	-	18	-
Salaried employees								
– lower level	15	-	3	-	13	23	8	17
– intermediate	11	17	7	12	10	10	6	16
– higher	6	11	6	9	10	14	8	11
Farmers, fishermen, etc.	16	35	13	30	-	-	-	-
Other self-employed	14	23	12	12	17	22	11	23
Average	12	22	8	15	12	21	8	18
(Sample N)	1394	825	1211	931	1096	627	1156	789

Source: Statistic Norway's Health Surveys 1985 and 1995, own analyses of data files. Subcategories with fewer than 25 respondents not reported.

As to self-assessed overall health (table 10), the same patterning of health is generally repeated, perhaps, however, with clearer social differences both among men and women. Contrary to what one would guess, it can be noted that although the number of reported chronic illnesses have increased from the early 1980s to the mid-/late 1990s, overall self-assessed health was hardly worse, indeed perhaps better, in 1995 than in 1985.

It should be underlined strongly that the figures given in tables 9 and 10 most probably underestimate the 'true' social differences, because they reflect health conditions among those currently working. Especially in the older groups (age about 40+), many, especially those who were placed far down on the occupational ladder, will have left work because of health problems, and analyses have repeatedly shown that if non-employed people are included according to their former class position, the social gradients turn out to be considerably larger (Dahl 1993b, Dahl and Birkelund 1999). It can be added that one study has suggested that long-standing conditions reported by male manual workers appear to be more serious than conditions reported by salaried employees (Elstad 1996), indicating that the figures in table 9 do not exaggerate the social differences in long-standing conditions, rather the contrary.

4. Social Differences in Working Conditions and Employment

A. *Working Conditions in Different Occupations*

An analysis of the social variations in working conditions examined job demands, job control (decision authority), job social support, muscular load and chemical and physical hazards in a number of specified occupations Andresen (1998). Using data from 1996, he showed that a number of adverse working conditions accumulated among workers. Especially industrial workers were often exposed to poor climatic conditions, pollution, and adverse ergonomic work environment. At the same time, industrial workers also had the lowest decision latitude regarding work tasks and had little job control. On the other hand, managers, and also usually teachers and nurses, clearly had a better physical and psychosocial work environment than factory workers, transportation workers, and workers in hotels and restaurants. This study also showed that from 1989 to 1996, more employees reported that their work was directed by deadlines, fixed routines, and demands from customers and clients, while the physical work environment changed only marginally during the same period. An emerging feature is that a number of "new" occupational groups, and especially groups that staff the welfare institutions, often have a burdensome, strenuous, demanding and potentially stressful work environment. Exposures to chemical and physical agents are rare, but exposures to different social-psychological stressors are common. It should be noted that nurses in particular also report heavy physical loads and a high degree of ergonomic problems.

B. *Variations Between Social Classes in Working Conditions*

The findings regarding different occupations indicate of course that also on the level of social classes, there are considerable differences as regards exposures to potentially unhealthy and harmful working conditions. The Surveys of Level of Living 1980-1995 had a remarkable consistency in how questions about working conditions were formulated, and this enables an estimation of the differences between socioeconomic groups, and provides some clues to appraise whether these differences have changed during recent decades.

Table 11: Physical working conditions. Average values on indices of harmful working environments and ergonomic strain, socio-economic groups, age 20-64, men and women, 1980-1983 and 1991-1995

Working conditions	Men				Women			
	Harmful environment index		Ergonomic strain index		Harmful environment index		Ergonomic strain index	
Period	80-83	91-95	80-83	91-95	80-83	91-95	80-83	91-95
Workers								
– unskilled	4.7	5.1	1.7	1.9	1.7	1.9	1.7	1.7
– skilled	4.5	5.0	1.4	1.6	2.9	2.5	1.7	1.5
Salaried employees								
– lower level	1.5	1.7	1.0	1.3	0.8	1.1	1.1	1.4
– intermediate	1.2	1.3	0.5	0.6	0.9	1.1	0.9	0.9
– higher	0.9	0.9	0.3	0.4	0.8	0.9	0.4	0.5
Farmers, fishermen, etc.	4.0	4.5	2.2	2.2	1.6	2.0	1.8	1.6
Other self-employed	2.8	3.0	1.4	1.4	0.6	1.0	0.8	0.9
Average	3.0	2.9	1.2	1.2	1.0	1.2	1.1	1.1
(Sample N)	2 559	2326	2559	2326	1798	1936	1798	1936

Source: Statistic Norway's Surveys of Level of Living, own analyses of data files. Harmful environment: Additive index, number of yes-answers to questions about work-places with draughts, temperatures above 30C or below 10C, moist, metal particles etc., smoke, damp, polluted air, vibrations, bad light, bad ventilation, working high above ground level, working with dangerous machines, acids etc., inflammable/explosive substances, other dangerous chemical substances (17 items). Ergonomic strain: Additive index, number of yes-answers to questions about monotonous physical work, strenuous working postures, daily lifting heavy things (3 items).

Table 11 analyses physical working conditions by utilising four Surveys of Living Conditions. The surveys have been pooled to make sample size larger and estimates more stable. Generally, although much has been written about the technological revolution and the coming of the service economy and how these trends have removed burdensome physical working conditions, it seems that little of this took place in Norway from 1980-1983 to 1991-1995. Actually, among men it seems that in each occupational class, physical working conditions tended to deteriorate. The average exposure to such negative working conditions was constant or even reduced, however, due to the fact that during the period there was a considerable reduction in the proportion of the employed population with particularly bad conditions (i.e., workers).

The second conclusion is that harmful environments (pollution, dangerous machines, etc., see legend below table 11) are much more prevalent among men than women, primarily because of high exposures among male workers and farmers. Self-reported ergonomic strain is however relatively equal among men and women. Furthermore, the very striking feature of table 11 is that workers, and also farmers etc., have much more harmful physical working conditions than salaried employees, and higher-level salaried employees have particularly favourable physical working conditions.

Table 12: Men's psychosocial working conditions. Decision latitude, variation, hectic working conditions, socio-economic groups, age 20-64, 1980-1983 and 1991-1995

Working conditions	Currently employed men, age 20-64							
	Decide own working speed to a high degree %		Plan own work schedule to a high degree %		Work is very varied %		Daily hectic work situations %	
Period	80-83	91-95	80-83	91-95	80-83	91-95	80-83	91-95
Workers – unskilled	43	45	28	32	31	33	14	24
– skilled	55	57	37	44	50	53	17	29
Salaried employees – lower level	48	42	46	39	40	38	17	30
– intermediate	60	57	61	59	58	54	22	26
– higher	73	62	72	67	70	67	23	26
Farmers, fishermen, etc.	75	75	68	65	61	53	11	10
Other self-employed	73	70	68	66	56	55	27	21
Average	58	57	50	52	50	51	19	25

Source: Same as table 11.

Table 13: Women's psychosocial working conditions. Decision latitude, variation, hectic working conditions, socio-economic groups, age 20-64, 1980-1983 and 1991-1995

Working conditions	Currently employed women, age 20-64							
	Decide own working speed to a high degree %		Plan own work schedule to a high degree %		Work is very varied %		Daily hectic work situations %	
Period	80-83	91-95	80-83	91-95	80-83	91-95	80-83	91-95
Workers								
– unskilled	56	52	40	46	8	7	9	12
– skilled	39	34	29	30	18	25	6	20
Salaried employees								
– lower level	37	31	31	29	27	26	11	20
– intermediate	36	42	40	41	44	49	16	21
– higher	41	47	55	50	57	60	20	20
Farmers, fishermen, etc.	74	68	41	53	24	37	6	11
Other self-employed	70	66	69	64	39	38	7	14
Average	43	42	39	40	32	39	12	19

Source: Same as table 11.

As regards psychosocial or organisational working conditions (men shown in table 12, women in table 13), the overall picture is that there have been no marked changes from the early 1980s to mid-1990s, except for the item 'experiencing daily hectic work situations', which was more prevalent in the latter period. Thus, according to these analyses, the alleged increasing flexibility, reorganisations, empowerment in the workplace etc. have hardly led to more decision latitude, more varied work, etc. in general, during the period analysed here. Overall, however, decision latitude and varied work seem more prevalent among men than women.

The social gradients are somewhat more complex regarding these organisational aspects of the working situation. Among *men* (table 12), intermediate – and especially higher-level salaried employees decide working speed, plan their own schedule, and have more varied work, than workers; however, to some extent, their daily working situation also seems more hectic. As could be expected, farmers and other self-employed people also have a relatively high degree of control over their own work. For *women* (table 13), the associations are more unsystematic.

C. Employment Status, Age, Education and Social Class

The extent, to which people in different socio-economic groups actually are employed, could be taken as a summarising indicator of a series of social forces and social conditions. The general level of unemployment (section 1.3) is one important factor, and one would assume that those with low qualifications generally would find it harder to get work, especially under conditions of high unemployment. Moreover, the higher level of health problems in disadvantaged socio-economic groups (section 3) will tend to restrict their employment activity if inclusion policies and practices are insufficient. A third factor is working conditions: less satisfactory working conditions in the 'lower' end of the occupational hierarchy could act to pressure those who usually have such occupations out of work.

Table 14: Percentages who are neither employed nor in education. Three age groups, gender, educational level, and social class. Health Survey 1995

	Men			Women		
Age groups	25-29	40-49	55-64	25-29	40-49	55-64
Average, all groups	5	6	23	18	11	34
Educational level						
– low up to 10 years	11	9	30	31	15	39
– medium 11-12 years	4	4	22	16	11	29
– higher 13+ years	1	3	10	9	4	17
Social class						
Workers						
– unskilled	8	16	49	33	20	46
– skilled	2	3	20	-	-	-
Salaried employees						
– lower level	-	-	-	30	16	44
– intermediate	2	3	24	9	9	19
– higher	0	3	19	9	1	15

Source: Statistic Norway's Surveys of Level of Living, own analyses of data file. Social class is based on current or (if not currently employed) most important previous occupation. Farmers/self-employed and unclassifiable excluded (i.e., never worked, always housewives, not left education yet, missing information, etc.) Estimates in subgroups with less than 25 respondents excluded.

A suggestion of how such forces acted in Norway in the mid-1990s is provided in table 14, reporting the percentages among men and women in different age groups who neither had employment nor were students in 1995 (among those aged 25-29, 8% were still in education). To indicate their position in the socio-economic hierarchy, both educational level and social class (based on current or previous occupation) are used.

Table 14 shows that non-employment (and not in education) was quite small among men up to their late forties, but somewhat higher for women (relatively many women in their late twenties are not working because of child care). In the age group 55-64, however, as many as about a quarter of the men and a third of the women were outside work. Furthermore, a remarkably steep socio-economic gradient in employment activity, both for men and women, and for all three age groups, can be observed. Those with low education had a much higher risk of being outside the labour market than those with high education. As to social class differences, it should be noted that these data suggest that the contrast is not primarily between workers and salaried employees. Rather, among men, the unskilled worker category was extremely disadvantaged, while skilled male workers had no worse employment chances than intermediate- and higher-level salaried employees. Similarly, among women, the great gap is between unskilled workers and lower-level salaried employees on the one hand, and intermediate- and higher-level salaried employees on the other hand.

5. Unionisation and the Role of the Trade Unions

A. Unionisation

According to the latest Survey of Level of Living, 57% of the occupationally active population were unionised. The highest rates were found in the civil service and education, where more than 80% are members of a union. The lowest percentages are found in industries like retail (23%) and service work in hotels and restaurants (32%). Over the last decade, there has been a slight drop in unionisation from 61% in 1989. Still, by far the largest organisation is the Norwegian Confederation of Trade Unions that has about 800,000 members.

B. How Powerful are the Trade Unions in Relation to Working Life Factors that may Affect Health?

Traditionally the main concerns of trade unions have been wages and earnings, working conditions and employment issues, and welfare policies and social security. In Norway, as in other Nordic countries, the trade unions are potentially powerful. Among other things, this is due to the high degree of unionisation as well as a developed institutional system that incorporates trade union representatives on important societal decision-making arenas. It is perceived that this kind of corporatism over the past decades has helped to smooth the economic development by curbing wages, and leading to higher economic growth than would have been possible without such an institutional framework. An important factor in this respect has been the moderate wage increases that occurred during the 1990s. In exchange for moderate wage claims, the members of the trade unions, and all other citizens as well, have experienced low inflation, and from the mid-1990s an economic boom accompanied by increasing employment rates and decreasing unemployment rates. It is also likely that collective and centralised wage bargaining have contributed to inequalities in wages and earnings being smaller in Norway than in many other countries in Europe, and certainly in the USA. Thus, by contributing to economic growth as well as to narrower income inequalities, the trade unions might have also played a role or the level and the social distribution of health.

Norway has had a Work Environment Act in effect for several decades. This Act is considered to be responsive and sensitive to the interests of workers and their well-being and health. It places the responsibility for the health of workers among the employees, and has a broad approach to a variety of aspects of the work environment such as psychosocial factors, ergonomic factors, physical and chemical factors and protection of workers from such hazards and exposures. This legislation also requires larger firms and corporations to establish administrative bodies, in which representatives from the trade unions or the employees participate, to monitor, and to check on the work environment. Employees' representatives are also involved in activities directed towards maintaining and improving 'Health, Environment and Safety' in the workplace. These efforts are likely to be conducive to many blue-collar workers' health. However, as shown above, a number of different aspects of the working environment are still worse for these groups than for white-collar workers.

In the same vein, the trade unions have had a long-lasting fight to maintain full income compensation during periods of sickness and have thus helped to 'decommodify' labour. However, the influence this has on health inequalities is hard to predict, since compelling evidence is lacking. One plausible argument is that when it is easy to opt out of work when sick, this will speed up recovery and help to maintain health in the long run. Another argument, which also has some credibility, is that especially long-term sick leave has detrimental effects on the likelihood of coming back to work and maybe also for health. Being long-term sick undermines self-confidence, erodes social bonds to the workplace, reduces well-being and might hinder the process of recovery.

The establishment of company-based health services for employees is also the result of pressures from the trade unions. But again, it is hard to assess the degree to which these health services have an impact on health inequalities.

C. Trade Union Policies on Social Class Differences in Health.

The theme 'social inequalities in health' has been of little concern to any of the trade unions in Norway. One will find few if any references to this term in the rhetoric, in publications and in statements made by trade union officials.

However, recently at least one programme has been launched that may be seen as particularly relevant for health inequalities. This is the programme for 'Inclusive Working Life'. This is a tripartite agreement (between the Government, trade unions, and employers' associations), which includes elements that may be beneficial to the employees' health. The three main objectives of the programme are to increase employment among older people, reduce sickness absence, and include more occupationally impaired people in the labour market. However, this programme only indirectly addresses health inequalities as such, since there is no mention of the issue, and no specific measures are proposed to tackle the problem. If successful, its impact on health inequalities is uncertain. On the one hand it might improve health among those who are worst off by improving their work environment and reducing exposures and health hazards. On the other hand, if the programme is too aggressive in bringing sick people back into 'bad' jobs, the result may be poorer health. Whether higher employment rates among older people and the occupationally impaired will result in better or worse health will among other things depend on what kind of work they are occupied in. This programme is currently being evaluated, but the results are yet to be seen.

6. Research and Policies Related to Health Inequalities

In this section we describe and discuss a number of issues that may provide a background for understanding and interpreting health inequalities in Norway, their size, trends and possible future developments. We focus on the relevant research efforts, policies and policy reforms and selected institutions.

A. Ongoing Research

Quite a number of research projects relevant for the study of socio-economic health inequalities are, or have been, in existence in Norway. Here, a few of those that are currently in progress will be briefly mentioned. The order of mentioning is random, and no claims are made that the list is complete or that the most significant projects are mentioned.

The Nord-Trøndelag Health Study (HUNT) surveyed practically the whole adult population in the county of Nord-Trøndelag in two waves (1984-1986 and 1995-1997, both screening and questionnaires), and a third wave is planned. Several studies relating to socio-economic health differentials have been published, for instance (Elstad and Krokstad 2003, Krokstad *et al.* 2002a Krokstad and Westin 2002). The Norwegian Institute of Public Health (and its predecessor the National Institute of Public Health) has been involved in a series of relevant projects, such as studies of the health of socially disadvantaged groups (Rognerud *et al.* 2000), of trends in social differences in mortality (Zahl *et al.* 2003), and population surveys in various Norwegian counties, for instance the large Oslo Health Study (the HUBRO project). This institution is also involved in a large cohort study of pregnancies and newborn babies (The Norwegian mother and child cohort study), which, in the decades to come, also will bring new data for the study of social variations in health. Relatively large nationwide health interviews surveys (sample approximately 3-4000) have been conducted by Statistics Norway in 1998 and 2002. A study on socio-economic differences in mortality 1990-1994 in Oslo is presently being conducted at the Institute of Community Medicine, University of Oslo (Claussen and Næss 2002, Claussen *et al.* 2003). A nationwide study of area differences in socio-economic patterns of mortality, trying to examine the impact of individual income and area characteristics (income inequality, social investments, social capital/social cohesion) on mortality, is in progress (Dahl *et al.* 2003). At the Research Centre for Health Promotion, University in Bergen, various relevant research projects have been conducted, some of them with a focus on socio-economic differences in health behaviours.

Generally, it appears that few of these research projects aim at studying the associations between working conditions and social inequalities in health. Certainly, they focus on social variations in health, but their explanatory variables are quite often health behaviours, diets, childhood influences, or more general social status indicators such as education, income, and occupation. Working conditions seem not to be regarded as the most prominent causal factor for health variations. However, the National Institute of Occupational Health has had many projects which examine exposures in workplaces and their aetiological role for specific diseases and health problems, but these studies usually focus on specific occupations and factories or other workplaces, and the results are seldom used to study the impact of working conditions on social class health differences on a more general level. Other studies could also be mentioned: one study in the Western part of Norway on the relationship between a large number of specific occupations and several health indicators (Moen *et al.* 2002), and a doctoral thesis on the relationship between manual work, socio-economic positions, and the risk of becoming a disability pensioner because of musculoskeletal diseases (Holte 2002).

B. Data Suitable for Comparative Analyses

The most suitable data which have a significant potential for comparative research are the periodic Surveys on Level of Living that Statistics Norway have conducted since 1973. Surveys were conducted approximately every fourth year during the period 1980-1995, and from 1996/97 they have been carried out annually. The surveys usually include questions on working conditions and work environment. Examples of areas covered are working times/hours; physical working conditions such as draughts, high temperatures, smoke, strong vibrations, dirty work, noise; hazardous environment/exposures such as working with dangerous machinery, acids, and chemical substances; ergonomic conditions such as repetitive movements, heavy loads, burdensome work positions; and psychosocial factors such as high pace, hectic work situation, and decision latitude.

Since 1996, two Surveys of Level of Living have been carried out annually, one cross-sectional survey including a main rotating theme, and one panel survey (repeated interviews with the same sample). In the 2000 cross-sectional survey the main theme was working conditions. All Surveys of Level of Living also include at least some questions on health, and also have information on socio-economic indicators such as income, education and social/occupational class. Hence these studies are well suited for analyses of the relationships between socio-economic status, working conditions and health, both in a snapshot perspective and in a longitudinal perspective. There are also other surveys carried out by Statistics Norway and other institutions that might be of interest, but the Surveys of Level of Living have several advantages: questions on work environment are often comprehensive, time series data exist, (many of) the surveys have standardised items which are repeated for several years, and panel data are available.

C. Public Policies on Health Inequalities

Until very recently, changing governments and health authorities had not been particularly concerned with social health inequalities. In an analysis of the relevant political documents on public health policies that were issued during the 1990s, Dahl (2002) concluded that Norway was located somewhere in the lower end of the so-called 'action spectrum' formulated by (Whitehead 1998). The action spectrum provides a framework for describing national policies pursued to tackle health inequalities, and stretches from a situation in which health inequalities are not even measured, to a one in which a comprehensive, committed and coordinated political action to deal with these challenges is implemented. Within the action spectrum, the analysis located Norway somewhere in the area around 'need for measurement', 'awareness raising', and 'indifference'. The author characterised Norway as a laggard in health policies when compared with the ways in which several other European countries have responded to this issue.

In 2002, however, a new Public Health Report was put forward by the current Center/Right coalition government. The White Paper is called *A Recipe for a Healthier Norway* (St. meld. No. 16, 2002-2003). This document may be seen as breakthrough for the health inequality issue on the political agenda in that it takes the issue more seriously than before. The document expresses a clear will to do something about the problem and introduces a set of several measures to deal with it.

The White Paper states that there are two broad aims for public health policy. The first is to contribute to more healthy life years for the entire population. The second is to "reduce differences in health between social strata, ethnic groups and gender". The Government declares that it is prepared to combat differences that are "unnecessary, unjust, and possible to influence". In particular it singles out health-damaging behaviour where opportunities are constrained, and where people are exposed to health-damaging and stressful living and working conditions, unequal access to health services and other services, and finally health-related mobility. The document argues that it important to have a long-term perspective and stresses the needs for increased efforts to monitor the situation, encourage more research in this field, and to increase administrative competence.

The Government announces that five concrete measures will be implemented:

- To assess policies that are aimed at changing lifestyles in terms of how this will influence health inequalities.
- To appraise new measures targeted at disadvantaged groups or geographical areas in the light of health inequalities.
- To include social inequalities in health as an important element in health impact assessments.
- To establish a new competence centre with the aim of developing policies in this area.
- To develop an Action Plan against Social Inequalities in Health during 2003.

What differentiates this White Paper from the previous official public health documents during the 1980s and 1990s is a recognition that health inequalities constitute a public health problem and that the Government commits itself to act. Obviously, the measures that are proposed will hardly change the actual situation much, but they may signal the start of a higher awareness and more active policies in this area in the years to come.

The fact that the Government has put the issue so high on the political agenda might lead to a more widespread public and professional debate on this topic, a debate that has hardly existed in Norway. Although working conditions are mentioned as one of the factors that may play a role, no concrete measures or policies are proposed for addressing the issue.

However, by this White Paper, one might say that Norway has taken a step up the ladder on the action spectrum, and now finds itself in a stage of concern and a willingness to take political action.

D. Policies to Increase Labour Market Participation among Older Workers

As described above, over the last three decades, labour market participation has been steadily declining among older people of a working age, i.e. those who are 55-67 years old. This trend has been particularly strong among men. Despite the fact that the official retirement age in Norway is 67, the average retirement age was about 62 years of age in the early 1990s. Because of the raised concern over this long-term trend, the aim of the official retirement policies over the past decade has been to increase the average retirement age. The policies and measures adopted have primarily focused on economic incentives, i.e. constructing incentive systems that reward those who stay longer, and 'punishing' those who leave earlier. These policies have not been particularly successful. Around the turn of the century the average retirement age had dropped further to slightly less than 60 years. A large proportion of the earlier exits are to disability pension. Today, about 10% of the population of a working age (16-67 years of age) receive disability pension. Another important pathway out of working life is a Contractual Pension, a semi-private early retirement scheme that covers all employees in the public sector, as well as the employees in the private sector where there is an agreement between the organisations of the employers and employees. The retirement age in this scheme has gradually gone down during the 1990s to today's 62 years. The trade unions have firmly expanded and defended this scheme despite the fact that different governments have recognised that the scheme hardly furthers the overarching goals and general policies in this field. It is abundantly clear that exit to disability pension is socially differentiated. The incidence of disability pension is many times higher – up to eight times – among groups with little education and lower occupational jobs than among groups who are better off in these respects (Krokstad *et al.* 2002b). The same pattern applies to the Contractual Pension, but it is perhaps not so marked. Nonetheless, people who have poorer jobs tend to take up a Contractual Pension significantly earlier than individuals who have better jobs (Midtsundstad 2001).

E. Commitment to Full Employment, Compensation Levels in Social Security Schemes

A paragraph in the Norwegian constitution grants its citizens the right to a job. Also after the Second World War and up to the seventies there was 'full employment' in Norway. For most political parties full employment is the first priority. This is seen as a human right, but it is also of vital importance for the viability of a welfare state of this type. A high volume of public transfers and benefits of high quality require a broad tax base and to maintain a broad tax base, full employment is a necessity. Thus, the high and increasing exit from the labour market of older workers and people with health problems, is an alarming sign. Also, when facing shifting business cycles, the aim of full employment is easier said than done.

Thus, in prevailing political rhetoric the commitment is high, but firm empirical evidence indicates that there is a gap between good intentions and reality. This applies in particular to social inequalities in the right to work. (See for example table 14, which indicates that whether people are in paid work or not depends to a high degree on their socio-economic status, here measured by education and social class.) People with low social status in all age groups are more often outside paid employment than are groups with higher social status. Research findings compellingly suggest that one important reason for this pattern is ill-health. People with lower social status tend to leave the labour market and remain outside because of health problems more than higher status groups do (e.g. Dahl and Birkelund 1997). It is likely that the work environment plays a role in these processes, but this is less well documented. This phenomenon may be judged in several ways. On the one hand it is a good thing, because low status people with poor health are able to leave a too demanding labour market and have the opportunity to lead a decent life on relatively generous benefits pro-vided by the welfare state. On the other hand it is a bad thing because the current labour market policies as well as employers' practices exclude disadvantaged socio-economic groups, who often suffer from poor health, from paid labour. Either way, there is a gap between the ideal of full employment and the actual employment rates, especially among groups with lower socio-economic status.

Norway is a member of the social democratic welfare state regime. The core-defining characteristic of this type of regime is, according to Esping-Andersen (1990), decommodification. This concept draws attention to the opportunities for 'all' to opt out of work and still be able to maintain the material means to lead a decent life. Universality and generosity are the major ingredients of decommodification: everyone is covered, and when they draw benefit, they can go on with the life they are accustomed to. By international standards sickness benefits, disability pension, and unemployment benefits are relatively high (Esping-Andersen 1990). In fact, sickness benefit ensures full-wage compensation from the very first day and for a full year, at least up to a ceiling. Under such circumstances most people do not have to fear selling their house or their belongings if health fails, or losing their job. Further, the opportunities granted by decommodification mean protection from fierce market forces. This protection also means freedom – freedom to choose to work or to choose not to work when circumstances are difficult.

In theory then, generous benefit levels are a good thing because they ensure a high degree of decommodification. Thereby they increase the freedom, for example relief from poor working conditions, and well-being among workers. On the other hand and according to the current economic orthodoxy, high benefits mean disincentives to work, and thereby create and sustain non-employment, social exclusion and reduced well-being. Further, high benefit levels may also tempt employers to lay off more people because they know that those sacked will not suffer from severe economic hardship. It should be noted that comparative research more than suggests that the social democratic welfare states perform among the best, not only in terms of the welfare and equality they produce, but also in terms of economic growth (Goodin *et al.* 1999). Nonetheless, it is hard to make a purely scientific judgement of the pros and cons based on hard facts, and whether today's balance is the optimal one.

7. Discussion: Do Working Conditions "Explain" Class Inequalities in Health?

How much of the relationship between social class and health may be explained by working conditions in the country? From the above exposition, it is clear that Norway has marked and consistent (perhaps even increasing) social class differentials in health, and no less marked social class differentials in terms of work environment, i.e., social

variations in exposures to harmful physical conditions and organisational aspects of the workplaces. But does this mean that working
conditions 'explain' the socio-economic variations in health? We will
now conduct two empirical analyses in order to shed some light on this
issue.

A. Class, Working Conditions and Health:
a Cross-sectional Approach

A possible (although problematic, see below) approach is to make a
cross-sectional analysis of the associations between health and social or
occupational class, and examine to what extent the class coefficients are
attenuated when working conditions and appropriate control variables
are included in multivariate analyses. Results from logistic regression
models are reported in table 15 a + b, using data from the five Surveys
of Level of Living 1980-1995. The response variable is the dichotomy
have/do not have a long-standing medical condition. The main explanatory variables are occupational class and three indices measuring current
working conditions. Estimates are adjusted for age group and survey
year. Two models are estimated – the first without, and the second with,
the three indices representing the burdens of disadvantageous working
conditions.

Table 15 a: ORs from logistic regression analyses of five Surveys of Level of Living 1980-1995, pooled. Long-standing medical condition (yes=1, no=0) regressed on current occupational class (model A) and current occupational class and current working conditions (Model B), adjusted for age group and survey year. Men

	Men			
	Model A		Model B	
	OR	p-val	OR	p-val
Workers				
– unskilled	1.68	<0.001	1.06	0.602
– skilled	1.52	<0.001	1.04	0.704
Salaried employees				
– lower level	1.29	0.091	1.09	0.588
– intermediate	1.17	0.075	1.11	0.249
– higher (reference)	1.00		1.00	
Working conditions indices				
– harmful environment			1.06	<0.001
– ergonomic strain			1.14	<0.001
– psychosocial strain			1.10	0.016
Age group				
– age 50-64	2.08	<0.001	2.27	<0.001
– age 35-49	1.23	0.002	1.30	<0.001
– age 20-34 (ref)	1.00		1.00	
Survey				
– 1995	1.30	0.004	1.26	0.012
– 1991	1.16	0.010	1.14	0.154
– 1987	1.17	0.073	1.15	0.124
– 1983	1.10	0.309	1.10	0.271
– 1980 (reference)	1.00		1.00	
Nagelkerke Rsquare	0.036	<0.001	0.055	<0.001
(N)	(5243)		(5243)	

Source: Statistic Norway's Surveys of Level of Living, own analyses of data file. Only currently employed are included, farmers and self-employed excluded. Indices of harmful environment and ergonomic strain: see table 11. Index of psychosocial strain in workplace: additive index of answer "very little" to three items: decide own working speed, decide working schedule, varied work (see table 12).

Table 15 b: ORs from logistic regression analyses of five Surveys of Level of Living 1980-1995, pooled. Long-standing medical condition (yes=1, no=0) regressed on current occupational class (model A) and current occupational class and current working conditions (Model B), adjusted for age group and survey year. Women

	Women			
	Model A		Model B	
	OR	p-val	OR	p-val
Workers				
– unskilled	1.21	0.145	0.92	0.563
– skilled	1.45	0.082	1.04	0.867
Salaried employees				
– lower level	1.06	0.623	0.96	0.737
– intermediate	1.00	0.970	0.95	0.638
– higher (reference)	1.00		1.00	
Working conditions indices				
– harmful environment			1.13	<0.001
– ergonomic strain			1.18	<0.001
– psychosocial strain			0.95	0.143
Age group				
– age 50-64	2.07	<0.001	2.28	<0.001
– age 35-49	1.30	<0.001	1.36	<0.001
– age 20-34 (ref)	1.00		1.00	
Survey				
– 1995	1.53	<0.001	1.47	<0.001
– 1991	1.34	0.004	1.28	0.017
– 1987	1.52	<0.001	1.46	0.001
– 1983	1.24	0.038	1.23	0.048
– 1980 (reference)	1.00		1.00	
Nagelkerke Rsquare	0.034	<0.001	0.058	<0.001
(N)	(4364)		(4364)	

Source: Statistic Norway's Surveys of Level of Living, own analyses of data file. Only currently employed are included, farmers and self-employed excluded. Indices of harmful environment and ergonomic strain: see table 11. Index of psychosocial strain in work-place: additive index of answer "very little" to three items: decide own working speed, decide working schedule, varied work (see table 12).

For men, the odds ratios (OR) for having a long-standing medical condition vary clearly with occupational class in the expected manner (model A). A striking result is that the effect of occupational class practically disappears when working conditions indices are included in the analysis (model B). Thus, it appears that very much of the social class variations among men in having (at least) one long-standing medical condition can be 'statistically explained' by the variations in working conditions. For women, however, the ORs for occupational class were rather small in model A, so there was not much class varia-tion to explain. Nevertheless, we note also here that working conditions

254

seem to have a considerable association with having or not having a long-term disease or illness.

This suggests, first, that variations in working conditions are quite strongly connected with variations in this health indicator (compared for instance with the age effect), and, second, among men (but not among women) that the social class variations in long-standing conditions can to a considerable extent be 'explained away' by the variations in their current working conditions. Two other health indicators can be formed from the same material, indicating psychological malaise and activity restrictions because of long-standing conditions, and the results are generally patterned the same way when these response variables are utilised.

But does this mean that the social variations in working conditions, at least for men, are a *major* factor behind the social class variations in health? A cross-sectional analysis of this kind has some obvious difficulties: first, that current health is a life-course result, and, second, that social class is not a fixed characteristic of a person. In the next section, we turn to a discussion of these problems.

B. Some Problems in Cross-sectional Analyses

The current health of any person is very seldom an instant effect of his/her contemporary circumstances, but should rather be seen in a life-course perspective. During a life course, a number of factors, many of which existed years or decades ago, will potentially have influenced current health status. A short list of such life-course factors will include material and social conditions during childhood and adolescence, health-related behaviours across the life course, material conditions and deprivation related to class situation at home rather than at work, life events, psycho-social circumstances during childhood, youth and adulthood, etc. – *and* the differential accumulation of exposures from good and bad working conditions across working life.

Moreover, many persons move between class locations during their life course. A significant proportion advance on the social ladder as they become older, and at the peak of their careers they often have less detrimental working conditions than before. At the point in their life course when previous unhealthy exposures become manifested in actual ill health, they will quite often be in a career phase far away from those working conditions that, in previous periods, were detrimental to their health development. Moreover, among many middle-aged people, one will often observe that those with rather health-damaging work conditions have surprisingly good health. This is hardly a 'proof' that the work environment is healthy. Rather, it arises because those who stay in such work are either lucky or especially healthy, and are therefore able to endure disadvantageous work environments. This phenomenon is known as 'the healthy worker effect'. On the other hand, those who failed to cope with exposures and strains have left and found less harmful or strenuous work. In fact, a very typical feature of Norway's current labour market is that severe, and also sometimes not-so-severe, health problems, which may have been the effect of their accumulated damaging working conditions, lead to exits from paid employment, making any cross-sectional correlation between health and working conditions potentially misleading. There is rather solid evidence of this kind of selection processes in Norway (Borgan 1996, Dahl and Birkelund 1997, Elstad and Krokstad 2003).

One would believe that such dynamics would generally tend to reduce cross-sectional associations between current health and current working conditions. These dynamics may in fact produce a 'reversed' association where good, and not bad, current health corresponds to unhealthy working conditions, at least in the later phases of a working career. In the light of these arguments, it is rather astonishing that the cross-sectional analysis reported in table 16 showed that the social class health variations among men could more or less be accounted for, in statistical terms, by the variations in currently reported working conditions.

C. Class, Working Conditions and Health among Middle-aged Men: A Life-course Approach

An attempt to take into account such dynamics has been made by (Elstad 2003). Using data obtained from retrospective interviews in a sample of 380 men aged 55, an index of burdensome working conditions across the working career was constructed, as well as indicators of lifestyle variations across the adult life course. Thus, variations in current self-reported health (an index based on several questions) among these 55-year-old men were predicted by unhealthy working conditions and poor health behaviours during their previous adult life course, adjusted for self-reported health at the age of 25. In the bivariate analyses, it turned out that both health behaviours and working conditions were associated with health at the age of 55, but in the multivariate regression analysis, only working conditions and especially physical working conditions, and not the lifestyle variables, retained a statistically significant effect (see table 16).

Table 16: Associations between an index measuring overall health status at age 55, and lifestyle factors, working conditions during adulthood, and health at the age of 25. Bivariate correlation coefficients (left) and OLS standardised regression coefficients from multivariate analyses (right). 380 Norwegian men, interviewed in 2001

	Bivariate correlations with health index age 55	OLS multivariate regression, response variable = health index age 55
Explanatory variables	Pearson r	Betas
Health at age 25	0.356[1]	0.293[1]
Smoking habits	0.125[3]	0.034[4]
Leisure time physical exercise	0.161[2]	0.033[4]
Weight problems	0.124[3]	0.077[4]
Physical working conditions	0.326[1]	0.240[1]
Psychosocial working conditions	0.201[1]	0.136[2]
Shift/night work	0.157[2]	0.058[4]
R^2		0.238[1]
Adjusted R^2		0.224

[1] $p<0,001$, [2] $p<0,01$, [3] $p<0,05$, [4] $p>0,05$.

Sources: Reproduced from Elstad (2003). Construction of health index: Zero/one long-standing illness = 0, two long-standing illnesses = 1, three long-standing illnesses = 2, four or more = 3. No/very few activity restrictions because of health problems = 0, some activity restrictions = 1, very much = 2. Very good self-perceived health = 0, good = 1, fair = 2, poor = 3. Values on these three items were added into each respondent's overall value on the health index. It can be argued that the index approximates an interval scale, which can therefore be analysed by means of OLS regression.

Immediately this suggests that, at least for this particular cohort of Norwegian men born in 1946 and observed in 2001, previous detrimental working conditions were more important for their current health problems than their degree of unhealthy lifestyles. Various problems connected to the validity of retrospective data, as well as possible bias in the analysed sample, e.g., response rate 64% (those in the cohort who had died could not be included in the gross sample), should not be overlooked. The response variable is 'biased' in a way, as it represents current self-reported ill health, but hardly the major causes of death.

Despite these problems, this suggests that previous variations in working conditions were quite strongly related to their current variations in health. A further suggestion is that the current emphasis on lifestyles in public health policies, although certainly not misplaced, could have been inspired to some extent by 'biased' studies which have often been interested in lifestyle factors but too often neglected work environments, so that the 'true' role of working conditions for the social patterning of health has been underestimated.

8. What About the Future?

The evidence presented here is of course in many ways fragmentary, but it suggests a viable hypothesis: the patterning of harmful working conditions has been disadvantageous for the health of those placed in the lower segments of the occupational hierarchy, and these social variations in working conditions are an important factor for social class differences in health, at least for men, but perhaps to a lesser degree for women.

This conclusion applies above all, however, to the middle-aged and older parts of the present-day male population. Although some working conditions may have instantaneous detrimental health effects (work accidents, for instance), the harmful influence of disadvantageous working conditions should in the main be seen as accumulated long-term effects. Relatively short stays in unhealthy work environments would perhaps seldom lead to drastically deteriorated health; thus, it seems not very plausible to explain social variations in health among men in their twenties or even thirties by their working conditions. Such a proposition seems much more probable as regards men in their forties and above.

Given that this suggested conclusion is correct: will working conditions continue to be a major factor for future social variations in health (among men), or in other words, for the cohorts born, say, after 1960?

To approach this question we will discuss four issues.

First, are exposures in working life (the general work environment) becoming less and less detrimental to health? Say, for instance, that there is a general trend, across all types of working environments, towards less exposures to ergonomic strain, unhealthy pollution, harmful psychosocial work milieu, etc. If so, the work arena will gradually lose its significance for the emergence of ill health. However, if the 10-year changes from the early 1980s to the mid-1990s demonstrated in tables 11-13 are representative for more long-term trends, it looks as if neither the physical nor the organisational working conditions on the whole are improving. This contrasts with what we often believe: that technological innovation together with political regulations of the work environment will gradually lead to a general improvement of the working environment. Spontaneously, we find it hard to believe that the physical working conditions have not improved, from, say, the 1950s till today. New technology and work environment regulations *must* have had some impact. But perhaps the changes have been less than has often been assumed? As for the *psychosocial* work environment, it is likely that it actually has become somewhat worse, because of increased competition in the private capitalist business sector, implementation of management reforms in the public sector, and efforts to speed up productivity by all kinds of employers, public as well as private. Data from recent surveys indicate that this is in fact the case.

Second, are the socio-economic *variations* in exposure to detrimental work environments becoming less and less marked? This is obviously related to the former question, but is not identical. If these variations become compressed, they will gradually become relatively less important for the emergence of socio-economic health disparities. Again, it is hard to answer this question, but tables 11-13 show that the social variations in potentially health-detrimental working conditions were no less marked in the early 1990s than ten years earlier. It should be noted that the social variations in working conditions seem more severe for the male than for the female working population – a fact which, when linked to the observation that social class health variations are less among women than among men, *could* be interpreted as indirect evidence that work environment variations are quite an important factor behind the male socio-economic health differences: where there are small socio-economic variations in work conditions, *in casu* among women, there are also smaller socio-economic health variations.

Third, is work becoming less and less prominent in people's life courses? In the cohorts born, say, around the First World War, many started to work in adolescence and continued (if their health allowed it) till they were 70 years of age (or even more), and they had weekly working hours of 48 or 45 and short holidays, during large parts of their working lives. The social variations in health which have been observed in mortality statistics and health surveys during the last third of the 20th century relate to a large extent to cohorts where work was paramount in people's life courses. Nowadays, education often continues into the twenties, actual retirement age is lower, holidays are longer, and the working week is considerably shortened (but the reduction in actual working hours has not been *so* great since the 1970s, cf. section 1.1). Even if health-detrimental work conditions and their social variations do not change, their health impact may be reduced in correspondence with a declining overall role of work in people's life circumstances. The other side of this coin would be that other circumstances (childhood influences, material conditions 'outside' work, health behaviours, etc.), formerly overshadowed by the impact of work, gradually become relatively more important determinants for health variations.

Fourth, are mobility regimes changing, with more frequent job shifts, career advancements, perhaps also more frequent occupational mobility downwards, more spells of career interruptions, periods with educational activity in adulthood, and numerous periods of unemployment which 'free' people from the influence of working conditions on their health? Such 'late modern' mobility regimes, *if* they are emerging, could disperse the exposures to unhealthy work environments both over the life course and across the social structure, and therefore imply that working conditions will be of less importance for health inequalities. Several of these decommodification processes were more legitimate in the 1970s and 1980s in many Western countries than they are today and have been for a while. Most policy reforms and initiatives during the 1990s aimed rather at re-commodifying labour. An analysis of social policy reforms that were implemented in Norway during the 1990s concluded that all but one reform referred to and furthered the so-called Work Approach (Dahl and Drøpping 2001). As data on employment rates in some subgroups, and disability rates show, the policies under the Work Approach umbrella fall short of being successful. But in most political camps the ideal of (paid) work is stronger than before, and most would like to strengthen the work ethic and increase participation rates in groups that are only loosely attached to the labour market. Programmes and measures that enhance work attachment in disadvantaged groups are popular. If current measures do not deliver the goods, and the work commitment prevails, which is likely, it might be that harsher remedies and measures will be introduced in the future. If both carrots and sticks are implemented, and both are used more aggressively than hitherto, the effects of work and working conditions on health may be more pronounced again. If more people are more or less forced to take up work where the working conditions are bad, this may have a detrimental impact on their health. But if the people who move to work get better and more rewarding jobs, their health may actually improve.

Summing up these arguments, we see that, on balance most of them point towards the suggestion that working conditions and the work environments will gradually attain a reduced role for the emergence of health inequalities and, by implication, for those socio-economic variations in health which will – or will not – be observed in the future. Needless to say, this discussion is speculative in nature; only time will tell.

Acknowledgements

Data collected by Statistics Norway and provided by the Norwegian Social Science Data Service have been analysed in this chapter. Neither of these two institutions is responsible for the analyses and interpretations of these data made in this chapter.

References

ANDRESEN Ø. 1998. Arbeidsmiljø: "Flere tidsfrister, rutiner og krav". *Samfunnsspeilet* 2.

ARNTZEN A., MOUM T., MAGNUS P., & BAKKETEIG L. S. 1996. "The association between maternal education and postneonatal mortality. Trends in Norway, 1968-1991". *International Journal of Epidemiology* 25: 578-584.

BIRKELAND E. 1999. "Stadig færre 60-åringer jobber". *Samfunnsspeilet* 5.

BORGAN J.-K. 1996. Socioeconomic trends i differential mortality among middle aged males in Norway 1960-1990. In Anonymous (ed.), *Yearbook of Population Research in Finland*. Helsinki: The Population Research Institute.

BORGAN J.-K., KRISTOFERSEN L. 1986. *Mortality by occupational and socioeconomic groups in Norway 1970-1980.* Oslo: Statistics Norway.

CLAUSSEN B., NÆSS Ø. 2002. "Mortality in Oslo by inequalities in occupational class". *Tidsskrift for Den norske lægeforening* 122: 1867-9.

CLAUSSEN B., SMITH G. D., THELLE D. 2003. "Impact of childhood and adulthood socioeconomic position on cause specific mortality: the Oslo Mortality Study". *Journal of Epidemiology and Community Health* 57: 40-45.

DAHL E. 1993a. "High Mortality in Lower Salaried Norwegian Men – the Healthy Worker Effect". *Journal of Epidemiology and Community Health* 47: 192-194.

—— 1993b. "Social Inequality in Health – the Role of the Healthy Worker Effect". *Social Science & Medicine* 36: 1077-1086.

—— 2002. "Health Inequalities and Health Policy": The Norwegian Case. *Norsk Epidemiologi* 12: 69-75.

DAHL E., BIRKELUND G. E. 1997. "Health inequalities in later life in a social democratic welfare state". *Social Science & Medicine* 44: 871-881.

—— 1999. "Employment, class, and health, 1980-1995: An analysis of five Norwegian surveys". *Tidsskrift for Samfunnsforskning* 40: 3-32.

DAHL E., DRØPPING J.A. 2001. The Norwegian Work Approach in the 1990s: Rhetoric and Reform. In Neil GILBERT and Rebecca A. VAN VOORHIS (eds.) *Activating the Unemployed. A Comparative Appraisal of Work-Oriented Policies*. New Brunswick: Transaction Publishers.

DAHL E., KJAERSGAARD P. 1993. "Trends in Socioeconomic Mortality Differentials in Postwar Norway – Evidence and Interpretations". *Sociology of Health & Illness* 15: 587-611.

DAHL E., ELSTAD J. I., HOFOSS D. 2003. Project: Social inequalities in health: social capital or social investments? *Project proposal*. Oslo: NOVA.

ESPING-ANDERSEN G. 1990. *The Three Worlds of Welfare Capitalism*. Cambridge: Polity Press.

ELSTAD J. I. 1996. "How large are the differences – really? Self-reported long-standing illness among working class and middle class men". *Sociology of Health & Illness* 18: 475-498.

—— 2003. "Livsstil, arbeidsmiljøbelastninger og helseulikheter blant 55-årige menn". *Tidsskrift for Den norske Lægeforening* 123: 2289-2291.

ELSTAD J. I., KROKSTAD S. 2003. "Social causation, health-selective mobility, and the reproduction of socioeconomic health inequalities over time: panel study of adult men". *Social Science & Medicine* 57: 1475-1489.

GOODIN R.E., HEADY B., MUFFELS R., DIRVEN H.-J. 1999. *The Real Worlds of Welfare Capitalism*. Cambridge: Cambridge University Press.

HOLME I., HELGELAND A., HJERMANN I., LEREN P. LUND-LARSEN P. G. 1980. "4-Year Mortality by Some Socioeconomic Indicators – Oslo Study". *Journal of Epidemiology and Community Health* 34: 48-52.

HOLME I., HELGELAND A., HJERMANN I. LEREN P. 1982. "Socioeconomic Status as a Coronary Risk Factor – the Oslo Study". *Acta Medica Scandinavica* 147-151.

HOLTE H. H. 2002. *Disability pensioning with musculoskeletal diseases in Norway*. Thesis. Oslo: Faculty of Medicine: University of Oslo.

KROKSTAD S., KUNST A. E., WESTIN S. 2002a. "Trends in health inequalities by educational level in a Norwegian total population study". *Journal of Epidemiology and Community Health* 56: 375-380.

KROKSTAD S., WESTIN S. 2002. "Health inequalities by socioeconomic status among men in the Nord-Trondelag Health Study, Norway". *Scandinavian Journal of Public Health* 30: 113-124.

KROKSTAD S., JOHNSEN R., WESTIN S. 2002b. "Social determinants of disability pension: a 10-year follow-up of 62,000 people in a Norwegian county population". *International Journal of Epidemiology* 31: 1183-1191.

KUNST A. 1991. "Cross-national comparisons of socio-economic differences in mortality". Thesis. Rotterdam: Department of Public Health: Erasmus University.

MIDTSUNDSTAD T. 2001. *Pensjonering i stat og skoleverk*. Fafo-notat 2001: 2: Oslo: Fafo.

MOEN B. E., RIISE T., HOLLUND B. E. & TORP S. 2002. *Arbeidsrelaterte plager i Hordaland.* Rapport 3/2002. Bergen: Seksjon for arbeidsmedisin: Universitetet i Bergen.

RAMM J. 2000. *Helseundersøkelsene 1968, 1975, 1985, 1995, 1998: dokumentasjon og spørreskjema*. Notater 2000/55. Oslo: Statistics Norway.

ROGNERUD M., STRAND B. H., HESSELBERG Ø. 2000. *The health of disadvantaged groups in Norway*. Oslo: National Institute of Public Health.

ROMMETVEIT A. 1997. *Levekårsundersøkelser 1981/ 1983/ 1987/ 1991/ 1995. Dokumentasjon og frekvensoversikter.* Bergen: Norsk samfunnsvitenskapelig datatjeneste.

SSB: 1982. *Statistical Yearbook 1982.* Oslo, Statistics Norway.

—— 2001. *Statistical Yearbook 2001.* Oslo, Statistics Norway.

—— 2002. *Statistical Yearbook 2002.* Oslo, Statistics Norway.

—— 2003. *Labour Force Survey 2001.* Oslo, Statistics Norway.

—— 2004. *Statistical Yearbook 2004.* Oslo, Statistics Norway.

—— www.ssb.no/emner/06/01/aku/, consulted January 17, 2005.

ST. MELD. 2002. Nr. 16 (2002-2003). "Resept for et sunnere Norge". *Folkehelsepolitikken.* Oslo: Det Kongelige Helsedepartement.

THÜRMER, H. 1993. "Risk factors for a, and 13-year mortality from, cardiovascular disease by socioeconomic status". Thesis. Tromsø: Institutt for samfunnsmedisin: Universitetet i Tromsø.

WHITEHEAD M. 1998. "Diffusion of Ideas on Social Inequalities in Health: A European Perspective". *The Milbank Quarterly* 76: 469-492.

ZAHL P.-H., ROGNERUD M., STRAND B. H. & TVERDAL A. 2003. *Bedre helse – større forskjeller. En analyse av hvordan inntekt, utdanning og husholdningsstørrelse har påvirket dødeligheten i befolkningen i periodene 1970-77, 1980-87 og 1990-1997.* Oslo: National Institute of Public Health.

Massachusetts, USA

John WOODING, David H. WEGMAN
& Kimberly RAUSCHER

Introduction

This chapter provides an introduction to the relationship between work, health and social inequality in the United States. As part of a collaborative overview of these issues between several European countries and the US, we face some special problems in equating knowledge and data between and across the various country studies. In this case we have chosen to focus only on Massachusetts. As a single state in a federated country, Massachusetts provides a fairly rough equivalency to the other countries under discussion here. As one of the oldest and most industrialized states in the US, Massachusetts is a good choice for this kind of comparative study. With a population of a little over 6 million and a land area of approximately 8000 square miles, Massachusetts is considerably smaller than other countries in this collaboration, yet its demographic and industrial features allow for rough comparisons and are reflective of some general trends in the US.

The United States is the only non-European country in this study. As such there are a number of specific peculiarities of the American experience that should be noted from the outset. Most obviously, Massachusetts is one of 50 states in a federated system of a very large country. While, like all American states, it maintains an independent legislature with control over state budgets, policies and laws, the federal system means that all policies, programs and economic actors are – to a greater or lesser degree – deeply affected by federal laws and public policy. Massachusetts is also part of an extensive and homogenous domestic market.

American culture and traditions are also worthy of note in a comparative context. The United States is a country of immigrants, and race continues to play a very significant role in all aspects of life and social policy. Founded under strong traditions of liberalism, inherited in part from the UK, but not augmented or mediated either by the influence of the socialist and social-democratic ideas so prevalent in Europe, or by the existence of strong labour organisations with formal political representation in the form of parties, the country has traditionally been seen as a "weak state". As a result, social welfare and social programs are fairly rudimentary by European standards. The population regards government and the public sector with some scepticism generally. The rights and protection of workers are fairly limited. Trade Unions represent only about 12% of workers in the private sector, about 14% if public employee unions are included. There is no national health care system and the vast majority of workers are covered by private insurers (although a very large number at any one time have no health insurance). Income tax rates are low compared with Europe, although some of this revenue is made up by a variety of indirect sales and property taxes that vary widely by state and locale. Many services that are provided by governments in Europe are provided privately in the US, and funded either through local government or directly paid by the consumer.

Massachusetts is one of the oldest states in the Union and was one of the earliest to become industrialised. It is traditionally regarded as among the more progressive politically and considered a Democratic stronghold, although in the last decade or so, governors have been Republican and the traditions of progressivism have faded rapidly. As is true of most countries with early industrialisation, Massachusetts today is dominated by its service sector economy, and possesses few physical resources other than its relatively highly skilled and educated population.

1. Social Class, Work and Health

One of the core questions posed by this work is the relationship between social class (variously described as social inequity, income differential, socio-economic status, etc.), the kind of work individuals are engaged in, and the health outcomes that result. Very little research has examined the intervening and specific role played by occupation (or the work environment) as mediating socio-economic status and health. The ways in which the workplace – and an individual's occupation – connects socio-economic position and health are poorly conceptualised and not well understood.

The relationship between "health and wealth", however, is pretty clear. Put simply, the assumption of much of the literature in this area is that the lower the social class status, the more likely an individual will suffer ill health and premature death. As Kaplan notes:

A substantial body of evidence demonstrates strong inverse associations between social class and health outcomes, with higher class being associated with lower risk. This pattern is generally found, regardless of what measure of social class is used, what outcomes are studied, and when and where the analyses are done (Kaplan 1996).

Numerous other studies support this central assertion, across a wide range of diseases. Social class position correlates with the incidence of death and disease (Winkleby *et al.* 1992, Kaplan & Lynch 1999, Syme & Berkman 1976, Pappas *et al.* 1993, Sorle *et al.* 1995, Streenland *et al.* 2004). However, this assertion does not capture the full complexity of the potential variables affecting the sets of relationships implicit in the "health and wealth" relation. The relationship between an individual's social class and risk of premature death or disease demands closer scrutiny. What factors play a role here? In what ways do income, education and occupation work together to determine health outcomes?

In the American context, the debate about the relationship between class and health has been framed as a debate about "social disparities and health" or "health disparities". Given the lack of class-based data and the paucity of information about general working conditions there has been surprisingly little research connecting class, work and health. A recent debate helps locate some of the issues, and might be applied not only to the question of the social class determinants of health, but also for thinking about the ways in which work affects these relations. Lynch has pointed out, for example, that we can interpret the association between income inequality and health in three ways: at the individual income level; as a result of the psychosocial environment; and at what Lynch defines as the "neo-material" level (Lynch 2000).

At the level of individual income it is clear that the association between income and health enables wealthier individuals to access the health-related resources that higher levels of income can buy. This is the basis for many of the conclusions of the major studies of social inequality and health. Lynch points out, however, that such results are not observable for aggregate level data, and that this raises questions about the usefulness of an interpretation or approach that cannot shed light on larger populations (Lynch 2000). Lynch's interpretation at the "neo-material" level provides an understanding of this relationship that relies on prior conditions, not simply individual wealth or income. These conditions involve, but are not limited to, such things as investment in education, health services, transportation, housing, etc. – in other words, those conditions which provide accessible resources for individuals. "The effect of income inequality on health reflects both lack of resources held by individuals, and systematic under-investment across a wide range of community infrastructure" (Lynch 2000).

The recent advocacy of a "psychosocial environment" approach takes a somewhat different view. As Lynch characterises this:

The psychosocial environment interpretation views health inequalities as the result of perceptions of relative income. These perceptions produce negative emotions like shame and distrust that are translated into poorer health at the individual level through psycho-neuro-endrocrine mechanisms, and health-damaging behaviours... under this view it is social rank *per se* that produces poorer individual and population health (Lynch 2000).

It is clear that level of income and social rank will have some effect on health outcomes across a range of related variables, and that the idea of the "neo-material" conditions of life are basic to income level, access to health, and to the perception of social rank with all the concomitant health consequences this may have. Further, as Lynch argues, many of these consequences will be mediated (positively or negatively) by the "social connectedness" of groups in a population or a community. We raise this discussion here, however, as a way of framing the following comments. If we are to understand how class, work and health interact we need to sketch out this relationship in a little more detail.

We know that socio-economic status impacts health in the broadest sense and that income levels directly affect an individual's access to health resources; that social rank (both socially constructed and individually internalised) will change health-related behaviours; and that a whole range of material conditions interact with social connections, psycho-social factors and, indeed, with cultural, historical and ideological contexts, to define the health of a given population (Coburn 2000). But what role does work have in all this?

As we noted above, there are no data available in the US that directly link social class, working conditions, occupation, and health outcome. What we do know (and is documented in the information gathered here) is that socio-economic position (defined in terms of income, race and education) will determine in part an individual's access to a given occupation. Typically, in the US as elsewhere, the lower the socioeconomic position the more likely the only work available will be lower paid, unskilled and consequently the more likely that the employee will be exposed to physical injury and to toxic chemicals.

A second dilemma resulting from the relationship between income, education and work is that occupation will frequently determine income as well as the resultant access (for families especially) not only to health resources, community support structures and information, but also to education and educational opportunity. This, in turn, will determine the accessibility of higher paid, safer and more meaningful work. Often, therefore, the circularity of relationship between socio-economic status and work and health is all too evident. This makes it particularly difficult to isolate work from other social, economic and cultural factors that may – in combination or individually – determine social class, access to a safer workplace and general health consequences.

In the light of the foregoing discussion, the remainder of this paper gathers together such data as is currently available that will identify class structure in Massachusetts by using income, education and race to illustrate broad demographic patterns. We pay particular attention to gender and race, the structure of the labour market (types of occupation, part-time versus full-time work), and the level of unionisation. The second section of the paper identifies and illustrates the relationship between health and social class in general, and in relation to occupation and work environment in particular. Some limited data are presented that are related to working conditions in the US as a whole. We conclude by considering the overall connection between class, health and work, and offer some preliminary recommendations for further work.

2. Education

While Massachusetts is historically among the better US states in terms of overall education of its population, its citizens are considerably better educated today than in years past. The percentage of all adults with a 4-year college degree has roughly doubled since 1980 (table 1). Following from greater participation in the workforce and congruent with international trends, women's educational attainment in Massachusetts has been rising over the last two decades. Today, many more women are earning post-secondary degrees. In 1980, approximately 9% of women earned a bachelor's degree and 6% earned an advanced degree. By 2000, these percentages had more or less doubled. The percentage of women who have at least attended college or who have earned an "associate's degree" (a lower-level degree) has also increased. Today, 26% of women have received some college education or gained a two-year degree, versus only 16% in 1980.

**Table 1: Size (%) of Educational Attainment Groups[1]
by Gender (ages ≥25), 1980-2000**

Level of attainment	Males			Females		
	1980	**1990**	**2000**	**1980**	**1990**	**2000**
Total population 25≥ years	1,585,096	1,846,603	2,003,520	1,878,160	2,115,620	2,269,755
Less than high school diploma	27.6	19.6	15.4	28.0	20.4	15.1
High school diploma/equivalency	32.0	27.2	26.7	40.1	31.9	27.8
Some college/ "Associate's" degree (lower level)	15.4	22.3	22.7	16.1	23.6	25.7
Bachelor's degree	11.8	17.8	20.0	9.1	15.5	19.0
Advanced degree	13.3	13.0	15.1	6.6	8.6	12.4

Note: Numbers may not total 100% due to rounding.
Source: US Census Bureau.

3. Race

While the United States is characteristically highly diverse, the population of Massachusetts is predominantly white. Racial diversity has increased in Massachusetts somewhat over the past 20 years for both males and females (table 2). The number of white males and females (of the working age population) has decreased by slightly less than 10% and the African American male population has increased modestly. The largest increase of any single ethnic category is among Asians, whose population in the state rose considerably from 1980 onwards, largely due to immigration from South East Asia during the late 1980s. The percentage of those who classify their race as "other" has also risen – from 0.2 in 1980 to roughly 4.0 in 2000 (for men and women). For whites and African Americans, the population shifts were identical within the general *and* the working age populations. However, Asians and those identified as members of some "other" race increased

---

[1] Some of the educational groupings in this table are classified differently in different time periods. For 1980, *High school diploma/equivalency* is classified by the US Census as "High School: 4 years" and does not include equivalency. *Some college/ "Associate's" degree* is classified as "College: 1 to 3 years"; and *Advanced degree* is classified as "College: 5 or more years". For 1990, *Advanced degree* is made up of the three Census classifications, "master's degree", "professional school degree", and "doctorate degree".

their representation within the working age population at a greater rate than they did in the overall population. The implications are clear: the Massachusetts workforce is now more diverse, but this diversity increasingly consists of people of Asian descent.

Table 2: Size (%) of Racial Groups by Gender
(working age population*), 1980-2000

Racial classification[2]	Males			Females		
	1980	1990	2000	1980	1990	2000
Total working age population	1,785,215	1,992,920	2,027,476	1,904,380	2,065,620	2,111,979
White	95.1	89.9	86.3	94.9	89.8	86.0
Black	3.7	4.9	5.4	4.0	5.1	5.6
Asian	1.0	2.6	4.3	1.0	2.5	4.2
Other[3]	0.2	2.6	4.0	0.2	2.6	4.1
Hispanic origin	N/A	4.60	6.8	N/A	4.50	6.8

*1990-2000=ages 15-64, 1980=ages 16-64. ^Does not include those classified as being of "two or more races". Note: N/A=data not available/reported. Numbers may not total 100% due to rounding. Source: US Census Bureau.

4. Income and Social Class

A. Education

Not surprisingly, the earnings of the working population in Massachusetts steadily improve with the years of education they have. Having less than a high school diploma puts one at the bottom of the earnings

---

[2]   For all tables with racial groups that use data from the US Census Bureau, White, Black, Asian and Other, may include persons classified as being "of Hispanic origin". Of Hispanic origin includes persons classified as being "of Hispanic origin" and they may be of any race. Please note that some groups are classified differently by the Census in different time periods. For 1980-1990, Asian is classified by the Census as "Asian and Pacific Islander". For 2000, the classification is "Asian", with Pacific Islanders classified under Native Hawaiian and Other Pacific Islander (for the tables in this chapter, included under Other). For 1980-1990, Black is classified as "Black". For 2000, the classification is "Black or African American". For 1990, Hispanic origin is classified as "of Hispanic origin". For 2000, the classification is "Hispanic or Latino".

[3]   For all tables with racial groups that use data from the US Census Bureau, the category *Other* is made up of a mix of different racial classifications in different time periods. For 1980, it is made up of the one Census classification, "American Indian, Eskimo or Aleut". For 1990, it is made up of the two classifications, "other race" and "American Indian, Eskimo or Aleut". For 2000, it is made up of "some other race", "American Indian and Alaska Native" (formerly, American Indian, Eskimo or Aleut) and "Native Hawaiian and other Pacific Islander" (formerly included with Asian).

scale. In terms of earnings, the benefit of this additional education is much greater today than it was 20 years ago. The situation of those without a high school education is grim, with annual and hourly earnings decreasing substantially since 1979. Over the last 20 years, it has been those with a college education who have realised earnings gains. Those with some level of graduate education have achieved the greatest increases. Clearly the shift from manufacturing to service industry and a concomitant increase in professionalisation has benefited those with college education, particularly at the post-bachelor degree level. As is clearly shown in table 3, in Massachusetts the earnings of both men and women have risen since 1980; however, women's earnings have increased much more substantially than those of men. Those with a post-graduate degree have benefited most.

Table 3: Annual Median Income[a] among Educational Groups by Gender (working age population*), 1980-2000

Level of attainment	Males			Females		
	1980	1990	2000	1980	1990	2000
Worked, with earnings						
For total working age population	15,671	32,141	45,862	7,452	17,641	27,802
Less than high school diploma	11,435	19,587	19,861	5,768	11,572	13,928
High school diploma/equivalency	13,667	24,952	33,079	6,864	14,119	20,341
Some college/ "Associate's" degree (lower level)	13,893	27,320	37,053	6,954	16,121	23,503
Bachelor's degree	21,004	40,775	66,668	9,529	22,499	37,650
Advanced degree	25,687	59,619	82,310	12,478	30,356	45,173
Worked full-time, year round, with earnings[4]						
For total working age population	18,884	40,252	45,041	10,844	25,337	39,990
Less than high school diploma	14,163	26,340	17,528	8,453	17,570	12,000
High school diploma/equivalency	15,976	30,416	34,866	9,975	20,472	20,065
Some college/ "Associate's" degree (lower level)	18,318	35,878	38,336	11,172	24,408	32,568
Bachelor's degree	24,023	47,524	51,441	12,932	30,226	55,315
Advanced degree	28,912	67,826	90,910	16,188	39,131	63,921

[a] *In dollars (figures for some educational groups are weighted averages).*
*2000=ages 16 and over, 1980-90=ages 18 and over.
Sources: 2000=Bureau of Labor Statistics, Current Population Survey. 1980-1990=US Census Bureau.

---

[4] For all tables with income figures, *Worked full-time, year round, with income* is defined by the US Census Bureau as follows: 1980, "usually worked 35 or more hours per week and 40 or more weeks per year"; and 1990-2000, "usually worked 35 hours or more per week for 50 to 52 weeks".

B. Race

In Massachusetts, income varies greatly by race and, as we have noted above, race may sometimes be used as a substitute for class in the American context. The income disparities between whites and racial minorities have increased steadily since 1980 (table 4). In the last 20 years, whites have had hourly and annual earnings increases of over 21%, yet Black and Hispanic workers have had overall losses. After experiencing increases in earnings during the 1980s, Black workers had earnings losses of approximately 2%; and Hispanic workers had earnings losses of nearly 10% by the end of the 1990s, taking them below 1979 earnings levels (Albelda & Kim 2002).

Table 4: Annual Median Income[a] among Racial Groups by Gender (ages ≥15), 1980-2000

Racial classification[1]	Males			Females		
	1980	1990	2000	1980	1990	2000
Worked, with income						
For total[+] population 15> years	12,244	24,215	32,406	5,309	12,155	19,173
White	12,462	25,226	35,007	5,317	12,318	19,825
Black	8,630	16,798	22,171	5,586	12,139	18,807
Asian	9,138	16,866	32,406	5,517	10,931	19,173
Other[b5]	9,186	12,976	18,065	4,904	7,710	11,585
Hispanic origin	N/A	13,417	18,430	N/A	8,242	12,153
Worked full-time, year round, with income[6]						
For total[+] population 15> years	17,215	32,749	45,130	10,773	23,090	33,281
White	17,401	33,656	46,663	10,817	23,413	34,683
Black	13,376	23,217	32,115	10,235	21,208	29,248
Asian	16,716	29,386	45,130	10,701	22,185	33,281
Other	14,447	20,581	26,565	9,311	17,405	22,677
Hispanic origin	N/A	20,664	26,606	N/A	17,737	24,150

[a] *In dollars.* [b]*Figures are weighted averages.*
Note: N/A=data not available/reported. + does not include those classified as being of "two or more races".
Source: US Census Bureau.

---

[5] For all tables with racial groups that use data from the US Census Bureau, the category *Other* is made up of a mix of different racial classifications in different time periods. For 1980, it is made up of the one Census classification, "American Indian, Eskimo or Aleut". For 1990, it is made up of the two classifications, "other race" and "American Indian, Eskimo or Aleut". For 2000, it is made up of "some other race", "American Indian and Alaska Native" (formerly, American Indian, Eskimo or Aleut) and "Native Hawaiian and other Pacific Islander" (formerly included with Asian).

[6] For all tables with income figures, *Worked full-time, year round, with income* is defined by the US Census Bureau as follows: 1980, "usually worked 35 or more hours per week and 40 or more weeks per year"; and 1990-2000, "usually worked 35 hours or more per week for 50 to 52 weeks".

In 1980, the *per capita* income for Blacks and American Indians was 65 and 69%, respectively, of what it was for whites. By 2000, those figures were down to 58 and 57%. The disparity between Whites and Asians is much smaller, yet it has still increased over the same period. In 1980, Asians' *per capita* income was 83% of that for whites, while in 2000 it was reduced to 77%.

5. Immigrant Workers and Social Class

A. Education

In general, we find immigrant workers at the lower levels of the social class pyramid. Typically less educated and denied easy access to further education by economic and social barriers, immigrant workers are only now beginning to gain a foothold in order to earn the privileges that come with education. While immigrant workers have shown some progress in gaining high school diplomas or the equivalent since 1994 (from 33% to 41% by 2004), the number of immigrants receiving some college education has declined since 2000. This is probably due to the rapid increase in the cost of such education, even in the public colleges and universities (table 5). Again, female immigrant workers have made notable gains in higher education.

Table 5: Proportion (%) of Employed Immigrants[7] (ages ≥16) within Educational Groups by Gender, 1994-2004

Level of attainment	Males			Females		
	1994	2000	2004	1994	2000	2004
Total non-citizen, employed population (n)	103,954	142,717	188,577	64,895	128, 969	97,744
Less than high school diploma	24	28	12	32	37	12
High school diploma/equivalency	33	22	41	15	31	26
Some college/"Associate's" degree (lower level)	16	26	13	23	20	14
Bachelor's degree or higher	28	25	34	30	11	49

Note: Numbers may not total 100% due to rounding.
Source: US Bureau of Labor Statistics, Current Population Survey.

---

[7] For all tables on immigrant workers using data from the Bureau of Labor Statistics, Current Population Survey, figures are for those classified as "foreign-born, non-US citizens" and who are employed members of the current labour force.

B. Race

Some of the differences between racial groups within the immigrant worker population become evident in the data from the last 10 years. By 2004, over 70% of the male, white non-citizen population and 50% of the female population were employed (table 6). The data for the non-white population clearly shows major distinctions for the employment opportunities of the immigrant population. Black and Asian immigrants clearly have much less chance of being fully employed than the white population, and only Asian women seem to have made notable progress over the last 10 years; the percentage of those women who are employed has doubled over this period. Black men and women have lost ground since 1994.

Table 6: Proportion (%) of Employed Immigrants[8] (age ≥16) within Racial Groups by Gender, 1994-2004

Total non-citizen, employed immigrant population	Males			Females		
	1994	2000	2004	1994	2000	2004
Racial classification (n)	103,954	142,717	188,577	64,895	128,969	97,744
White	62	70	72	64	57	50
Black	16	23	13	15	30	18
Asian	10	7	13	16	13	32
Other	12	0	1	5	0	0
Hispanic origin	21	28	26	11	34	15

Note: Numbers may not total 100% due to rounding.
Source: US Bureau of Labor Statistics, Current Population Survey.

6. Labour Market Position

A. Labour Force

The Massachusetts civilian labour force (people over 16 who are working or looking for work) was estimated to be about three and a quarter million in 2000. In 2001, about 70% of men over 16 years of age and about 57% of women were working – levels that have remained fairly stable over the last 20 years, the only notable increase being female workforce participation during the 1980s. Of those working,

---

[8] For all tables on immigrant workers using data from the Bureau of Labor Statistics, Current Population Survey, figures are for those classified as "foreign-born, non-US citizens" and who are employed members of the current labour force.

about 55% of the men and 45% of the women were salaried and waged workers in the private sector (see table 7).

Among the differing age groups, some notable developments have clearly characterised workforce participation rates. The number of both male and female workers under 19 years of age has declined in the last 20 years, while the number of workers in their earlier 2000s has remained fairly steady. The key age group, those between 24 and 54, remain employed at a relatively constant rate, with some decline since 1980 in the percentage of men employed. As the population ages, employment rates, for men in particular, are slowly declining, and gradually increasing for women (see table 8). As is the case for many advanced industrial societies, the working population is ageing, and the number of retirees in Massachusetts will increase significantly over the next 20 years. Nevertheless, it is interesting to note that nearly one third of males over the age of 65 in Massachusetts are still working. Indeed, 13% of males over 70 years of age are still employed. The number of government workers and the number of self-employed (both men and women) has remained fairly consistent over the last 20 years.

Table 7: Labour Market Positions (%) by Gender (ages ≥16), 1980-2000

Employment status	Males			Females		
	1980	1990	2000	1980	1990	2000
Total population 16≥ years (n)	2,076,546	2,268,095	2,370,006	2,383,663	2,541,677	2,640,235
Civilian labour force	75.0	75.6	72.4	52.8	60.2	60.4
Employed	71.0	69.9	69.0	50.4	56.7	57.8
Private wage & salary workers	55.2	55.7	55.5	39.7	45.7	46.0
Government workers	10.7	8.8	8.1	9.2	8.4	8.8
Self-employed workers	4.9	5.2	5.3	1.2	2.4	2.9
Unpaid family workers	0.1	0.1	0.1	0.2	0.2	0.1
Unemployed	4.0	5.7	3.4	2.4	3.5	2.6
Not in labour force	22.6	23.8	27.4	44.5	39.7	39.6

Note: Numbers may not total 100% due to rounding and the omission of the armed forces population.
Source: US Census Bureau.

B. Employment and Unemployment

Unemployment rates differ by gender, yet they have become more similar over the last 20 years. In 1980, 4% of men were unemployed and 2.4% of women were without work. By 2000, 3.4% of men and 2.5% of women were unemployed. During the long economic boom of the 1990s the general unemployment rate went down, although for the last 20 years the unemployment rate of men has generally been higher than that of women. The unemployment rate of young workers (men and women between 16 and 24) has tended to be consistently higher than that of the more mature worker (table 8 a + b).

The gender makeup of the employed population has shifted to include more women. The percentage of women who are employed today (58) rose by almost 7.5 percentage points from what it was during the late 1970s. For the last two decades those who work for themselves have mainly been men; however, we can see that the gender gap among the self-employed has been narrowing.

Table 8 a: Proportion (%) Working in Different Age Groups, 1980-2000. Males

Age group		1980	1990	2000
16-19 years	Total population (n)	221,074	170,349	167,270
	Employed	46.7	44.7	43.4
	Unemployed	6.7	10.0	8.6
	Not in labour force	45.9	44.6	47.9
20-24 years	Total population (n)	270,376	251,143	199,216
	Employed	71.8	68.3	68.2
	Unemployed	6.5	9.6	7.4
	Not in labour force	19.8	20.6	24.0
25-54 years	Total population (n)	1,038,518	1,292,959	1,403,579
	Employed	89	86	84
	Unemployed	3.9	5.8	3.1
	Not in labour force	6.8	7.6	12.2
55-64 years	Total population (n)	275,819	241,277	258,884
	Employed	74.3	69.5	68.7
	Unemployed	2.9	4.1	2.6
	force	22.8	26.5	28.6
65-69 years*	Total population (n)	270,759	112,439	99,649
	Employed	19.0	N/A	32.4
	Unemployed	1.2	N/A	1.0
	Not in labour force	79.8	67.2	66.5
≥70 years	Total population (n)	--	199,928	241,408
	Employed	--	N/A	13.37
	Unemployed	--	N/A	0.4
	Not in labour force	--	86.7	86.2

*1980 figures are for those 65 years and over (includes ≥70 years).
Notes: N/A=data not available/reported. Numbers may not total 100% due to rounding.
Source: US Census Bureau.

Table 8 b: Proportion (%) Working in Different Age Groups, 1980-2000. Females

Age group		1980	1990	2000
16-19 years	Total population (n)	222,854	169,161	163,557
	Employed	48.4	51.1	46.9
	Unemployed	4.8	6.9	7.5
	Not in labour force	46.8	42.5	45.6
20-24 years	Total population (n)	282,649	256,896	206,923
	Employed	68.4	70.1	69.1
	Unemployed	3.7	5.3	5.9
	Not in labour force	27.7	24.4	24.9
25-54 years	Total population (n)	1,104,050	1,334,655	1,465,801
	Employed	64	74	75
	Unemployed	2.7	4.0	2.6
	Not in labour force	33.1	21.8	22.7
55-64 years	Total population (n)	318,750	273,405	285,410
	Employed	48.3	51.4	56.9
	Unemployed	1.8	2.6	1.7
	Not in labour force	49.9	46.0	41.3
65-69 years*	Total population (n)	455,360	142,322	117,626
	Employed	8.0	N/A	22.7
	Unemployed	0.5	N/A	0.6
	Not in labour force	91.5	70.3	76.7
70> years	Total population (n)	--	365,238	400,918
	Employed	--	N/A	5.79
	Unemployed	--	N/A	0.3
	Not in labour force	--	94.5	93.9

*1980 figures are for those 65 years and over (includes 70> years).
Notes: N/A=data not available/reported. Numbers may not total 100% due to rounding.
Source: US Census Bureau.

C. Full- and Part-time Workers

The rate of employment is not always captured realistically by the data. For example, among the total working-age male population (≥16 years old) in 2000, 78% worked at least 1 week in the previous year, of whom 85.3% were employed full-time (worked ≥35 hours/week). Many people who would like to work full-time cannot find full-time work, and therefore work part-time or in a temporary capacity; and, although they could have worked as little as 1 hour in 1 week (a rare possibility) they are recorded as working. The proportions of full- and part-time workers help to shed light on the real employment situation in Massachusetts, as in other countries and states. The number of men and women working part-time (less than 35 hours per week) has remained steady over the last 10 years, but over twice as many women as men are engaged in part-time work. Again, this has remained consistent over the last two decades. Just over 11% of men were working between 15 and 34 hours per week in 2000. In contrast, nearly 30% of women were working this number of hours per week (see table 9 a + b).

Table 9 a: Proportion (%) of Full- and Part-time Workers by Gender for the Working-age Population who Worked, 1980-2000. Males

Usual hours worked per week	Males		
	1980	**1990**	**2000**
Total working-age population* (n)	1,967,198	2,268,095	2,370,006
Total who worked (n)	1,607,034	1,840,377	1,853,473
Full-time (≥35)	88.1	85.4	85.3
Part-time (1-34 hours)	11.4	14.6	14.7
(15-34 hours)	N/A	11.7	11.5
(1-14 hours)	N/A	3.0	3.3

1990-2000=ages ≥16, 1980=ages ≥18.
Notes: "Total who worked" includes the civilian and non-civilian population.
N/A=data not available/reported. Numbers may not total 100% due to rounding.
Source: US Census Bureau.

Table 9 b: Proportion (%) of Full- and Part-time Workers by Gender for the Working-age Population who Worked, 1980-2000. Females

Usual hours worked per week	Females		
	1980	**1990**	**2000**
Total working-age population* (n)	2,277,749	2,541,677	2,640,235
Total who worked (n)	1,332,161	1,672,948	1,746,551
Full-time (35>)	63.7	64.2	65.7
Part-time (1-34)	35.8	35.8	34.3
(15-34)	N/A	28.9	27.9
(1-14)	N/A	6.9	6.4

1990-2000=ages 16 and over, 1980=ages 18 and over
Notes: "Total who worked" includes the civilian and non-civilian population.
N/A=data not available/reported. Numbers may not total 100% due to rounding.
Source: US Census Bureau.

D. *Employment by Industry and Occupation*

In common with other industrial countries, employment by industry in Massachusetts reflects the general trend away from traditional manufacturing into service work. The number of men working in manufacturing is nearly half of what it was in 1980, and the figures for women are even clearer: the proportion working in manufacturing has declined from 20% in 1980 to just over 8% by 2000. As is to be expected, services make up the last proportion of employment in 2000: over one third of the men and over half of the women are currently employed in the service sector. There has been a slight increase in the number of men working in construction since 1980, and the number of men and women working in the retail sector has dropped by nearly one third between 1990 and 2000 (see table 10[9]). When examined by occupational groups (available only for 2000) a much higher proportion of construction workers and a somewhat higher proportion of manufacturing workers are males (table 11[10]). By contrast, females are much more likely to be employed in sales or office occupations. Note, for tables 10 and 11 "employed" refers to those who were at work at least 1 hour during the reference week at interview, in contrast to table 9 where "worked" refers to any work in the previous year.

---

[9] For tables 10 and 11 data are for the *employed population* only, defined as "All civilians 16 years old and over who were either (1) "at work" – those who did any work at all during the reference week as paid employees, worked in their own business or profession, worked on their own farm, or worked 15 hours or more as unpaid workers on a family farm or in a family business; or (2) were "with a job but not at work" – those who did not work during the reference week, but who had jobs or businesses from which they were temporarily absent because of illness, bad weather, industrial dispute, vacation, or other personal reasons". Table 9 data are based on report of work at any time in the past year, while data in tables 10 and 11 refer to employment during the reference week identified at the time of the interview.

[10] For all tables with branches of industry, please note that some branch labels differ from year to year. In 1980 and 1990, *Agriculture, forestry, fishing and* hunting did not include the words "hunting"; *F.I.R.E., insurance, real estate and rental and leasing* did not include the words "and rental and leasing"; and *Transportation, warehousing and utilities* was labelled "Transportation, communications and other public utilities".

Figures collected from the 2000 US Census were not for the service industry as a whole. The Census figures reported were for newly specified, narrower branches of *Services*. These include: "Professional, scientific, management, administrative and waste management services", "Educational, health and social services", "Arts, entertainment, recreation, accommodation and food services", and "Other services (except public administration)". The figures for *Services* in 2000, are the sums of employees in all of these new branches.

Table 10: Employees (%) in Different Branches of Industry by Gender (ages ≥16), 1980-2000

Branch of industry	Males			Females		
	1980	1990	2000	1980	1990	2000
Total, all branches (n)	1,473,622	1,585,698	1,635,535	1,200,653	1,442,252	1,525,552
Agriculture, forestry, fishing and hunting	1.1	2.0	0.5	0.5	0.6	0.2
Mining	0.1	0.1	0.1	0.02	0.03	0.01
Construction	7.0	9.4	9.6	0.7	1.2	1.1
Manufacturing	30.6	22.5	16.8	20.3	13.2	8.6
Wholesale trade	5.0	5.4	4.4	2.2	2.7	2.0
Retail trade	13.8	15.2	11.2	17.1	17.2	11.1
Transportation, ware-housing and utilities	8.2	8.1	5.9	3.6	4.1	2.3
Information	N/A	N/A	3.9	N/A	N/A	N/A
F.I.R.E.* and rental and leasing	4.7	6.1	7.2	8.3	10.1	9.3
Services	23.5	26.7	35.6	42.8	47.1	58.1
Public administration	5.9	4.8	4.8	4.5	3.7	3.6

Finance, insurance, real estate.

Notes: Includes civilian population only. N/A=data not available/reported. Numbers may not total 100% due to rounding. Source: US Census Bureau.

Table 11: Employees (%) in Different Occupations[11] by Gender (≥16 years), 1980-2000

Occupation	Males			Females		
	1980	1990	2000	1980	1990	2000
Total (n)	1,473,622	1,585,698	1,635,535	1,200,653	1,442,252	1,525,552
Managerial and professional occupations	28.1	31.3	38.3	23.8	32.8	40.9
Technical, sales, and administrative support Occupations	20.4	23.3	19.0	45.1	43.3	36.2
Service occupations	11.2	11.2	12.3	16.1	14.7	15.9
Farming, forestry and fishing occupations	1.3	1.5	0.5	0.3	0.3	0.2
Precision production, craft and repair occupations*	18.8	17.1	13.9	2.2	2.2	0.6
Operators, fabricators and labourers	20.2	15.7	16.0	12.5	6.7	6.2
Self-employed (included in above categories)	6.9	7.5	7.6	2.5	4.3	5.0

Source: US Census Bureau.

---

[11] For all tables including occupations, Bureau of Census changes in subgroupings of occupations in the year 2000 have been adjusted by the authors to maintain consistency for comparisons with previous decades.

7. Unionisation

With the decline of manufacturing in the US, there has been a de-cline in general union membership, as traditional blue-collar jobs – where unions were historically strong – have been replaced with non-union service sector work. The decrease in unionisation is perhaps one of the most significant features of the American work experience and of the American economy. Unions have never played the economic or political role they have played in Europe. In the 1950s close to a third of Americans were union members; today approximately 14% of workers are unionised. There have been some increases in public sector unioni-sation in the last 10 years, but this has not compensated for the overall decline in the last third of the 20th century. Recently this trend may be reversing in Massachusetts (table 12).

It is also true that unions have never had the direct political role they have had in Europe – in England or Sweden for example. While charac-teristically supporting the Democrat Party, the political power of the central union organisation, the American Federation of Labor and the Congress of Industrial Organisations (AFL-CIO), does not play the equivalent role that similar central labour organisations do in Europe. In Massachusetts the state AFL-CIO has had somewhat greater influence than other state-level labour organisations because of strong Democratic traditions.

Table 12 a: Union Membership* among
the Employed Population by Gender, 1994-2004. Males

Membership status	Males		
	1994	2000	2004
Total employed population with earnings (n)	1,208,074	1,410,924	1,480,588
Union member (%)	14	14	19

* Defined as "member of a labour union or similar association".
Note: Numbers may not add up to 100% due to rounding.
Source: US Bureau of Labor Statistics, Current Population Survey.

Table 12 b: Union Membership* among the Employed Population
by Gender, 1994-2004. Females

Membership status	Females		
	1994	2000	2004
Total employed population with earnings (n)	1,313,424	1,399,581	1,477,597
Union member (%)	13	14	13

* Defined as "member of a labour union or similar association".
Note: Numbers may not add up to 100% due to rounding.
Source: US Bureau of Labor Statistics, Current Population Survey.

8. Health and Social Class

As we have noted, data on social class or socio-economic status is not generally available in the US. Relating social class to health is therefore problematic. Once again we use ethnic and racial identity as a substitute for class in seeking to assess this relationship. We also provide insights based on the combination of income and occupation as indicators of social class.

One of the most important aspects of the relationship between social class and health for the issues under discussion here is the impact this has in terms of workplace injury and exposure.

In 2000, the rate of fatal occupational injuries was 5.5 per 100,000 workers, with these events occurring about ten times more frequently among males. Overall, the rate is down, although only slightly, from what it was in 1990. After declining from 1993 to 1996, the rate began to increase again.

The annual rate of occupational fatalities in Massachusetts is lower than in most states in the US, as well as lower than many developed nations. Although the reasons for this are not completely understood, several observations are helpful in understanding these differences. General factors include possible underreporting of occupational fatalities and the reporting practices for commuting fatalities. While occupational fatalities are the most reliably reported adverse work-related events, there is concern about the completeness of illness, injury and fatality reporting in the US (Azaroff *et al.* 2002, Azaroff *et al.* 2004). Furthermore, the total number of occupational fatalities reported in Massachusetts (as well as in other states) does not include motor vehicle fatalities while commuting to or from work.

One specific factor contributing to the relatively low rate for Massachusetts is the industrial composition of the workforce. For example, the service sector is about 20% larger in Massachusetts compared with the nation (32% vs. 27%). Also, proportionately more workers were employed nationally in higher-risk industrial sectors such as Agriculture, Construction, and Transportation and Public Utilities.

Another specific factor is that homicide and motor-vehicle-related fatalities at work, two important contributors to the occupational fatality burden, are comparatively low in the general population of Massachusetts.

Other specific factors may include the comparatively high levels of education and socio-economic status in Massachusetts, the higher proportion of unionised workers in the state (15%), and greater access to emergency medical services.

Rates of occupational fatalities by educational groups are not available, but in 1990 the number of fatalities occurred most commonly among those with only a high school education, whereas in 2000 the numbers were more equally distributed by educational groups (table 13). However, rates of occupational fatalities were higher among men than women but did not appear to differ much by race (table 14).

Table 13: Number of Fatal Occupational Injuries among Educational Groups by Gender, 1990-2000

Level of attainment	Male		Female	
	1990	2000	1990	2000
Total number of fatalities	59	41	2	9
Less than high school diploma	11	9	0	0
High school diploma/equivalency	36	14	1	4
Some college/ "Associate's" degree (lower level)	4	7	0	2
Bachelor's degree or higher	6	10	1	3
Advanced degree	N/A	--	N/A	--
Unknown	2	1	0	0

Note: -- rates are not available.
Sources: Massachusetts Department of Public Health.

Table 14: Rates* (number) of Fatal Occupational Injuries among Racial Groups[12] by Gender, 1990-2000

Racial classification	Male		Female	
	1990	2000	1990	2000
Total population	2.0 (59)	1.3 (41)	0.1 (2)	0.3 (9)
White	2.0 (53)	1.4 (37)	0.1 (2)	0.3 (9)
Black	2.2 (3)	1.2 (2)	0.0 (0)	0.0 (0)
Asian	0.0 (0)	0.0 (0)	0.0 (0)	0.0 (0)
Other	N/A (1)	N/A (0)	N/A (0)	N/A (0)
Hispanic origin	1.1 (2)	.6 (2)	0.0 (0)	0.0 (0)

* Age-adjusted per 100,000 workers.
Note: N/A=data not available/reported.
Sources: Massachusetts Department of Public Health.

---

[12] For all tables with racial groups using data from the Massachusetts Department of Public Health, *White, Black, Asian*, and *Other*, are classified as "non-Hispanic". *Hispanic origin* includes persons classified as being "of Hispanic origin" and they may be of any race. *Asian* is classified by the MDPH as "Asian/Pacific Islander, non-Hispanic". *Other* is made up of a mix of races and includes the classifications, "American Indian, non-Hispanic", "Other", and "Unknown" (a group distinguished by the MDPH of people for whom no racial data were available).

9. Overall Mortality and Social Class

There were 56,591 deaths in Massachusetts in 2000 (Massachusetts Department of Public Health 2002). The age-adjusted mortality rate for this year was 816.5 per 100,000 residents, which is lower (6%) than the national rate, a consistent finding throughout the 1990s. Since 1990, the mortality rate has dropped by 7% with a slightly higher total number of males than females. The rates for both genders have been steadily dropping over the last 10 years. In 1991, the mortality rate (per 100,000 residents) was 1134 for males and 720.7 for females, dropping to 988.5 and 697.8 respectively in 2001. Among the total population of Massachusetts, heart disease was the number one cause of death (26.7% of all deaths), followed by cancer (24.2%).

A. *Mortality by Education and Race*

Mortality rates by educational attainment were not available for Massachusetts until 2002. Results for that year support the common finding that mortality is inversely associated with educational attainment. The age-adjusted death rate for those with no more than a high school education was 539.4 per 100,000, which is 3 times higher than the rate of 174.4 for those with 13 years of education or more. The relative mortality advantage for further education persists as the population ages; however, the differential advantage decreases from 4.6 to 2.8 across the working years.

**Table 15: Death Rates (all causes) among
Educational Groups by Age, 2002**

Years of school completed (Both sexes)	Age-Specific Rates 2002			Age-Adjusted Rates
	25-34 years	35-44 years	45-64 years	25-64 years
High School or Less	159.2	306.8	941.8	539.4
13+ education	34.6	75.0	332.5	174.4

Source: Massachusetts Department of Public Health.

B. *Race*

Mortality by race showed consistently higher rates for blacks compared with whites. Over the past 10 years, mortality has fallen for both racial groups and the differences have somewhat narrowed (table 16). Results are also reported for persons of Hispanic origin but this designation is a mix of Black and White, and it is difficult to interpret these rates without further demographic detail. It is worth noting that the leading causes of death varied by race. Among Asians, Blacks and Hispanics, cancer was the leading cause of death, while for Whites the leading cause was heart disease. Heart disease was the second leading killer among all minority groups. HIV/AIDS remained the third leading cause of death among Hispanics, and for the third consecutive year, more Hispanics died of HIV/AIDS than black, non-Hispanics.

Table 16: Age-Adjusted All-Cause Mortality Rates*
among Racial Groups by Gender, 1990-2000

Female racial classification	Male		Female	
	1990	2000	1990	2000
For total population	1 140.1	999.4	711.4	686.8
White	1 137.2	999.8	708.7	685.7
Black	1 494.4	1 248.7	888.2	824.8
Asian	695.0	478.4	495.4	371.9
Other*	-	-	-	-
Hispanic origin	509.1	706.3	333.0	526

* *Rates cannot be calculated due to a lack of data for some races within this aggregate group.*
Note: A lack of available data prevents the reporting of gender-specific rates by race for 1980.
Sources: Massachusetts Department of Public Health.

The low mortality rate for those self-identified as of Hispanic origin is puzzling, especially in the light of the fact that, among tabulated groups, those of Hispanic origin have the highest proportion reporting less than good or poor self-rated health (see table 19). This observation, termed the "Hispanic Paradox", is not new and is likely to have many causes. Many hypotheses have been proposed to explain this paradox, including the assumption that it is an artefact of the data, a result of migration, and due to cultural or social buffering effects. It appears that part of the differential mortality can be attributed to return migration, or the "salmon-bias" effect. A complete explanation is still being sought (Franzini *et al.* 2001, Palloni & Arias 2004, Palloni & Morenoff 2001).

C. *Mortality by Occupation*

No data are available for Massachusetts that directly relate mortality to occupational class or to working conditions. Recently, Steenland, *et al.*, published a report based on death certificates for working-age adults (35-64 yrs) from 27 states over the period 1984-1997 (Massachusetts was not included) (Steenland *et al.* 2004). Over this period, there was a general trend for improved mortality experience in the population for most causes of death. In this study, social class (socio-economic status), based solely on usual occupation, was assigned by employing a method that associated education and income with occupational titles. The mortality findings are therefore related to occupation but not to working conditions. Socio-economic status was considered in four quartiles. The report studied summary risks by SES for selected major causes of deaths, as well as trends in cause-specific mortality over the study interval (table 17).

**Table 17: Annual Percentage Change in Mortality Rates
for Total Population and by SES Quartile: 1984-1997**

	All Causes	CHD	Stroke	COPD	External Causes	Lung Cancer
Total population	-0.6	-3.3	-1.3	0.0	-0.5	-0.8
SES quartile, men						
1 (lowest)	-0.4	-2.6	-1.1	0.1	-0.6	-0.4
2	-1.0	-3.5	-1.2	-1.3	-0.3	-1.8
3	-1.7	-4.7	-2.2	-1.5	-1.4	-2.4
4 (highest)	-1.9	-4.9	-2.0	-1.7	-1.6	-3.6
SES quartile, women						
1 (lowest)	0.2	-2.0	-1.8	3.9	0.1	1.8
2	-0.3	-2.5	-0.1	2.7	0.2	1.1
3	-0.9	-3.4	-1.4	0.0	-1.7	0.3
4 (highest)	0.2	-2.2	-1.1	1.5	-0.5	0.3

*Note. CHD = coronary heart disease; COPD = chronic obstructive pulmonary disease; SES=socio-economic status quartile; NA = not available.
Steenland and Walker 2004.*

The findings demonstrated consistent increases in mortality with de-creasing SES, which was strongest for males and most striking for COPD and external causes. When the findings were examined for trends over the study interval, the SES-related differences were observed to be growing; again this was more evident in the males. Over this same interval there was also evidence of increasing economic disparity be-tween the highest and lowest SES groups in the US.

While these findings do not include Massachusetts deaths, the inves-tigators examined regional groupings of states for mortality differences but were not able to find any important impact of regional groups on SES findings. Thus, it is reasonable to assume that the mortality experi-ence of working people in Massachusetts is likely to be similar.

10. Self-reported Overall Health and Social Class

In 2001, 12% of the Massachusetts population reported having "fair or poor health" (Massachusetts Department of Public Health 2003). Just over 5% reported that their health (either physical or mental) had limited their activities for 15 or more days in the previous month, and 7% reported having been in pain for 15 or more days in the previous month. The percentage of people reporting overall fair or poor health has increased by over 1/3 over the ten-year period, 1992-2001. In 2001 women were slightly more likely than men to report that their health limited their activities (5.7% v 5.2%) or that they were in pain for 15 or more days in the previous month (7.4% v 6.1%).

A. Education

The pattern of differences in self-reported health measures among those with different levels of education is similar to that found among those will different levels of income. As seen in table 18, almost 40% of those with the lowest levels of education (less than a high school education) report being in fair or poor health in 2000, and this has increased by almost 25% since 1994 (the first year of the survey). This is in contrast with the results among those with 4 years or more of college education, where less than 6% report being in fair or poor health. Similar results were found when educational attainment was evaluated according to responses to questions about pain 15 days or more in the previous month and activity limitations in the past month, although the differences by educational attainment were much smaller (data not shown).

Table 18: Percentage Reporting Less than Good or Poor Health among Educational Groups by Gender, 1994-2000

Level of attainment	Males		Females		Total	
	1994	2000	1994	2000	1994	2000
Less than high school diploma	30.6	38.8	33.7	40.8	32.4	39.8
High school diploma/equivalency	8.8	17.8	15.5	17.4	12.4	17.6
Some college/"Associate's" degree (lower level)	6.8	11.4	7.3	10.4	7.1	10.8
Bachelor's degree or higher	6.7	5.9	5.9	5.6	6.3	5.8

Source: Massachusetts Department of Public Health.

B. Race

The percentage of Massachusetts residents reporting fair or poor health differs markedly by race (table 19). In both 1994 and 2000, a substantially larger proportion of Hispanics reported fair or poor health (30.4%) compared with both Whites and Blacks (range 10-14%). Differences among the racial groups for activity limitations were minor, while reports of pain 15 days or more in the previous month were least common among those of Hispanic origin (data not shown).

288

Table 19: Percentage Reporting Less than Good or Poor Health among Racial Groups by Gender, 1994-2000

Racial classification	Males		Females		Total	
	1994	2000	1994	2000	1994	2000
White	8.6	12.0	11.3	11.4	10.1	11.7
Black	NA	14.7	13.4	16.3	10.6	13.6
Hispanic origin	NA	28.5	32.1	32.2	30.4	30.4

Note: "NA" means data are not available (see footnote for further explanation).
Source: Massachusetts Department of Public Health.

11. Self-reported Mental Health and Social Class

In 2002, 9% of the Massachusetts residents surveyed reported having "poor mental health" for 15 days or more in the previous month, a proportion that has been fairly consistent over the years since 1993. The percentage of people who reported that they were sad for 15 or more days in the previous month was 7.1%. 70% of the population reported that they were full of energy for 15 or more days in the previous month. Women in the state (11%) were more likely than men (7.2%) to report experiencing poor mental health for 15 days or more in the previous month. The percentage of those reporting sadness varied very little by gender.

A. Education

Education also has a marked effect on the self-reported mental health of the people of Massachusetts. Those with less education are more likely to report having poor mental health and depression for 15 days or more in the previous month. Nearly 11% of those with less than a high school education reported having poor mental health, while only 6.6% of those with 4 years or more of college reported their mental health as poor. The results are similar for depression: nearly 10% of those without a high school education reported being depressed, while only 4.9% of those with a college education reported experiencing depression in the past month.

Hispanics (12%) and Blacks (8.2%) were most likely, and Asians (5.3%) least likely, to report having poor mental health in the previous month. Hispanics (9.1%) and Blacks (8.8%) were also the most likely to report being depressed for 15 or more days in the previous month. Asians (6.4%) and Whites (6.1%) were the least likely to report being depressed.

B. Workplace Exposures

There is no routine survey of working conditions in Massachusetts or any other state. Nationally there have been two surveys sponsored by the National Institute for Occupational Safety and Health: the National Occupational Hazards Survey, 1972-1974 (NIOSH 1974), and the National Occupational Exposure Survey, 1981-1983 (Sieber 1990) to estimate exposures by industry (Sieber 1990). Both efforts surveyed a national sample of employers for potential occupational exposures to chemical, and a limited number of physical, and biological agents. These surveys were designed to assess industries, however, and not occupations.

NIOSH subsequently sponsored a supplement to the 1988 National Health Interview Survey (NHIS) to collect detailed information from participants on their work histories and on selected work exposures. NHIS is the principal source of information on the health of the civilian non-institutionalised population of the United States, through the regular collection and analysis of data on a broad range of health topics. A major strength of this survey lies in its ability to display these health characteristics by many demographic and socio-economic characteristics. To date, only the 1988 survey has included substantial information about population exposure to work-related risk factors and detailed assessment of the occupational nature of selected conditions. Regular population-based information on the distribution of common workplace exposures that can be assessed by interview is essential in order to understand the relationship between these risk factors and health data contained within NHIS.

Using this survey, in 1997 Wagener *et al.*, assessed selected exposures by occupational class (table 20)(National Institute for Occupational Safety and Health 1974, Wagener *et al.* 1997). Some of the differences cited in that report are quite striking, e.g. industrial chemical exposure is twice as common in blue- compared with white-collar jobs, and exposures to cleaning and disinfectant agents are highest among service workers and farm workers. Differences are also noted in the self-assessment of hazardous exposures, although in these reports a low proportion of exposures among those in white-collar jobs is most notable. The physical exposures assessed follow predictable patterns.

Table 20: Percentage Distribution of Currently Employed Adults≥ 18 Years of Age, by Sex and Selected Reported Exposures[13]

	Major occupational group				
	Total	**White-collar**	**Service**	**Blue-collar**	**Farm**
Reported Exposure to Selected Substances					
Industrial chemicals					
Women	26	21	32	43	52
Men	52	32	44	74	76
Soaps, detergents, or disinfecting solutions					
Women	32	23	72	28	53
Men	38	25	59	48	56
Agricultural products					
Women	22	14	56	14	74
Men	21	12	48	18	86
Substances believed to be harmful if breathed or on skin					
Women	23	18	36	42	43
Men	39	25	44	56	50
Reported Exposures to Specific Types of Work Activity					
Repeated strenuous physical activity					
Women	10	6	19	22	23
Men	22	7	17	38	44
Repeated bending, twisting, or reaching					
Women	24	16	42	45	35
Men	35	14	36	56	56
Bending or twisting of hands or wrists					
Women	36	30	43	64	37
Men	40	23	39	60	53
Hand operation of vibrating machinery					
Women	4	2	5	14	6
Men	12	3	7	22	24

Source: Wagener et al. 1997.

Not until 2001 did Massachusetts begin to collect limited information on work exposures, and these were ones that related only to the physical demands of work. Women report that they experience demanding physical work 1/3 as often as men; similarly, Asians experience

---

[13] These data come from the National Health Interview Survey. This continuous survey follows a *multistage* area probability design that permits the representative sampling of households, permitting the results to be projected to estimates for the US population. Proportions reported in the table are therefore based on the 1988 sample of households that have been projected to the entire population of workers.

much less of this type of work compared with the three other races. Differences by race and gender are present, but are much less striking for the other types of work activity. Overall, under 20% report work that requires mostly walking, while 70% report sitting or standing at work. Future surveys would benefit from more specificity (e.g., asking about sitting and standing work separately) as well as questions about a greater range of workplace exposure types.

12. Conclusion

The information and data presented here provide a snapshot of the demographic, economic and social aspects of the working population of Massachusetts. From the data on health that we have gathered there are clear indications of some significant relationships between the health of individuals, the educational level they have achieved, their ethnic and racial background, and the occupations they have.

These findings for Massachusetts, and for the United States in general, indicate a significant lack of information critical to understanding the role of working conditions in determining health equity or health disparities. This is true, despite the evidence documenting an effect of socio-economic status on health inequities. Since working conditions are subject to intervention, it is important to have information that permits changes to be introduced, with priority given to alterations that will promote health and eliminate inequities. Surveys of working conditions similar to the European Surveys of Working Conditions undertaken by the European Foundation seem most appropriate. These might be undertaken by adding relevant modules in the National Health Interview Survey and updates of the Quality of Employment Surveys at least every five years. Inclusion of some elements of these modules in the Behavioral Risk Factor Surveillance System (BRFSS) instrument that is used in most states would enhance specificity at the state level. These surveys are currently undertaken on an annual basis in Massachusetts and, in 2000, included more than 8000 subjects in the state survey. Limited survey elements have already been included in the most recent surveys. Samples large enough to associate exposures or health conditions with groups of occupations would enhance the value of such data.

The question we asked from the outset was: what is the connection between social class, work and health? In what ways can we identify how social class, mediated by the work environment, results in poor health in Massachusetts? The answer to this question in the US presents a particular problem. Data on social class are not collected directly, and we are therefore not able to provide even a cross-sectional analysis over time of the relationship between social class, occupation and health.

What we have used instead is race and educational achievement as a substitute for class. In doing so we can, at the very least, identify that educational achievement is different among the races, and that this, in turn, limits the kinds of jobs available to the different racial groups. Obviously, many of those with only a high school diploma (or less) end up in occupations that are poorly paid and frequently more dangerous to the health of the worker. The lower incomes available to those working in unskilled or semi-skilled jobs will also limit the opportunities available for living in healthy and safe communities, access to decent housing and nutrition, and the knowledge and resources to make use of whatever health care services are available. In contrast, an individual with higher income, a well-paid job with high status, a good education, and high social rank, has more life opportunities and better access to those resources necessary for a healthy life. But it is also clear that these individuals emerge (or not) from a set of material conditions (Lynch's "neo-materialism") that may or may not be collectively available. In other words, in Massachusetts and in the US in general, we can conclude that the ways in which occupation and working conditions mediate the relationship between social class and health will be intimately dependent on social class, and the social and economic context in which an individual grows up and lives – determining life chances, education and occupation. In this sense, the data provide good evidence that social class appears to be strongly related to, and seems likely to influence, the kinds of occupations available; and those occupations tend to maintain the social class structure and related health disparities.

References

Albelda R., Kim M. 2002. "A tale of two decades. changes in work and earnings in Massachusetts, 1979-1999". *Massachusetts Benchmarks. The Quarterly Review of Economic News & Insight* 5: 12-17.

Azaroff L.S., Lax M.B., Levenstein C., Wegman D.H. 2004. "Wounding the messenger: the new economy makes occupational health indicators too good to be true". *International Journal of Health Services* 34(2): 271-303.

Azaroff L.S., Levenstein C., Wegman D.H. 2002. "Occupational injury and illness surveillance: conceptual filters explain underreporting". *American Journal of Public Health* 92: 1421-1429.

Coburn D. 2000. "Income, inequality, social cohesion and the health status of populations: the role of neo-liberalism", *Social Science and Medicine* 51: 139-150.

Franzini L., Ribble JC., Keddie AM. 2001. "Understanding the Hispanic paradox". *Ethnicity and Disease* 1: 496-518.

Kaplan G.A., Lynch, J.W. 1999. "Socioeconomic considerations in the primordial prevention of cardiovascular disease". *Preventive Medicine* 29: S30-S35.

Kaplan G.A. 1996. "People and places: contrasting perspectives on the association between social class and health". *International Journal of Health Services* 26: 507-519.

Lynch J. 2000. "Income inequality and health: expanding the debate". *Social Science and Medicine* 51: 1001-1005.

Massachusetts Department of Public Health. September 2003. "A Profile of Health Among Massachusetts Adults, 2001: Results from the Behavioral Risk Factor Surveillance System", 78 p.

Massachusetts Department of Public Health. April 2002. "Massachusetts Deaths 2000", 99 p.

National Institute for Occupational Safety and Health (NIOSH) 1974. *National Occupational Hazard Survey – Vol. I Survey Manual.* DHHS (NIOSH): 74-127.

Palloni A., Arias E. 2004. "Paradox Lost: Explaining the Hispanic Adult Mortality Advantage" . *Demography* 41: 385-415.

Palloni A., Morenoff J.D. 2001. "Interpreting the paradoxical in the hispanic paradox: demographic and epidemiologic approaches". *Annals of the New York Academy of Science* 954: 140-74.

Pappas G., Queen S., Hadden W., Fisher G. 1993. "The increasing disparity in mortality between socioeconomic groups in the United States, 1960 and 1986". *New England Journal Of Medicine* 329: 103-109.

Sieber W.K. 1990. *National Occupational Exposure Survey: Sampling Methodology.* DHHS (NIOSH): Publication No. 89, 102 pp.

Sorlie P.D., Backlund E., Keller J.B. 1995. "US mortality by economic, demographic and social characteristics: the National Longitudinal Mortality Study". *American Journal of Public Health* 85: 949-956.

Steenland K., Hu S., Walker J. 2004. "All-cause and cause-specific mortality by socioeconomic status among employed persons in 27 US states, 1984-1997". *American Journal of Public Health* 94(6): 1037-42.

Syme S.L., Berkman L.B. 1976. "Social class, susceptibility, and sickness". *American Journal of Epidemiology* 104: 1-8.

Wagener D.K., Walstedt J., Jenkins L. and Burnett C. 1997. Women: Work and health. Vital & Health Statistics: Series 3: *Analytical & Epidemiological Studies* 31: 1-91.

Winkleby M.A., Jatulis D.E., Frank E., Fortman S.P. 1992. "Socioeconomic Status and Health: how education, income and occupation contribute to risk factors for cardio-vascular disease". *American Journal of Public Health* 82: 816-20.

Spain

Joan BENACH, Marcelo AMABLE, Carles MUNTANER,
Lucía ARTAZCOZ, Imma CORTÉS, María MENÉNDEZ,
& Fernando G. BENAVIDES

Introduction

In the last three decades the Spanish economic, political and social structure has changed dramatically (Harrison 1985, Etxezarreta 1991, Salmon 1995). This includes the transformation from a rural to an urban society, the political and cultural changes that took place during the initial period of democracy after the end of Franco's dictatorship, a new migration pattern (internal migration, migration of Spaniards to other countries, the return of Spanish migrant workers, and the arrival of foreign migrants), and the ageing of the Spanish population.

From an economic perspective, the developments changed the outlook of the country during the 1960s and the early 1970s. Spain went from being a rural society to being an urban country with a decreasing number of salaried rural workers and a large industrial working class. These decades witnessed a very high economic growth (about 6-7% per year), second only to Japan in the 1960s, due to rapid industrialisation. This growth subsequently slowed down (to about 2-3% per year) in the period 1973-1985, when unemployment increased sharply as the Spanish economy was affected by the slowdown that characterised most developed capitalist countries. In the early 1980s a profound restructuring of the industrial sector took place under the socialist government, when unemployment rose again very rapidly. The 1986-1992 period was dominated by the integration of Spain into the European Community, and more widely into the world economy, through the dismantling of barriers to the movement of commodities and financial capital, as well as the incorporation of Spanish businesses into foreign multinational corporations (Salmon 1995). At the end of 1992 the Spanish economy entered into its deepest recession of the last decades and the unemployment rate rose to 23% in 1995. Since 1996 the economy has rebounded modestly; there was a freeze on public sector wages and the government accomplished its objective of meeting the Maastricht criteria of low inflation, low debt by sharply reducing social welfare expenditure (Navarro & Quiroga 2004). The regressive taxation system with a large amount of fiscal fraud, Spain's less developed welfare state, and the failure to implement redistribution through social and economic policies at the regional level have contributed to sharp regional inequalities. Regional nationalism has also contributed to this trend by empowering a number of conservative governments that reduced social welfare spending.

Since the 1960s Spain's economy has grown at rates consistently above the European Union (EU-15) average, but in spite of this, other indicators such as income, unemployment, or poverty are worse than in most EU-15 member states. Like other southern European countries, Spain is still poorer than many European countries, with a Gross Domestic Product which is only about 85% of the EU average, while income inequality remains high. In comparison with richer European countries Spain has consistently shown higher deprivation indicators such as poverty or unemployment rates. One out of every five households is poor, according to European Union standards, with eight million Spaniards living in poverty, while general population surveys have consistently estimated the Spanish poverty rate at around 20%, and over 44% among those below 25 years of age (Benach & Amable 2004). Moreover, social inequalities in Spain are more pronounced. For example, income *per capita* in the most affluent regions is more than twice that of the most disadvantaged regions, and similar differences are also evident in unemployment, educational level, and other socio-economic and labour market indicators (Benach *et al*. 2004).

Spain has undergone thorough political decentralisation over the last twenty years. Today, Spain's 17 regions have very high levels of legislative and political autonomy, including responsibility for health issues, with a potential for generating inter-regional differences within the country. Spain has rapidly evolved from its recent role as a source of immigrants, to a receiver of foreign labourers. In the 1970s more than a million Spaniards migrated to other European countries, and at the end of this decade three million Spaniards were living abroad (García Ballesteros *et al*. 1992). Yet, in the 1980s migration sharply declined, and in the 1990s a new phenomenon started with the arrival of large numbers of legal and illegal immigrants, mostly from Northern Africa, Latin America and Eastern European countries, and smaller contingents of well-to-do immigrants from other EU countries, such as retirees from Germany or the UK. The number of foreign residents in Spain has significantly increased in recent years and these new migrants are changing the demographic structure, with the result that immigration has become an important social and political issue. For example, in 2001 the immigration growth was the highest in the EU, with a total number of more than 1 million foreign residents (2.5% of the total population) (Jansà *et al.* 2003).

Traditionally, the participation of Spanish women in the labour market has been much lower than in other countries of the European Union (EU-15). Still in 2001 the women's activity rate was 39%, whereas the mean of the EU was 47%, and there were countries such as Denmark where the proportion was nearly 60%. On the other hand, social services for families are underdeveloped, there are minimal publicly funded day care places, and involvement of men in domestic work is very low (Artazcoz *et al.* 2001).

In Spain, research on work-related inequalities in health is very limited. Reasons for this situation include the small number of research groups focusing on this field, and that information on social and occupational inequalities in health is scarce (Benach *et al.* 2002, Artazcoz *et al.* 2003). The aims of this chapter are twofold: first, to characterise Spanish labour force participation and the labour market structure; second, to review current evidence on occupational and social class inequalities in Spain; and third, to comment on some of the key policy factors related to the improvement of the work environment and the reduction of work-related inequalities.

To accomplish these aims, we review major findings available in studies on health inequalities, and we present new information drawn from a number of secondary data sources. Social and economic data on labour force participation and the labour market structure have mainly been provided by the Labour Force Surveys and the Ministry of Labour and Social Affairs. Data from the last available Spanish Surveys on Working Conditions (1997, 1999) are useful to analyse inequalities of working conditions by gender and occupational class (manual vs. non-manual workers) and type of contract (permanent vs. temporary). Data on mortality, injuries caused by occupational accidents, and from the last Spanish Health Surveys (1993, 1995, 1997, 2001), are useful to analyse occupational and social class inequalities in health. Additionally, information from the last Barcelona Health Survey (2000) makes it possible to analyse other work-related health inequalities by gender and social class.

1. Structure of the Labour Market

During the last few decades, the transformation of the production sector, the loss of importance of the agrarian sector, as well as the economic and social changes previously mentioned, have produced important changes in the labour market. We focus here on two key subjects: labour force participation and labour market structure.

A. Labour Force Participation

People's participation in the labour market depends on a variety of economic, technological, political and cultural factors. The high level of unemployment, the progressive deterioration in the quality of the employment and the growth of female labour force participation are perhaps the most important differential features of Spain in comparison with other European countries.

Economic Participation and Unemployment

The low rate of labour market participation of the Spanish population in the last few decades can be seen in table 1. In spite of a slight increase in recent years, Spain has yet to reach the employment levels of the European Union (68.9% in 2002). The difficulties of the Spanish economy to generate high levels of employment have been observed since the beginning of the period in 1980, with the partial exception of the last few years. However, activity and unemployment rates show a remarkably different behaviour by gender. Thus, the female participation rate has significantly increased throughout the period considered, with a growth of more than 14 points, whereas male participation has decreased almost continuously during the period, except in the last year. This is due to the concentration of women in the growing service sector: according to the Labour Force Survey, 3,700,000 in the period 1992-2003, the employees being 85% in the service sector, of which more than 65% were women (Consejo Económico y Social 2003). On the other hand, the 2003 data show an increase both in activity rates and in employment rates in both sexes (table 2).

**Table 1: Population of 16-year-olds and older (in thousands)
in relation to the economic activity, Spain. 1980-2003**

Situation of economic activity	Years			
	1980	1990	2000	2003
Population ≥ 16-years old (n)	26,691.7	30,407.8	33,270.1	34,175.5
Active (n)	13,380.1	15,410.4	17,763.5	18,751.1
Activity rate (%)	50.1	50.7	53.4	54.9
Employed (n)	11,892.7	12,906.8	15,306.1	16,666
Employment rate (%)	44.6	42.4	46.0	48.8
Unemployed (n)	1,487.5	2,503.6	2,457.5	2,085
Unemployment rate (%)	11.1	16.2	13.8	11.1
Inactive (n)	12,986	14,767.8	15,415	15,424.4
Inactivity rate (%)	48.7	48.6	46.3	45.1

Source: EPA [LPS], 2° trimester.

298

**Table 2: Activity and employment rates (%) of 15-64 year-olds
by gender (Spain, 1980-2000)**

Rates	Years											
	1980		1985		1990		1995		2000		2003	
	Men	Women	Men	Women	Men	Women	Men	Women	Men	Women	Men	Women
Acti-vity	74.2	27.7	70.6	28.5	68.3	34.2	64.9	37.5	66.3	41.2	67.3	43.2
Em-ploy-ment	66.3	24.3	56.4	21.4	60.2	25.8	53.3	26.0	60.0	32.8	61.9	36.3

Source: EPA [LPS], 2° trimester.

Unemployment began to rise in the mid-1970s and continued rising until the mid-1980s, when Spain reached the highest rates within the EU with nearly 3 million Spaniards unemployed. Since the mid-1980s and until recent years, unemployment has consistently been about twice that of the EU average (around 20% of the economically active persons or more than 3 million out of 39 million people). Indeed, the scale of unemployment was the most serious social problem Spain faced during the 1990s. There were about 250,000 long-term unemployed persons with dependent relatives, and 800,000 unemployed persons without any financial aid. Moreover, large differences in unemployment are shown across regions and small areas. For example, in 1996 two poor regions in southern Spain, Andalusia and Extremadura, had unemployment rates of 32.4% and 30.2% respectively (Ministerio de Trabajo y Asuntos Sociales 2002), while northern regions such as Navarre had about 11%. In addition, important differences on the small-area scale have also been reported (Benach *et al.* 2001). Moreover, Spain has the highest percentage of temporary employment within the EU (Franco & Winqvist 2002), a new public health research topic that must be investigated further (Benach *et al.* 2000).

The increase in unemployment rates apparently stopped in 2000, a trend decrease that was also observed in 2003 (table 3). In spite of this reduction, the country is still severely hit by unemployment (11% in 2002) with high levels of unemployment among women (16.2% in 2002) and young people (21.5% in those younger than 25 years in 2002) (table 3), with large regional and small-area differences (Benach *et al.* 2004). Together with Greece and Italy, Spain shows the highest gender differences in unemployment of the EU-15. The high unemployment rates among under-25-year-olds, the great majority of whom are looking for their first job, show fewer gender differences than the general rates.

It is in the group of youngsters that we observe the greatest gender equality – in labour market participation. However, unemployment rates in the last few years show that women still have greater difficulty in finding a job than men. In addition, the long-term unemployment has been 42.9% for men and 52.2% for women (49.2 on average). Women showed the highest unemployment rates in all occupational categories, but the widest differences are found in the less qualified occupations; female unemployment was 67.7% among unskilled workers and 59.6% among operators, while male unemployment in these sectors was 15.2% and 4.8%, respectively.

The social and health impact of these poor employment figures may partially be buffered by the fact that about one third of those unemployed have some coverage against unemployment (Artazcoz *et al.* 2004). On the other hand, many young people are 'protected' by their families since they live in their parents' homes until adulthood, and 'real' (although unregulated) employment is likely to be higher than stated by statistics, due to the importance of the underground economy.

Table 3: Unemployment rate by gender and age 1980-2003

Gender	Years					
	1980	1985	1990	1995	2000	2003
Men	10.6	20.1	11.9	17.9	9.5	8.0
Aged 16-25	27.2	45.6	25.7	36.4	19.6	19.0
Women	12.4	24.9	24.4	30.6	20.4	15.8
Aged 16-25	27.0	50.1	39.1	48.3	32.1	26.7
Total	11.1	21.5	16.3	22.7	13.8	11.1
Aged 16-25	27.1	47.6	31.9	41.9	25.3	22.3
Those looking for their first job	68.1	84.3	73.1	83.8	82.7	69.3

Source: EPA [LPS], 2° trimester.

Employment Arrangements

One of the most significant changes of the European labour market in the last two decades has been the generalisation of new forms of work organisation and flexible labour markets, with the emergence of new forms of non-standard employment arrangements, precarious work and various types of underemployment, including involuntary part-time employment and insecure employment (Benach *et al.* 2002). Non-standard work arrangements refers to temporary work, informal work, and other arrangements characterised by reduced job security, lower compensation and impaired working conditions (Muntaner *et al.*, submitted). Precarious work has been broadly used to signal that new work and employment forms tend to reduce social security and social protection (Rodgers 1989). Other terms in common use are 'contingent employment', which refers to jobs that are structured to be short-term or temporary, including employees working on limited duration contracts, independent contractor jobs, work on demand working through temporary work agencies or self-employed (Muntaner *et al.* submitted).

Figure 1: Temporary workers (%) in EU countries (1985-2000)

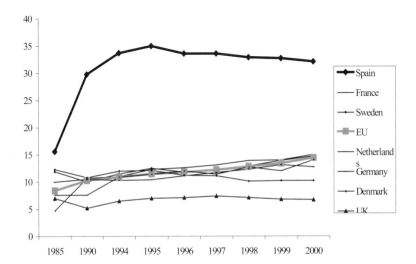

In Spain the EU economic integration and the big changes in the labour market have resulted in widespread non-standard work arrangements. Thus, the initiatives to create employment (except for the last few years), have not substantially reduced unemployment rates (especially among women), while underemployment has increased, and new types of flexible employment have deteriorated the quality of employment. Additionally, the underground economy accounts for about 21% of the Gross Domestic Product (GDP) (Alañón & Gómez de Antonio 2003), with a large part of the active population working under these precarious circumstances. While in the EU, precarious employment (fixed-term contracts and temporary work associated with low job security, lack of benefits and lower pay) accounts for 15% of paid employment, Spain shows the highest percentages of all (figure 1). Thus, in the second half of the 1990s an endless number of forms of 'self-employed' productive activity appeared, dependent on a percentage of temporary work much larger than the EU (31.3% vs. 13.4% in 2002). In 2001, 91% of the new 14 million contracts were temporary contracts, with more than two thirds of workers having contracts lasting less than six months. About 5 million workers revolve incessantly around temporary jobs that have poor working conditions and few labour rights (Ministerio de Trabajo y Asuntos Sociales 2002).

Temporary work arrangements are unevenly distributed by gender, the percentages of women in temporary work being higher than among men. In 2002, 34.2% of salaried women had a temporary contract (compared with 14.5% in the EU-15) and the figure was 29.2% for salaried men. When considering the employment of the youngest, 81.3% of the employed among under-20-year-olds and 63.4% of the employed among under-25-year-olds had a temporary contract for the year 2000.

A significant increase in the percentage of salaried employees was observed in the 1980s when the levels of salaried employees were low, while in the 1990s, they grew to 80%. The most substantial impact on the growth of salaried employees was caused by a surge in women's employment (table 4). On the other hand, self-employment levels were approximately 30% in the 1980s and 19.7% in the 1990s.

In Spain, although part-time employment increased over the last decade it does not have the same importance in quantitative terms as in other EU countries (table 5). However, there is a convergence with other EU and OECD countries, which is the relevance of the part-time job as a means of labour insertion for women, reaching 17% of female employment. Considering the reasons for part-time employment, how-ever, those women who do not want full-time employment accounted for 7.9% in 1987 and 8.2% in 2002, whereas those who could not find full-time employment were 31.3% and 19%, respectively.

Table 4: Salaried employees (%) by gender 1980-2003

	Years					
	1980	1985	1990	1995	2000	2003
Men	72.5	70.5	74.0	73.7	77.9	79.1
Women	64.7	66.2	73.7	76.6	83.3	85.2
Total	70.3	69.2	73.9	74.7	79.9	81.4

Source: EPA [LPS], 2° trimester.

Table 5: Part-time employment (%) 1987-2003

	Years				
	1987	1990	1995	2000	2003
Men	2.3	1.6	2.6	2.8	2.6
Women	13.7	12.1	16.5	17.1	17.0
Total	5.7	4.9	7.4	8.0	8.1

Source: EPA [LPS], 2° trimester.

B. Labour Market Structure

Economic Activity and Occupational Stratification

In recent decades an increase in the tertiary sector has been observed with a marked decrease in the primary sector. Between 1960 and 1970 the percentage of farmers and stockbreeders decreased from 39.5% to 24.5%, while construction, mining, industrial and transport workers increased from 31.6% to 40.7% of the working population (table 6). The increase in office work modified the composition of the salaried working classes, increasing their weight in the service sector, while industrial work was reduced by half a million workers between 1977 and 1992. In these same years a great transformation in rural employment took place, in which a million jobs among the small agrarian businessmen without salaried workers were lost.

Table 6: Active population by occupation (percentages, 1950-2001)

Occupation or Profession	1950	1960	1970	1981	1991	2001[*]
Professionals and technical personnel	3.3	4.1	5.4	9.2	13.2	15.2
Public administration personnel, managers and directors	7.3	1.0	0.9	1.6	1.7	4.5
Administrative personnel and related workers	a	5.1	8.3	12.1	13.7	20.0
Merchants, salesmen and related workers	3.3	6.5	8.2	9.3	11.6	5.5
Hotel services, domestic and Security workers	7.3	7.2	9.3	10.0	12.1	15.5
Agricultural, husbandry, fishing, Hunting and related workers	48.5	39.5	24.5	15.4	6.3	5.8
Manufacturing, building and transport workers	27.5	31.6	40.7	40.5	28.3	27.6
Personnel with unspecified occupation	0.9	3.6	1.5	1.1	12.3	5.3
Armed forces	1.9	1.4	1.2	0.8	0.8	0.5
Total	100	100	100	100	100	100

*Source: a, Included in the previous 'Public administration personnel'; * Based on the Active Population Survey; Classification according to the Clasificación Nacional de Ocupaciones 1979; Del Campo S., 2002.*

One of the most characteristic features of the changes occurring in the Spanish economy during this period is found in the labour market structure. Trends towards employment growth in the service sector, a relative decrease in the industrial sector (mostly manufacturing and capital goods) and constant employment contraction in the agrarian sector continued in the late 1970s and throughout the 1980s (figure 2). For example, between 1977 and 1993, employment in services increased 32%, whereas in industry and agriculture it decreased by 74% and 48%

respectively. In the process of expanding services, the State has played an important role as an employer. For instance, between 1972 and 1988 the employees in the public sector increased from 7.7% to 15.8%. Between 1970 and 1991, construction, industrial, mining and transport workers went from 40.8% to 28.1% of the total active population, whereas the number of professionals and office workers increased (from 5.4% to 13.2%, and from 8.3% to 13.7%, respectively) (Durán & Benavides 2004).

Figure 2: Proportion (%) of the working population in different branches 1980-2003

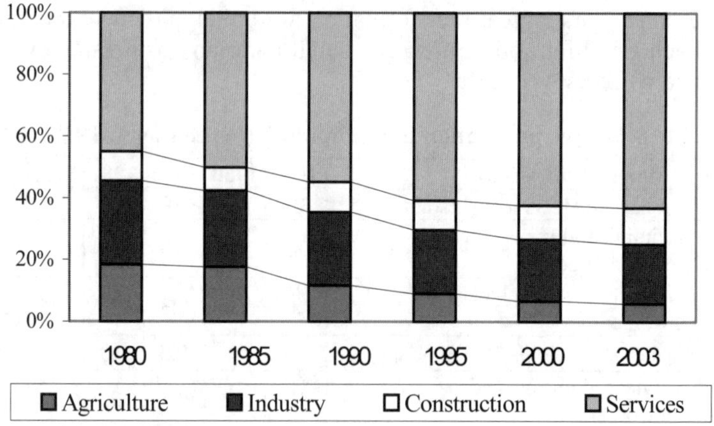

Source: Active Population Survey, 2° trimester.

Although female labour participation has significantly increased, there is a clear occupational segregation by gender, in which women and men constitute two separate workforces with very different jobs (table 7). Women are concentrated among non-manual workers with low qualifications: administrative (15.8%), in restoration (13.1%) and in commerce (8.9%), and among unskilled workers in services (13.8%). On the other hand, men are grouped among skilled manual construction (13.7%) and industrial (8.6%) workers, facilities and machinery operators (13.9%) and unskilled labourers (8.8%). Moreover, we can also observe a clear segregation in the management and administration posts with much higher percentages of men.

There has been a greater occupational insertion of women in the new middle stratum of employees (46%), whereas their inclusion in the industrial working class is much less pronounced (27%). In the early 1990s, while women were concentrated in occupations related to services with a generally low level of qualifications (office workers or commerce employees with 19.7% and 14.5%, respectively), the largest occupations among men with most workers permanently employed were artisans and skilled industrial workers (13.3%), building workers (11.1%) and farm workers (9.1%) (data not shown). These labour changes had a different impact by gender. For example, the increase of employment in the private sector until the early 1990s entailed a reduction of 300,000 jobs as a result of a decrease of more than 600,000 jobs among men, and a growth of more than 260,000 jobs for women. In spite of these changes, equality at work between women and men is still far from being achieved. For example, in 2000 the pay of Spanish women was 30% lower on average than that of men, which is double the average gender pay gap in the European Union (Martin Artiles 2003).

**Table 7: Employment in occupational groups in 2001
according to gender**

Occupation	Men	Women	Total
	%	%	%
Management and public administration	8.4	6.5	7.7
Technicians and university professionals	9.8	15.9	12.1
Supporting technicians and professionals	9.7	11.7	10.5
Office workers	6.0	15.8	9.7
Personal service workers and commerce	9.2	22.2	14.1
Skilled workers – agriculture and fishing	4.9	2.4	4.0
Skilled workers – manufacturing, construction and mining industries	26.0	3.4	17.5
Operators of facilities and machinery	14.0	3.9	10.3
Unskilled workers	11.8	18.2	14.2
Total	100	100	100

Source: EPA [LPS], 2° trimester.

Social Class

Social class can be defined by positions in society stemming from relations of ownership or control over different types of assets. On the other hand, social stratification refers to the ranking of individuals according to control over socially valued resources and the distribution of the burdens and rewards of life (Muntaner *et al.* 1998, Muntaner *et al.*, submitted). Occupational social stratification provides an easy and available approach to understanding the evolution of social class structure in a given country.

In Spain the evolution in the occupational structure and in the composition of job positions shows the proliferation of non-manual jobs and jobs that require higher levels of qualifications, such as administrative, commercial or technical skills. Between 1971 and 1991, for example, the increase in the service sector from 17.6% to 30.8% of all people employed was mainly accounted for by salaried professionals and office workers. The occupations that shaped the existing social stratification in the 1990s can be grouped as follows: about two thirds are workers (a third correspond to salaried manual workers, and another third part is composed of salaried office, commercial and service workers); almost a fourth is made up of self-employed workers (businessmen without salaried workers) and independent professionals. Finally, people belonging to the management and businessmen with salaried workers constitute a small minority (table 8).

Table 8: Structure of social classes (percentages) (Spain, 1988-1991)

Class	1988a	1991b
Owners		
Capitalist	4.8	6.0
Businessmen with salaried workers	3.6	3.9
Managers and directors	1.2	2.1
Self-employed and independent	23.3	21.1
Professionals	1.3	2.2
Businessmen without employees	13.6	15.7
Agricultural proprietors without salaried workers	8.4	3.2
Salaried workers		
Employees	36.1	41.4
Dependent professionals and service workers	11.8	16.9
Commercial, technical and administrative workers	24.3	24.5
Manual workers	32.9	29
Skilled	23.5	16.7
Unskilled	5.1	10.8
Farmers	4.3	1.5
Unclassified	2.9	2.5

Source: a) Del Campo, 2002; b) FOESSA, 1994.

Temporary work is more frequent among manual salaried workers. While in 1991 among non-manual workers the proportions of men and women working with temporary contracts were 29.8% and 39% respectively. The corresponding percentages in manual workers were 46.7% and 36.8%.

An income concentration in the most privileged social classes and an increase in the most deprived social classes took place during the growth period of the 1960s and in the beginning of the 1970s (table 9). Although table 9 points to a reduction in income differences from the early 1970s to the early 1990s, income inequalities have tended to increase in the 1990s. These trends are closely related to the economic recession, to the high level of unemployment and to conservative government policies since the mid-1990s (not shown in table). Income distribution shows clear geographical differences at both regional and small-area levels. Thus, southern regions of Spain such as Extremadura and Andalusia only have about 76% and 80% of Spain's average household income.

Table 9: Income distribution by households deciles, 1964-1993
(% of total household income)

Deciles	Years							
	1964	1970	1974	1980	1981	1986	1991a	1993b
1	1.4	1.4	1.8	2.4	2.5	2.7	2.7	3.7
2	3.3	3.1	3.8	3.9	4.1	4.1	4.3	4.9
3	4.7	4.3	4.5	5.2	5.4	5.3	5.6	5.6
4	6.1	5.3	5.1	6.3	6.7	6.4	6.8	6.8
5	7.2	6.4	6.3	7.5	7.9	7.5	7.9	8.3
6	8.5	7.9	8.0	8.8	9.2	8.5	9.2	9.6
7	9.2	8.6	9.1	10.0	10.7	9.9	10.7	10.7
8	10.4	9.9	10.1	11.5	12.6	11.4	12.5	12.1
9	12.4	12.3	12.4	15.1	15.5	15.0	15.5	15.7
10	36.9	40.8	39.6	29.2	25.4	29.1	24.7	22.5

Sources: Del Campo S., 2002; a) FOESSA, 1994; b) Argentaria, 1995.

2. Occupational and Social Class Inequalities in Working Conditions

We found considerable differences between occupational classes with regard to exposures to unhealthy and damaging working conditions. In the next examples we illustrate some physical, chemical, ergonomic and psychosocial risk factors.

Tables 10 a and 10 b present selected results from the IVth Spanish National Survey on Working Conditions conducted in 1999 for men and women respectively. Physical risks are in general reported most frequently among male manual workers. For example, almost 52% of male manual workers were exposed to noise (30.5% for female manual workers) as compared with 32% in male non-manual workers (20.5% in female non-manual workers).

In the city of Barcelona we found a strong social class gradient for an overall measure of physical hazards (level of noise at work, air pollution at work, moving loads at work and repetitive movements with hands or arms) in both men and women (figure 3). Social class, assigned according to the respondent's current occupation, was measured with a widely used Spanish adaptation of the British classification (Domingo & Marcos 1989). Class I includes managerial and senior technical staff and freelance professionals; class II intermediate occupations and managers in commerce; class III, skilled non-manual workers; class IV, skilled (IVa) and partly skilled (IVb) manual workers; and class V, unskilled manual workers. In order to test whether gender patterns were the same for manual and non-manual workers, the six original classes were collapsed into these two categories: non-manual workers (classes I, II and III) and manual workers (classes IVa, IVb and V).

For both genders, manual workers (classes IV and V) show a higher prevalence of physical and chemical hazards. In particular, working class men are more exposed to physical hazards than their non-working-class counterparts.

For Spain, results also show a higher rate of exposure to musculoskeletal load among manual working classes (classes IV and V) and among women (table 10). Repetitive hand and arm movements were particularly prevalent among women. For example, almost 46.3% of female manual workers were exposed to repetitive hand or arm movements (34.4% for men) as compared with 28.2% in female non-manual workers (29.2% in men).

Figure 3: Mean of an index of physical risk factors[1] by occupational social class and sex in the working population (95% CI). Barcelona, 2000

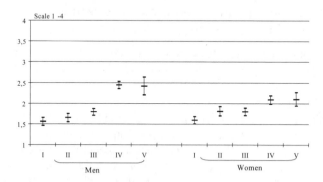

Source: Barcelona Health Survey, 2000.
[1] *The overall measure of physical hazards was created through a 4-point Likert scale using four risk factors: level of noise at work that does not enable one to speak with others, air pollution at work, moving loads of more than 14 kg at work and repetitive movements with hands or arms.*

Regarding psychosocial and organisational working conditions, psychosocial job demands were higher among non-manual workers, while gender differences were small within the class. Among manual workers psychological demands were generally more frequent among women, except for requirements of sustained attention, which were more frequent among men (table 10 a + b). On the other hand, social support showed minimal differences by class. Lack of job control, however, was two to four times more common among manual workers as compared with non-manual workers. Male and female manual workers reported control items to the same extent, except for lack of opportunities to develop own skills, which was twice as common among female manual workers. For the city of Barcelona, figure 4 shows that an overall measure of psychosocial risk factors (not doing varied work, not having autonomy at work, having excessive work and social isolation at work) was more common in the lower occupational social classes, especially in classes IV and V. This is especially noticeable among working-class women.

Finally, it is important to consider the vulnerable position of many employees to health hazards. There has been an overall increase in risk factors among both permanent and temporary workers, especially for the latter. Prevalence rates for all risk factors are higher among temporary workers. In 1999, for example, 5.8% of permanent workers worked on unstable surfaces, whereas that figure doubled for temporary workers (11.6%). Differences between contracts are more evident in work organisation exposures. For example, regarding not having control over job breaks, rates were 27 and 39% for permanent and temporary workers, respectively. Despite the fact that workers have legal protection from hazardous working conditions, temporary workers may be especially reluctant to use this protection for fear of losing their jobs (Amable *et al.* 2001). Regarding unions and immigrants' rights, non-governmental organisations have reported that illegal immigrants often work for sub-standard pay and in sub-standard working conditions, mainly in agriculture and construction. For example, in 2001 the Labour Inspectorate reported 7,501 cases of labour rights violations related to immigrants (US Department of State 2003).

Table 10 a: Proportion (%) of male non-manual an manual workers (25-64 years) exposed to selected physical, chemical, ergonomic and psychosocial risk factors

	Non-manual (N=831)	Manual (N=1241)
Physical risks		
Uncomfortable temperature in summer	21.7	36.6
Uncomfortable temperature in winter	20.9	27.0
Uncomfortable humidity	18.4	17.2
Noise	32.2	51.8
Vibrations	5.4	12.1
Toxic products	11.4	25.4
Musculoskeletal risks		
Painful or tiring positions > ½ day	6.9	9.7
Staying in the same position > ½ day	29.8	25.1
Carrying heavy loads > ½ day	3.2	7.3
Making an important effort > ½ day	2.2	4.8
Repetitive hand or arm movements > ½ day	29.2	34.4
Psychosocial risks		
Working with high demands of attention > ½ day	66.2	57.5
Working with high speed > ½ day	43.7	31.3
Repetitive tasks > ½ day	28.8	32.2
Too heavy workload	19.4	10.5
Doing overtime during the working day without any financial compensation	32.2	18.1
Poor relations with superiors	7.5	8.8
Poor relations with colleagues	2.4	2.4
Unable to change the order of tasks	9.2	28.9
Unable to change methods of work	16.9	39.5
Unable to change the pace	15.7	35.4
Unable to change the order of breaks	17.7	36.7
Lack of opportunity to develop own skills	3.6	13.7
No promotion since started working in the company	41.4	42.7

Source: ENCT IV [SNSWC], 1999.

Table 10 b: Proportion (%) of female non-manual an manual workers (25-64 years) exposed to selected physical, chemical, ergonomic and psychosocial risk factors

	Non-manual (N=695)	Manual (N=468)
Physical risks		
Uncomfortable temperature in summer	19.1	24.3
Uncomfortable temperature in winter	18.3	16.3
Uncomfortable humidity	14.2	10.0
Noise	20.5	30.5
Vibrations	2.5	5.2
Toxic products	9.4	17.8
Musculoskeletal risks		
Painful or tiring positions > ½ day	7.2	11.5
Staying in the same position > ½ day	36.1	36.0
Carrying heavy loads > ½ day	0.9	4.3
Making an important effort > ½ day	0.7	2.6
Repetitive hand or arm movements > ½ day	28.2	46.3
Psychosocial risks		
Working with high demands of attention > ½ day	64.7	42.9
Working with high speed > ½ day	40.1	28.8
Repetitive tasks > ½ day	27.9	43.2
Too heavy workload	19.3	15.8
Doing overtime during the working day without any financial compensation	29.2	23.5
Poor relations with superiors	5.1	8.0
Poor relations with colleagues	2.6	2.0
Unable to change the order of tasks	8.8	30.0
Unable to change methods of work	21.3	39.9
Unable to change the pace	20.1	35.9
Unable to change the order of breaks	17.5	36.7
Lack of opportunity to develop own skills	5.8	22.8
No promotion since started working in the company	51.8	65.7

Source: ENCT IV [SNSWC], 1999.

**Figure 4: Mean of psychosocial risk factors[1] (95% CI) by occupational
social class and sex in the working population in Barcelona 2000**

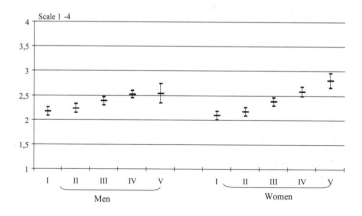

Source: Barcelona Health Survey, 2000.
[1] *The overall measure of psychosocial hazards was created through a 4-point Likert
scale using four risk factors: not doing varied work, not having autonomy at work,
having excessive work and social isolation at work.*

3. Occupational and Social Class Inequalities in Health

A. *Mortality*

Most research on socio-economic inequalities in health, including
occupational class health inequalities, has been based on mortality
statistics, and mainly on ecological studies. Most of these studies are
descriptive; there are very few investigations on trends, and almost no
analyses have attempted to investigate specific determinants of such
inequalities in health (Borrell & Pasarín 1999). Individual-based studies
are few, due to the absence or poor quality of information on socio-
economic characteristics in death certificates. In fact, the only individually based Spanish studies have been conducted in eight provinces
where occupation was more consistently available in the death certificates, and in a few cities where it was possible to link local census
socio-economic information with the death register (Borrell *et al.* 1999).
These studies have shown a higher mortality in men 30-64 years of age
for most causes of death among the more deprived occupational social
classes in comparison with professionals and managers, and these class
differences have increased over the period from 1980-1982 to 1988-
1990 (figure 5) (Regidor *et al.* 1995).

312

Figure 5: Ratio of SMRs of male manual workers compared to professionals, 30-64 years for selected causes of death in 8 provinces

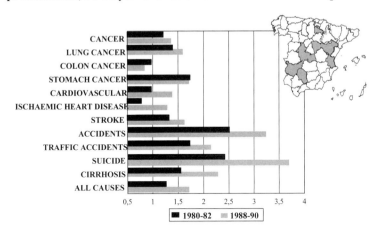

Source: Regidor E., et al. 1995,"Increased Socioeconomic Differences in Mortality in Eight Spanish Provinces". Soc Sci Med 41(6): 801-807.

A study on trends in socio-economic differences in the economically active male population grouped in four categories (professional/managerial, clerical/sales/service workers, farmers, and manual workers) aged 25-64 years in Spain (table 11) has shown mortality differences from ischaemic heart and cerebrovascular diseases (Lostao *et al.* 2001). In 1980-1982 professionals and managers aged 25-44 years had the lowest risk of mortality due to ischaemic heart disease, and by 1988-1990 the socio-economic differences in mortality had increased. In 1980-1982, professionals and managers aged 45-64 years had higher mortality from ischaemic heart disease than the other occupational groups. For cerebrovascular disease, manual workers experienced the highest mortality in the 25-44 year age group in 1980-1982, and the differences seemed to increase by 1988-1990 in comparison with all other groups. Manual workers also had the highest mortality from cerebrovascular diseases between 45 and 64 years in 1980-1982, and the difference in comparison with non-manual employees increased to 1998-1990. These findings could be the result of the adoption of healthier lifestyles (e.g., reduced smoking and increased physical activity) in the higher socio-economic classes, and an increase in smoking and sedentary lifestyle in the lower socio-economic classes. Likewise, changes in the exposure to risk factors at the workplace, especially to psychosocial factors, might have played a significant role. Nevertheless, as the authors point out, caution needs to be exercised, since a number of potential limitations may have compromised these findings. Thus, results are derived from only eight provinces (mostly rural) which do not necessarily represent the whole country. The high mortality risk in manual workers may be attributed to the small sample size, and results of unlinked cross-sectional studies may be compromised by the bias derived from excluding the economically inactive population and the numerator/denominator bias.

Table 11: Ischaemic heart disease and cerebrovascular disease mortality by occupational class: Rate ratio (95% CI) for occupationally active men aged 25-44 and 45-64 years at death, 1980-1982 and 1988-1990

	Ischaemic heart disease		Cerebrovascular disease	
	1980-1982	1988-1990	1980-1982	1988-1990
25-44 years				
Professional and managerial	1.00	1.00	1.00	1.00
Clerical/sales/service workers	1.34 (0.74-2.43)	1.20 (0.58-2.49)	1.07 (0.77-1.47)	2.02 (0.58-7.00)
Farmers	1.27 (0.69-2.33)	2.10 (1.02-4.33)	0.89 (0.65-1.21)	2.99 (0.84-10.61)
Manual workers	1.28 (0.73-2.25)	1.81 (0.93-3.49)	1.39 (1.03-1.87)	4.30 (1.35-13.74)
45-64 years				
Professional and managerial	1.00	1.00	1.00	1.00
Clerical/sales/service workers	0.74 (0.60-0.91)	0.80 (0.61-1.05)	0.95 (0.68-1.33)	1.00 (0.66-1.52)
Farmers	0.51 (0.42-0.63)	1.25 (0.98-1.60)	0.82 (0.60-1.13)	1.68 (1.14-2.47)
Manual workers	0.78 (0.64-0.94)	1.37 (1.08-1.74)	1.28 (0.94-1.75)	1.52 (1.04-2.23)

Source: Lostao L., Regidor E., Aiach P., Dominguez V., 2001.

B. Self-perceived Health Status and Other Health-related Factors

Poor self-perceived health (measured through a single question: "Would you say your overall health is very good, good, fair, poor or very poor?") is more common in lower than in higher social classes, as summarised below. 40% of those in manual classes and 27% of those in professional classes in 1995 reported less than good self-perceived health, and those differences had increased in the period 1987-1995 (Urbanos 1999). Additionally, another study showed that poor self-perceived health status increased in the low-income regions during the period 1987-1993 (Navarro & Benach 1996) (figure 6).

Figure 6: Odds ratios of poor self-perceived health by occupational class and region in men (National Health Surveys 1987 and 1993). Class I is used as reference category

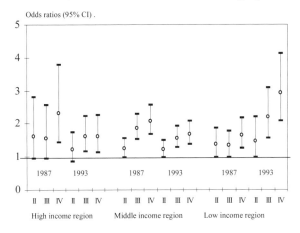

Source: Navarro V., Benach J. and the Scientific Commission for the study of health inequalities in Spain Desigualdades sociales en salud en España (Social Inequalities in health in Spain). Madrid: Ministerio de Sanidad y Consumo, 1996.

In the last national health survey, conducted in 2001, there was a gradient in poor self-perceived health by social class and gender (Daponte, in press) but the gradient was steeper among women than men (figure 7). Indeed, the occupational and social conditions of working-class women are very deficient in Spain: Working class women are more often unemployed, and they have high family demands that require taking care of children and elderly dependents in a context of few public services. A study in Catalonia showed that poor self-perceived health was three times more common among working-class female cleaners than among non-manual employees (Artazcoz *et al*. 2003).

Moreover, the more deprived social classes are more likely to experience chronic illnesses such as asthma, chronic bronchitis, hypertension or diabetes and worse health-related behaviours like smoking, lack of physical exercise and alcohol abuse. For example, in 1993, working social class women were 2.5 times more likely to be diagnosed with diabetes than women of the most privileged social class (Navarro & Benach 1996).

**Figure 7: Odds ratios (95% CI) of reporting poor self-perceived
health by social class among men and women 2001.
Class I is used as the reference category**

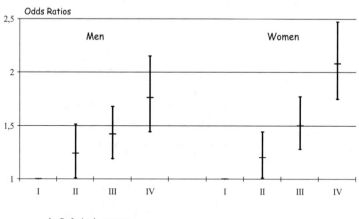

I Professionals, managers
II Intermediate occupations, salesman
III Skilled workers
IV Non skilled workers

*Source: Daponte A. Socioeconomic environment and trends in inequalities in health in
Spain. PhD Dissertation, 2005.*

C. Injuries

Spain has the highest European incidence of occupational injuries
resulting in more than three days of job leave and one of the highest
incidences of fatal injuries on the job. For example, in comparison with
the EU average in 1999, Spain showed a 71% excess of injuries leading
to more than 3 days of leave and a 35% excess of occupational injuries.
The distribution of injuries by occupation shows large differences. For
example, regarding fatal injuries caused by occupational accidents on a
working day, the occupations with the highest incidences were among
non-skilled and skilled construction workers (204 and 168.8 per 1,000
workers respectively in 2000-2001) and metal workers (160.1) (Durán
& Benavides 2004).

Figure 8: Incidence of non-fatal occupational injuries, resulting in leave of absence, per 1,000 workers according to type of contract, 1989-2001

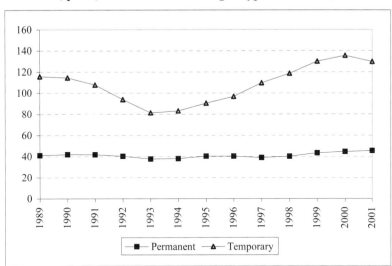

Source: MTAS, Statistics of Occupational Accidents; Statistics of Affiliation to Social Security.

Figure 9: Incidence of fatal occupational accidents per 100,000 workers according to type of contract, 1989-2001

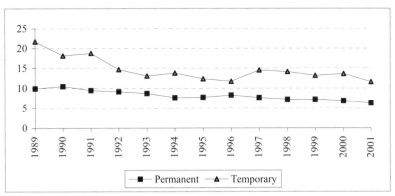

Source: MTAS, Statistics of Occupational Accidents; Statistics of Affiliation to Social Security.

Type of contract is one of the key factors associated with a higher incidence of occupational injuries. From 1989 to 2001, temporary workers have shown a risk of non-fatal injury between two and three times higher than that for permanent workers (figure 8). The relative risk was around two in the case of fatal injuries (figure 9). A more refined analysis by sex and occupation confirms these findings (table 12) (Benavides *et al.*, submitted). Thus, temporary workers show significantly higher relative risks of traumatic occupational injuries, particularly among men (more than three times the risk among permanent workers). In all occupational categories, temporary workers have a significantly higher risk of non-fatal occupational injuries than permanent employees. In relation to fatal occupational injuries, strong associations were found in elementary occupations (RR=3.5), among machine operators (RR=2.8), and trades workers (2.2). Finally, the analysis of occupational injuries by two large occupational classes and type of injury also showed a much higher incidence among manual workers (table 13).

Table 12: Incidence and relative risk (RR) of fatal and non-fatal occupational injuries in temporary and permanent employment by sex and occupation 2000-2001. The results are adjusted for age, length of employment, and economic activity

	Non-fatal Incidence[1]			Fatal Incidence[2]		
	Perma-nent	Tempo-rary	RR	Perma-nent	Tempo-rary	RR
Sex						
Males	57.6	185.4	3.22*	6.2	17.1	2.74*
Females	22.5	54.9	2.44*	0.3	0.5	1.70
Occupations (ISCO-88)						
Legislators, senior officials and managers	5.9	17.2	2.91*	3.0	0.0	0.00
Professionals	5.0	10.4	2.08*	0.8	1.0	1.22
Technicians and associate professionals	10.7	23.8	2.22*	2.6	4.7	1.81*
Clerks	12.3	30.7	2.49*	0.7	1.0	1.47
Service workers and shop and market sales workers	44.3	85.1	1.92*	1.4	1.1	0.79
Skilled agricultural and fishery workers	63.1	120.5	1.91*	25.9	11.3	0.44*
Craft and related trades workers	104.7	232.9	2.22*	7.4	15.7	2.13*
Plant and machine operators and assemblers	67.4	128.8	1.91*	11.5	32.0	2.78*
Elementary occupations	73.8	185.0	2.50*	3.1	10.9	3.47*
Total	44.6	131.6	2.95*	4.00	10.2	2.57*

[1] *per 1,000 workers* [2] *per 100,000 workers* * *statistically significant with p <0.05.*
Source: Durán F., Benavides F.G., 2004.

Table 13: Occupational injuries with leave of absence from work, by occupational class and type of injury. Rates per 1,000 workers (minor, serious, and total), 10,000 workers (fatal) and relative risk (RR)

	Non-manual	Manual	RR
Minor	8.81	88.53	10.05
Serious	0.21	1.09	5.10
Fatal	0.27	0.87	3.21
Total	9.05	89.71	9.91

Source: Durán F., Benavides F.G., 2004.

D. Work-related Diseases

Data on work-related diseases by occupational class and severity of illness show much higher incidences among manual than non-manual workers for both minor and serious illnesses (table 14). Likewise, large differences can be observed with regard to different occupations and classes (0.7 per 100,000 for chief executive officers vs. 469.2 for construction workers, 482.7 for manual textile workers and 696.5 per 100,000 for qualified workers in the extractive and metallurgical industries, in 2002) (Durán & Benavides 2004). In Spain there has not been any systematic attempt to verify the completeness and accuracy of occupational disease registries (usually very susceptible to underreporting). Therefore the quality of the data remains a serious concern in these studies.

Table 14: Work-related diseases by occupational class and type. Rates per 1,000 workers (minor, serious, and total), 10,000 workers (fatal) and relative risk (RR)

	Non-manual	Manual	RR
Minor	1.30	17.53	13.50
Serious	0.49	1.45	2.95
Total	1.35	17.67	13.12

Source: Durán F., Benavides FG., 2004.

E. The Impact of Working Conditions on Social Inequalities in Health

An approach to explore the key question of the impact of work on health inequalities has been attempted, by analysing cross-sectional associations between occupational class and health, using data from the 2000 Barcelona Health Survey which includes data on occupational social class, age, and sex, as well as on physical and psychosocial working conditions. The response variables were less than good self-perceived health and mental health (using the GHQ-12 questionnaire).

For both health outcomes, occupational class gradients are stronger for women than for men. With regard to self-assessed health, a substantial proportion of the variation is explained statistically by working conditions in the case of men (42%), whereas among women that proportion is significantly lower (7%) (table 15 a + b). Moreover, whereas among men the contribution of working conditions to the class differences in health increases as social class decreases, there is not a consistent pattern among women.

Table 15 a: The effects of physical and psychosocial working conditions on social inequalities in self-perceived health among men [a][b]

	Model 1		Model 2			Model 3			Model 4		
	ORa	(95% CI)	ORa	(95% CI)	Difference (%)	ORa	(95%CI)	Difference (%)	ORa	(95% CI)	Difference (%)
Age	1.06	(1.04-1.07)	1.06	(1,05-1,07)	(%)	1.06	(1,05-1,07)	(%)	1.06	(1,05-1,07)	(%)
Social class 1											
Social class 2	0.69	(0.29-1.65)	0.64	(0.27-1.55)	-16	0.66	(0.27-1.57)	-10	0.62	(0.26-1.49)	-23
Social class 3	2.32	(1.40-3.83)	2.05	(1.24-3.41)	20	2.19	(1.32-3.63)	10	1.97	(1.18-3.28)	27
Social class 4	3.57	(2.19-5.81)	2.54	(1.51-4.27)	40	3.24	(1.98-5.31)	13	2.39	(1.41-4.03)	46
Social class 5	4.37	(2.20-8.68)	3.18	(1.56-6.45)	35	3.49	(1.68-7.24)	26	2.95	(1.45-6.01)	42
Physical risk			1.88	(1.36-2.60)					1.8	(1.30-2.50)	
Psychoso-cial risk						1.5	(1.12-2.01)		1.41	(1.05-1.90)	

[a] *Class I includes managerial and senior technical staff and freelance professionals; class II intermediate occupations and managers in commerce; class III, skilled non-manual workers; class IV, skilled (IVa) and partly-skilled (IVb) manual workers; and class V, unskilled manual workers. In order to test whether gender patterns were the same for manual and non-manual workers, the six original classes were collapsed into these two categories: non-manual workers (classes I, II and III) and manual workers (classes IVA, IVB and V).*

[b] *Physical risk factors were created using four items: level of noise at work that does not enable one to speak with others, air pollution at work, moving loads of more than 14 kg at work and repetitive movements with hands or arms. Psychosocial risk factors were created using four items: not doing varied work, not having autonomy at work, having excessive work and social isolation at work.*

Source: Barcelona Health Survey, 2000.

Table 15 b: The effects of physical and psychosocial working conditions on social inequalities in self-perceived health among women [a][b]

	Model 1		Model 2			Model 3			Model 4		
	OR a	95% CI	OR a	95% CI	Diffe-rence (%)	OR a	95% CI	Difference (%)	OR a	95% CI	Diffe-rence (%)
Age	1.05	1,04-1,06	1.05	1-04-1,06		1.05	1,04-1,07		1.05	1,04-1,06	
Social class 1											
Social class 2	1.85	0.88-3.89	1.75	0.83-3.69	12	1.85	0.88-3.89	0	1.75	0.83-3.69	12
Social class 3	2.2	1.18-4.10	2.16	1.16-4.04	3	2.19	1.17-4.09	1	2.17	1.16-4.05	3
Social class 4	4.25	2.29-7.91	3.87	2.07-7.23	12	4.22	2.26-7.89	1	3.88	2.07-7.29	11
Social class 5	6.86	3.62-13.0	6.31	3.32-12.0	9	6.78	3.54-12.98	1	6.36	3.31-12.20	9
Physical risk			1.42	1.06-1.90					1.42	1.06-1.91	
Psychosocial risk						0.98	0.73-1.33				

[a] *Class I includes managerial and senior technical staff and freelance professionals; class II intermediate occupations and managers in commerce; class III, skilled non-manual workers; class IV, skilled (IVa) and partly-skilled (IVb) manual workers; and class V, unskilled manual workers. In order to test whether gender patterns were the same for manual and non-manual workers, the six original classes were collapsed into these two categories: non-manual workers (classes I, II and III) and manual workers (classes IVA, IVB and V).*

[b] *Physical risk factors were created using four items: level of noise at work that does not enable one to speak with others, air pollution at work, moving loads of more than 14 kg at work and repetitive movements with hands or arms. Psychosocial risk factors were created using four items: not doing varied work, not having autonomy at work, having excessive work and social isolation at work.*

Source: Barcelona Health Survey, 2000.

Interestingly, the contribution of working conditions in explaining social class gradients in mental health is substantial and similar in both sexes (39% among men and 35% among women) (table 16 a + b). While these potentially interesting findings suggest that occupational class inequalities in health may be partially explained by working conditions, these results should be examined in the future with more refined analyses.

Table 16 a: The effects of physical and psychosocial working conditions on social inequalities in mental health among men [a] [b]

	Model 1		Model 2			Model 3			Model 4		
	ORa	(95% CI)	ORa	(95% CI)	Diffe-rence	ORa	(95% CI)	Diffe-rence	ORa	(95% CI)	Diffe-rence
Age	1.00	(0.99-1.01)	1	(0,99-1,01)	(%)	1.00	0,99-1,01	(%)	1	(0,99-1,01)	(%)
Social class 1											
Social class 2	1.45	(0.84-2.48)	1.41	(0.82-2.42)	9	1.44	0.84-2.46	3	1.41	(0.82-2.41)	9
Social class 3	1.29	(0.83-2.01)	1.23	(0.79-1.92)	21	1.28	0.82-2.00	3	1.23	(0.78-1.92)	21
Social class 4	1.31	(0.84-2.04)	1.12	(0.7-1.79)	61	1.29	0.83-2.02	5	1.11	(0.69-1.79)	65
Social class 5	1.69	(0.86-3.31)	1.43	(0.71-2.87)	38	1.66	0.84-3.27	4	1.42	(0.71-2.86)	39
Physical risk									1.35	(0.98-1.86)	
Psychosocial risk						1.06	0.79-1.42		1.03	(0.77-1.38)	

[a] *Class I includes managerial and senior technical staff and freelance professionals; class II intermediate occupations and managers in commerce; class III, skilled non-manual workers; class IV, skilled (IVa) and partly-skilled (IVb) manual workers; and class V, unskilled manual workers. In order to test whether gender patterns were the same for manual and non-manual workers, the six original classes were collapsed into these two categories: non-manual workers (classes I, II and III) and manual workers (classes IVA, IVB and V).*

[b] *Physical risk factors were created using four items: level of noise at work that does not enable one to speak with others, air pollution at work, moving loads of more than 14 kg at work and repetitive movements with hands or arms. Psychosocial risk factors were created using four items: not doing varied work, not having autonomy at work, having excessive work and social isolation at work.*

Source: Barcelona Health Survey, 2000.

Table 16 b: The effects of physical and psychosocial working conditions on social inequalities in mental health among women [a] [b]

	Model 1		Model 2		Difference (%)	Model 3		Difference (%)	Model 4		Difference (%)
	ORa	(95% CI)	ORa	(95% CI)		ORa	(95% CI)		ORa	(95% CI)	
Age	1.00	0.98-1.01	0.99	0,98-1,01		1.00	0,98-1,01				
Social class 1											
Social class 2	1.6	0.94-2.73	1.49	0.87-2.55	18	1.59	0.93-2.71	2	1.49	0.87-2.55	18
Social class 3	1.33	0.84-2.10	1.30	0.82-2.05	9	1.28	0.81-2.03	14	1.26	0.80-1.99	21
Social class 4	1.93	1.21-3.06	1.68	1.05-2.69	27	1.75	1.10-2.79	20	1.56	0.97-2.51	40
Social class 5	2.33	1.38-3.93	2.08	1.23-3.53	19	2.02	1.19-3.44	23	1.86	1.09-3.17	35
Physical risk			1.56	1.19-2.03		1.47	1.13-1.92	16	1.49	1.14-1.95	-4
Psychosocial risk									1.4	1.07-1.84	

[a] *Class I includes managerial and senior technical staff and freelance professionals; class II intermediate occupations and managers in commerce; class III, skilled non-manual workers; class IV, skilled (IVa) and partly-skilled (IVb) manual workers; and class V, unskilled manual workers. In order to test whether gender patterns were the same for manual and non-manual workers, the six original classes were collapsed into these two categories: non-manual workers (classes I, II and III) and manual workers (classes IVA, IVB and V).*

[b] *Physical risk factors were created using four items: level of noise at work that does not enable one to speak with others, air pollution at work, moving loads of more than 14 kg at work and repetitive movements with hands or arms. Psychosocial risk factors were created using four items: not doing varied work, not having autonomy at work, having excessive work and social isolation at work.*

Source: Barcelona Health Survey, 2000.

4. Policy Considerations

Among the many factors that may play a role in improving the work environment and reducing work-related health inequalities, some of the most relevant include the development of legislation, the role of key social actors, the production of knowledge, and the implementation of effective actions. We highlight here the following four key issues: recent legislative changes, the role of the trade unions, and the development of research and policy interventions.

A. Legislation

Because of 40 years of dictatorship during the 20th century, labour laws emerged in Spain much later than in other European countries. For example, the right to collective bargaining and the right to strike did not appear in the Spanish legislation until the Constitution of 1978. The basic modern rules governing health and safety at work containing an extensive list of regulations and prescriptions were set only in 1971, later supplemented by other regulations directed specifically at certain industries, occupations or types of work, many of which implemented European Directives and Regulations. In November 1995, the Prevention of Occupational Hazards Act (Law 31/1995) established a modern and general framework of health and safety at work that regulated, among other things, the general obligations or duties of employers, employees and the manufacturers and suppliers of machinery and equipment with regard to the prevention of risk, and the consultation and participation rights of workers and employee representatives. This law on the prevention of occupational risks and its corresponding regulations led to the universal legal protection of health at work (except workers in the informal sector), and the integration of prevention into management structures of companies.

The implementation of this legislation, however, took place in a situation where companies and the Spanish government sought more flexible forms of labour market organisation. Thus, a deep-reaching reform of labour legislation took place in 1994. This extensive reform, (followed by other minor reforms in 2001 and 2002), sought the amendment of many of the precepts of the major labour laws (e.g., the Workers' Statute, the Labour Procedure Act or the Labour Offences and Sanctions Act), and included the adoption of a number of new laws such as an Act on temporary employment agencies, and the revision of regulations on temporary/fixed-term contracts, training contracts and redundancy procedures that established the foundations for a revised regulation of the collective bargaining system. Some of the major aspects of this reform included: a significant transfer of regulatory powers regarding pay and conditions from the law to collective agreements; the decentralisation of collective bargaining, especially in the form of firm agreements; a lifting of the public monopoly on job placement, to allow the operation of private employment agencies and temporary employment agencies; and the reduction of the costs of individual dismissal, through a restriction of the cases in which back pay awards after dismissal appeal hearings are to be paid by employers. Under these conditions, more and more often previously illegal situations that harmed workers were made legal. By and large, these changes led to the progressive segmentation of the labour force, with a core of permanent workers and a group of precarious workers with greater insecurity of employment.

Given the agreements between representatives of the government, employers' organisations and trade unions (January 2003), important legislative reforms of the Prevention of Occupational Hazards Act are expected during 2004 and 2005. Two of the main legislative issues to be reformed include the integration of prevention into the structure and line management of companies with implementation of proper internal preventive resources, and a number of measures to put into force inspectorate mechanisms of control, surveillance and penalisation (Durán & Benavides 2004).

B. Trade Unions

After having been suppressed during Franco's regime, trade union freedom was restored in Spain by the 1978 Constitution and developed in the Trade Union Freedom Act. The two main labour federations are the Workers' Commissions Confederation (*Comisiones Obreras*, CC.OO.) and the General Workers' Confederation (*Unión General de Trabajadores*, UGT), which tend to describe themselves as class-based trade unions.

Although no official figures are available, according to several sources it is estimated that only between 18 and 20% of the Spanish employed labour force is unionised (about 2.6 million people out of 13.1 million) (US Department of State 2003, Bonet 2004). The highest rates of unionised workers are found in the industrial sector (21%), while the lowest percentages are found in the construction sector (11.2%) (Van der Meer 1997).

Trade Union Policies on Workplace Health Factors

Similarly to other southern European countries, trade unions in Spain are weaker than in many Northern European countries. Traditionally, the main concerns of Spanish trade unions have been wages, earnings and employment issues, and it is only more recently that working conditions, welfare policies and some occupational health issues have been on their agenda. Nevertheless, in recent years a number of valuable actions and interventions may have helped to improve the work environment for the majority of workers, some of which may have even improved the working conditions of the most vulnerable workers. First, the new Prevention of Occupational Hazards Act and its corresponding regulations have increased worker participation through the action of trade union representatives and delegates who can play a specific role in the implementation of Occupational Health Prevention plans. Second, thanks to the social dialogue established in the Social

Dialogue Table for the Risk Prevention of Occupational Hazards among the Government, employers' organisations (the Spanish Confederation of Employers' Organisations and the Confederation of Employers of Small- and Medium-Sized Enterprises) and the main trade union confederations (the Workers' Committees and the General Union of Workers), a number of needs and insufficiencies have been detected and several agreements have been reached to fulfil them. These agreements, approved in the National Commission of Health and Safety at the Workplace (January 2003), try to improve the current legislation on Prevention of Occupational Hazards. Also, it has emphasised the integration of prevention into the structure and line management of companies, requiring a major commitment and participation of the employers in the process. Third, given the high incidence of occupational injuries and hazardous working conditions, trade unions have heavily criticised the Government for devoting insufficient resources to inspection and enforcement. In particular, trade unions have underlined the low level of application of the prevention law, and the importance of subcontracting, temporary employment and the increasing instability of the labour market as the main factors behind occupational injuries. Fourth, given the lack of trade union representatives in many small- and medium-size firms, and in sectors such as construction, where many workers have temporary contracts, trade unions have proposed the creation of 'regional safety delegates' who will function as prevention delegates (Miguélez 2000). This proposal has already reached the construction sector in some regions such as the Canary Islands or Catalonia. Finally, in Spain collective bargaining agreements are widespread in both the public and private sectors; in the latter they covered about 83% of workers in 2003, even though only a relatively small number of workers were union members (Durán & Benavides 2004). The collective bargaining process is an important potential space that trade unions may use to improve the work environment, workers' rights and occupational health for all workers. However, today it is not possible to assess the degree to which these processes may have had an impact on the reduction of health inequalities.

Trade Union Actions regarding Health Inequalities at the Workplace

Work-related inequalities in health have not been specifically addressed by any of the Spanish trade unions. In fact, specific references or discussions on this subject are rarely found in trade union publications. However, it is important to note the efforts made by the Trade Union Institute of Work, Environment and Health (ISTAS), an independent non-profit technical foundation created by the Workers' Committees (CC.OO.) to promote occupational health and environmental protection serving the interests and needs of all workers. The main activities of ISTAS include the following: the production of information; design of training programmes to improve the capabilities of trade union safety delegates and representatives; coordination of a regional network of technical offices that advise safety delegates and Health and Safety Committees as well as other union officers and bodies; promotion of lines of research that are of interest to the trade union movement in cooperation with universities and scientific organisations; and dissemination of knowledge and the promotion of public debate around the issues of occupational health and environmental problems. However, these activities have only indirectly addressed health inequalities, and no specific measures proposed to deal with health inequalities at work have been suggested.

C. Research

Spain has moved rapidly from having no monitoring of social inequalities in health to having a small but active programme in that research area. While in the 1970s and early and mid-1980s social inequalities in health constituted a 'non-issue', an increase in the number of studies took place in the late 1980s and remarkable progress has been achieved in the 1990s (Benach *et al.* 2002). The so-called Spanish Black Report was published in 1996, providing an extensive review of class, gender and geographical health inequalities in Spain, and documenting considerable inequalities in mortality, health status, health behaviours and utilisation of health services (Navarro & Benach 1996). In addition, this report also documented the effects of various social and health policy interventions on health inequalities, and made specific recommendations to tackle those inequalities. Thus, the report made four major recommendations: the urgent need to monitor health inequalities, the development of both social and health data on health inequalities, the establishment of a Scientific Commission to study health inequalities on a permanent basis, and the urgent need to implement interventions to tackle health inequalities in all social groups rather than only in the worst-off sectors of the population. Similarly to the *Black Report* or the *Health Divide* in the UK, the new conservative government did not show much enthusiasm for the Spanish report. The report was 'buried'; its findings were not considered, and its recommendations dismissed. In spite of the progress achieved in the last few years in understanding socio-economic inequalities, the number of research groups focusing on health inequalities, as well as the public health institutions and funding sources to support them, are very limited (Benach *et al.* 2004). Moreover, most of these research projects do not aim in particular to study the role played by working conditions on social inequalities in health. Indeed, the first study on occupational health inequalities has only recently been published in the region of Catalonia (Artazcoz *et al.* 2003) as part of a Catalonian Black Report (Borrell & Benach 2003). Therefore, we may say that today, in an overall evaluation, research on social inequalities in health is located in a "denial/indifference" phase (Benach *et al.* 2002), while research on work-related inequalities may be located in what has been called the "need for measurement" phase (Whitehead 1998).

D. Policy

Work-related health problems in Spain imply enormous costs in terms of both money and health to workers and their families, as well as to companies and society as a whole (Durán & Benavides 2004). The high level of occupational injuries, for example, reflects important deficiencies in the prevention systems that a developed European country should not allow itself to have. Norms and regulations on prevention of occupational hazards have been only partially applied and budgets have been limited. Moreover, many interventions targeting traditional occupational hazards, and thought to be implemented for those holding permanent jobs and working for medium-to-large-size firms, are unlikely to meet the demands of the new work-flexible environment. Indeed, the growth in precarious working conditions constitutes one of the main obstacles to reduce work-related health inequalities. In Spain only a few specific interventions such as special employment programmes, employment quotas and preferential employment directed particularly at young workers, female employment, disabled workers and older workers have been implemented. Nevertheless, the success of these interventions is limited and its impact on health inequalities has not been evaluated.

In order to face the emergent health problems imposed by labour mobility and precarious employment, integral policies, which take technical, economic, cultural and political factors into account, are needed. Some of the main challenges lying ahead are the following. First, we need to improve our knowledge of new occupational health hazards, with special attention to class- and gender-based work-related health inequalities. Second, we need to give more priority to efficient forms of intervention that tackle the needs of the most vulnerable workers, helping to increase their level of participation in preventing occupational injuries and illnesses. Problems of women, migrants, precarious employees and manual workers, as well as those of small enterprises, deserve special attention. Third, and very importantly, it is crucial to ensure the proper enforcement and evaluation of actions and interventions. Knowledge, priorities and interventions should be adapted to each type of worker, workplace and firm, with an understanding of their socio-economic position. In an increasingly deregulated labour market, a key political challenge is the need for generating social and political forces that help to strengthen the labour rights of workers.

The airing of social inequalities in health research has so far produced little reaction with regard to health policies and interventions, and there are no specific national or regional policies or interventions aiming to reduce social health inequalities. The health of the working population has yet to become a top priority of the Spanish policy agenda. Policies or interventions to reduce work-related health inequalities have not been formulated as one of the main goals of the national and regional health strategies. This crucial gap is a serious and a major concern to reduce inequalities in health. The main reasons for the lack of official reaction include both the weakness of public health groups, trade unions, social organisations, and other social groups, and the lack of political will of the national conservative government as well as of many regional governments. Until now in Spain no national or regional policies have been formulated seeking to reduce health inequalities with the specific goal of reducing work-related inequalities in health. If work-related inequalities in health are to be reduced, it is essential both to increase our knowledge and to carry out a wide range of interventions and policies implemented and evaluated at all levels. The labour movement, labour-based political organisations, social organisations, and, especially, governments at the national and regional levels, have the responsibility of defining and being accountable for occupational health policies that enforce legislation and firm compliance that leads to occupational health for all. Indeed, the most important policy issue today is that of putting the need to understand and reduce work-related health inequalities on the agenda of governments, unions and other social institutions.

References

ALAÑÓN A., GÓMEZ DE ANTONIO M. 2003. Una evaluación del grado de incumplimiento fiscal para las provincias españolas. Instituto de Estudios Fiscales, dependiente del Ministerio de Hacienda: http://www.minhac.es/ief/principal.htm. [Page visited 19-11-03].

AMABLE M., BENACH J., GONZÁLEZ S. 2001. "La precariedad laboral y su impacto sobre la salud: conceptos y resultados preliminares de un estudio multi-métodos". *Arch Prev Riesgos Laboral* 4, 169-184.

ARGENTARIA. 1995. *Las desigualdades en España. Síntesis Estadística*. Madrid: Argentaria.

ARTAZCOZ L., BORRELL C., BENACH J. 2001. "Gender inequalities in health among workers: the relation with family demands" . *J Epidemiol Community Health* 55: 639-647.

ARTAZCOZ L., CORTÈS I., BENACH J., BENAVIDES FG. 2003. "Les desigualtats en la salut laboral". [Occupational health inequalities] In: BORRELL C., BENACH J. (coords). *Desigualtats en salut a Catalunya* [Health inequalities in Catalonia]. Barcelona: Mediterránea: 251-282.

ARTAZCOZ L., BENACH J., BORRELL C., CORTÈS I. 2004. "Unemployment and mental health: understanding the interaction between gender, family roles and social class". *Am J Public Health* 94: 82-88.

BENACH J., BENAVIDES FG., PLATT S., DIEZ-ROUX AV., MUNTANER C. 2000. "The health-damaging potential of new types of employment: a challenge for public health researchers". *Am J Public Health* 90: 1316-7.

BENACH J., YASUI Y., BORRELL C., ROSA E., PASARÍN MªI., BENACH N., ESPAÑOL E., MARTÍNEZ JM., DAPONTE A. 2001. *Atlas of mortality in small areas in Spain (1987-1995)*. Barcelona: Universitat Pompeu Fabra.

BENACH J., MUNTANER C., BENAVIDES FG., AMABLE M., JÓDAR P. 2002. "A new occupational health agenda for a new work environment". *Scand J Work Environ Health* 28: 191-6.

BENACH J., BORRELL C., DAPONTE A. 2002. "Social and economic policies in Spain with potential impact on reducing health inequalities". In: MACKENBACH J.P., BAKKER M. (eds.). *Reducing inequalities in health: A European perspective*. Routledge: 262-273.

BENACH J., AMABLE M. 2004. Las clases sociales y la pobreza [Social classes and poverty]. In: BORRELL C., GARCÍA CALVENTE Mª DEL MAR, VICENTE J., (eds.) *Informe de la Sociedad Española de Salud Pública y Administración sanitaria (SESPAS) 2004: La salud pública desde la perspectiva de género y clase social* [Public health from a gender and social class perspective]. *Gac Sanit* 18: Suppl 1: 16-23.

BENACH J., DAPONTE A., BORRELL C., ARTAZCOZ L., FERNÁNDEZ E. 2004. Las desigualdades en la salud y la calidad de vida en España [Inequalities in health and quality of life in Spain]. In: NAVARRO V (coord.). *El Estado de Bienestar en España* [The Spanish Welfate State]. Madrid: Tecnos: 375-410.

BENAVIDES FG., BENACH J., DELCLÓS G., AMABLE M., MUNTANER C. Temporary employment and risk of traumatic occupational injuries (submitted).

BONET X. (Centre d'Estudis i Recerca Sindicals [Trade Union Research and Studies Centre], CERES). 2004. Personal communication.

BORRELL C., REGIDOR E., ARIAS LA., NAVARRO P., PUIGPINÓS R., DOMINGUEZ V., PLASÈNCIA A. 1999. "Inequalities in mortality according to educational level in two large Southern European cities". *Int J Epidemiology* 28: 58-63.

BORRELL C., PASARÍN MI. 1999. "The study of social inequalities in health in Spain: where are we?". *J Epidem Community Health* 53: 388-9.

BORRELL C., BENACH J. (eds.). 2003. *Desigualtats en salut a Catalunya* [Health inequalities in Catalonia]. Barcelona: Mediterránea: 251-282.

CONSEJO ECONÓMICO Y SOCIAL. 2003. *Segundo informe sobre la situación de las mujeres en la realidad sociolaboral española.* Madrid: Consejo Económico y Social.

DAPONTE A. 2005. "Socioeconomic environment and trends in inequalities in health in Spain (1987-2001)". PhD Dissertation. Baltimore: The Johns Hopkins University.

DEL CAMPO S. 2002. "Social Stratification and Inequalities in Spain: The State of The Art". In: LEMEL Y., NOLL H. *Changing Structures of Inequality: A Comparative Perspective.* London: Mc Gill-Queen's University Press.

DOMINGO A., MARCOS J. 1989. "Propuesta de un indicador de la "clase social" basado en la ocupación". *Gac Sanit* 3: 320-6.

DURÁN F., BENAVIDES FG. (eds.). 2004. *Informe de salud laboral. Los riesgos laborales y su prevención. España, 2003.* [Occupational Health Report. Occupational risk hazards and its prevention. Spain, 2003] Barcelona: Zurich Prevención.

ENCUESTA DE POBLACIÓN ACTIVA [Labour Population Survey]: Instituto Nacional de Estadística [page visited: 27-10-03] Accessible in: http://www.ine.es/inebase/cgi/um?M=%2Ft22%2Fe308&O=inebase&N=&L.

ENCUESTA NACIONAL DE CONDICIONES DE TRABAJO IV [IV Spanish National Survey on Working Conditions]. 1999. Instituto de Seguridad e Higiene en el Trabajo.

ETXEZARRETA M. (ed.). 1991. *La reestructuración del capitalismo en España, 1970-1990.* Barcelona: Icaria.

FIELD CENSUSES S. 2002. "Social Stratification and Inequalities in Spain: The State of The Art". In: LEMEL Y., NOLL H. *Changing Structures of Inequality: A Comparative Perspective.* London: Mc Gill-Queen's University Press.

FRANCO A., WINQVIST K. 2002. *At the margins of the labour market? Women and men in temporary jobs in Europe. Statistics in focus.* Eurostat: European Communities.

FOESSA. V. 1994. *Sociological Report on the Social Situation in Spain.* Madrid.

GARCÍA BALLESTEROS A., BOSQUE J., CARRERAS C., 1992. *A Geographical Outline of Spain.* Madrid: Real Sociedad Geográfica.

HARRISON J. 1985. *The Spanish Economy in the Twentieth Century.* New York: St Martin's Press.

JANSÀ J.Mª., GARCÍA DE OLALLA P. 2003. Desigualtats en la salut i la immigració [Health inequalities in immigrants]. In: BORRELL C., BENACH J. (coords). *Desigualtats en salut a Catalunya.* [Health inequalities in Catalonia]. Barcelona: Mediterrània: 217-250.

LOSTAO L., REGIDOR E., AIACH P., DOMINGUEZ V. 2001. "Social inequalities in ischaemic heart and cerebrovascular disease mortality in men: Spain and France, 1980-1982 and 1988-1990". *Soc Sci Med* 52: 1879-87.

MARTÍN ARTILES A. 2003. *Equal opportunities bargaining slow to develop* [page visited: 08-01-04]. Accessible in: http://www.eurofound.eu.int/emire/ spain.html.

MIGUÉLEZ F. 2000. *Strike over accidents and subcontracting in construction sector.* Accessible in: http:www.eiro.eurofound.eu.int/2000/04/word/es0004 282fes.doc [page visited: 08-01-04]

MINISTERIO DE TRABAJO Y ASUNTOS SOCIALES (MTAS). 2002. *Anuario de estadísticas laborales y de asuntos sociales 2000* [page visited: 08-01-04]. Accessible in: http:www.mtas.es/Estadisticas/anuario00.

MUNTANER C., EATON WW., DIALA C., KESSLER RC., SORLIE PD. 1998. "Social class, assets, organizational control and the prevalence of common groups of psychiatric disorders". *Soc Sci Med.* 47: 2043-53.

MUNTANER C., BENACH J., HADDEN W., GIMENO D., BENAVIDES FG., A Glossary for the social epidemiology of work organization (submitted).

NAVARRO V., BENACH J. and THE SCIENTIFIC COMMISSION FOR THE STUDY OF HEALTH INEQUALITIES IN SPAIN. 1996. *Desigualdades sociales en salud en España* [Social Inequalities in health in Spain]. Madrid: Ministerio de Sanidad y Consumo.

NAVARRO V., QUIROGA A. 2004. "Políticas de estado de bienestar para la equidad". In: BORRELL C., GARCÍA CALVENTE Mª DEL MAR, VICENTE J., (eds.) *Informe de la Sociedad Española de Salud Pública y Administración sanitaria (SESPAS) 2004: La salud pública desde la perspectiva de género y clase social. Gac Sanit* 18: Suppl 1: 147-57.

REGIDOR E., GUTIÉRREZ-FISAC JL., RODRÍGUEZ C. 1995. "Increased socioeconomic differences in mortality in eight Spanish provinces". *Soc Sci Med* 41: 801-7.

RODGERS G., Precarious work in Western Europe. In: Rodgers G., and Rodgers J. (eds.). 1989. *Precarious jobs in Labour Market regulation: The growth of Atypical Employment in Western Europe.* Belgium: International Institute for Labour Studies 1-16.

SALMON K. 1995. *The Modern Spanish Economy. Transformation and Integration into Europe* (2ⁿᵈ edition). London: Pinter.

URBANOS RM. 1999. "Análisis y evaluación de la equidad horizontal interpersonal en la prestación pública de servicios sanitarios. Un estudio del caso español para el período 1987-1995" [Analysis and evaluation of horizontal equity in public provision of health services. A case study of Spain in 1987-1995]. PhD Dissertation. Madrid: Universidad Complutense.

US DEPARTMENT OF STATE. *Country Reports on Human Rights Practices. Spain* [page visited: 22-12-03]. Accessible in: http://www.state.gov/g/drl/rls/hrrpt/ 2002/18392.htm.

VAN DER MEER M. 1997. *Trade union development in Spain.* Mannheim Center for European Studies.

WHITEHEAD M. 1998. Diffusion of ideas on social inequalities in health: A European Perspective. *The Milbank Quarterly* 76: 469-92.

Sweden

Mona BACKHANS & Peeter FREDLUND

Introduction

The last few decades have seen quite remarkable changes in the Swedish labour market, concerning both labour demand, work organisation and the scope of labour market policies. The recession of the 1990s has had long-lasting consequences, as it turned Sweden from a society with full employment to one where large parts of the working population are outside the labour force. It amplified the ongoing restructuring of the labour market and the gradual shift in the class structure, and it had a profound impact on working conditions during this period. While an increased work pace and deteriorating psychosocial working conditions indicate a potentially increased effect of working conditions on health and social inequalities in health, the labour force has diminished, leaving especially the less educated groups struggling to get into the labour market. Due to a 'healthy worker' effect, this might leave us with a non-significant effect of deteriorating working conditions on health inequalities. This chapter is constructed around four central themes. The first section describes major changes in the Swedish labour market during the last twenty years, giving a background to the changing world of work and its impact on health inequalities. Second, trends in work environment characteristics in different classes, occupations and sectors are described, with a focus on the development since the 1990s. Third, previous studies of class differentials in mortality and morbidity in Sweden since the 1960s have been reviewed, and complemented with analyses on the Swedish Survey of Living Conditions (ULF) of health inequalities from 1980-2001. This is followed by a section where the contribution of working conditions on class differentials in health have been assessed, also using the ULF survey. Finally, a concluding discussion aims to bring previous sections together. Here, we introduce a focus on policy measures as a means for reducing health inequalities.

1. Labour Market Changes

Earlier studies of the labour market development point to a number of structural changes during the last few decades which have altered the demand for labour (Castells 2000, Magnusson & Ottosson 2002, The Working Life Delegation 1999: 69). Technological development, especially within information technology, has meant rationalisation and restructuring of work within both industry and the service sector. There has been a growth of international trade due to decreasing transport costs, deregulation of financial markets, gradual lowering of trade tariffs and the establishment of regional common markets such as the EU. One consequence has been the emergence of a global division of labour, where manufacturing jobs are being relocated to countries with a large supply of cheap labour. Changes in work organisation, promoted by IT development and higher demands on productivity, have often meant both an enlargement of job tasks and an intensification of work. Both formal education and factors such as work experience, as well as communicative and social skills are said to be more essential. Overall, demand has shifted from low to highly skilled labour – a shift that could lead to both increasing wage gaps as well as higher levels of unemployment for those with lower education. However, there has been a marked upgrading of educational qualifications in the population, and a growing number of employees are overqualified for their jobs, so supply has shifted as well (le Grand *et al.* 2001a).

On the supply side, the most dramatic change is the growth in female labour force participation since the mid-1960s, when the female participation rate was about 50%. Today it is slightly under 80%. Factors that encouraged a growing participation in the labour market were the introduction of separate taxation for married couples in 1971, the rapid expansion of public subsidised childcare facilities and the right to paid parental leave for 6 months since 1974 (today 15 months) (Sundström 2003). Another important reform was the right for parents to have reduced working hours until the youngest child is seven, which has contributed to the large share of part-time work among women. The reforms should be seen in the light of the permanent shortage of labour during the boom years of the 1960s, which led to efforts from the Government to increase the supply of female labour, as well as the struggle for economic independence and equality among Swedish women who were relatively well represented in government (Bergqvist 2001).

A. The 1990s Unemployment Crisis

Unlike many other European countries that have experienced high unemployment since the 1970s, Sweden had a long period of low unemployment, which was broken only in the early 1990s. The recession started with an international downturn in the economy, which primarily affected the export-oriented industries and led to massive downsizing. This was accompanied by a crisis on the Swedish real estate market, and a subsequent major collapse of the banking system. The sharp reduction in consumption and demand for labour spread the crisis to the home market. Within a few years, 600,000 people lost their jobs, the majority of which in the private sector. The loss of tax revenue put a heavy strain on public finances. During the later phase of the recession, reconstruction of state finances meant tax increases and cuts on public expenditure, as well as layoffs and frequent restructuring of the public sector (Lundborg 2000, Magnusson 1999, Lundberg *et al.* 2001). At most, the total unemployment (open unemployment + labour market programmes) was as much as 16% of the labour force (Source: The Labour Market Board). Groups especially hit by unemployment were those who were establishing themselves in the labour market, such as young people and recent immigrants/refugees, while middle-aged people (45-54 years) were less exposed to the consequences of the economic crisis (The Welfare Commission 2002: 32). During the late 1990s there was a marked growth in employment, especially in the private service sector. But still in 2000, the labour force participation rate was 8 percentage points lower than in 1990 (SCB 2001). The 1990s recession amplified the ongoing restructuring of the labour market and the gradual shift in the class structure (The Welfare Commission 2002: 32). It also had a profound impact on working conditions during this period.

B. Labour Force Participation

Between 1990 and 2000, the labour force participation rate for men declined from 91 to 84% of the population aged 20-64 (table 1). The continuing growth in female participation came to a halt during the economic crisis; at 79% it is almost back to the same level as in 1980. The participation rate has declined especially in the youngest age group (20-34) (not shown). This reflects the high and rising proportion of students in this group[1]. The proportions who are on disability benefits

---

[1] The categories in the group "outside the labour market" have changed, which means that data is generally not comparable between 1980 and later years, except for students and housewives. It has not been possible to categorise the material in the same age groups, which also hampers comparison.

has risen, while the group of 'voluntary' early retirees has declined (not shown). This could partly be an effect of new regulations in 1997, stating that only medical reasons are grounds for a disability pension – earlier also labour market conditions could be applied (www.rfv.se). It also mirrors the rise in sickness absence since 1997, leading to a subsequent rise in disability pensions (Socialdepartementet 2002: 5). The only group that has not experienced a drop in labour force participation between 1980 and 2000 is older women, due to a decreasing proportion of housewives.

According to the Survey of Living Conditions (ULF), for men all classes have had a gradually declining trend in those currently employed since 1980, slightly more among manual than non-manual workers (table 2). Today, 88% of unskilled manual workers compared with 96% of higher non-manual employees are currently employed. For women, there was an increase between 1980 and 1990, followed by a clear drop. Women's class differentials are even more pronounced[2]. There has been a marked decline of employment (7-8 percentage points) for female unskilled workers and lower non-manual employees. From 1980 to 1990 there was a marked decline in the proportion of women who were not possible to classify according to occupational class, while this group has increased for both men and women during the most recent period. The rate of open unemployment increased from less than 1.5% in 1990 to 4% for women and 5% for men in 2000 (table 1). Also, the group who see themselves as job seekers but who are not included in the official definition has grown between 1990 and 2000. If these were to be included among the unemployed, the figure would rise to 6-7%.

As mentioned earlier, women's growing labour force participation has often taken the form of part-time work (table 1). Part-time employment is often seen as non-standard, precarious labour, but this may be less true in Sweden, where part-time employees enjoy the same employment rights and are included in the social security system if they work at least 17 hours a week (Sundström 2003). The majority of part-time work in Sweden is over 20 hours per week. Part-time employment has decreased by 13 percentage points among women during the last 20 years, while for men it has risen slightly. In both 1980 and 1990, part-time work increased with age, but today, around 1/3 of women in all age groups work part-time. Among men, the proportion in part-time work has doubled in the two youngest age groups, but it is still the case that less than 10% of men in any age group work part-time.

---

[2]   Housewives will normally be classified according to their husband's occupation. This may not accurately reflect the individual's labour market position, and these have therefore been excluded from the analysis.

Table 1: Proportion part-time, self-employed, unemployed and labour force participation rate, by sex and study period, men and women 20-64 years (N in hundreds)

	Employed part-time (%)	Self-employed (%)	In employment (n)	Unemployed (%)	In the labour force (n)	Labour force participation	Population 20-64 years (n)
Men							
1980	5.2	9.8	21,537	1.5	21,857	90.8	24,073
1990	6.1	13.0	22,389	1.4	22,708	90.6	25,061
2000	8.0	14.7	21,130	4.9	22,207	84.2	26,388
Women							
1980	47.0	4.9	17,783	1.9	18,130	76.9	23,571
1990	40.0	5.3	20,554	1.3	20,828	85.5	24,352
2000	33.7	5.8	19,304	4.1	20,134	78.6	25,608

Source: Labour force survey (AKU).

An international trend that has attracted considerable attention is the growth of so-called atypical, non-standard or flexible labour, including temporary employment, but there are large national differences (Goudswaard & Andries 2002, Felstead & Jewson 1999). It is contested whether this development reflects structural changes or is mainly a result of the downturn in the economy (le Grand *et al.* 2001a). Labour legislation underwent some minor changes in 1997, which has opened up for more fixed-term employment (Svensson 2002). The labour force survey has data on type of employment since 1987. If we compare the figures for 1990 with 2000, it is clear that there has been a marked growth of fixed-term employment during the period in all age groups and for both men and women (table 3). This trend is stronger for men than for women, but the proportion in fixed-term employment is still greater for women. This is especially true in the youngest age group, where 1/3 of women are on fixed-term contracts compared with 1/5 of men. The only type of temporary employment that is more common among men is those working on a project basis or on trial contracts (not shown), jobs that are more likely to lead to permanent employment and that have been shown to be more similar to standard jobs in terms of job content and work environment (Wikman *et al.* 1998). The most precarious types of temporary employment, work on demand and seasonal jobs, have increased the most, about threefold during the period. These types of jobs are often associated with financial difficulties and little chance of obtaining permanent employment (Aronsson 1999, Aronsson *et al.* 2000, Håkansson 2001).

Table 2: Employment rate in different socio-economic groups (Erikson-Goldthorpe schema) and % not classifiable, by sex and study period, men and women 20-64 years

Period	1979-80	1989-90	2000-2001
Men			
Unskilled manual	92.4	90.5	87.7
Skilled manual	94.3	91.8	88.5
Lower non-manual	96.7	65.0	92.4
Intermediate non-manual	96.6	93.9	92.0
Higher non-manual	98.0	98.3	96.3
% not classifiable	4.6	5.1	9.0
N	5,404	4,008	3,773
Women			
Unskilled manual	90.4	89.4	82.1
Skilled manual	90.9	92.1	88.2
Lower non-manual	94.8	94.7	86.4
Intermediate non-manual	96.1	97.6	94.4
Higher non-manual	98.7	97.7	94.7
% not classifiable	22.7	10.2	13.9
N	6,038	4,306	4,150

Source: Survey of Living Conditions (ULF).

Table 3: Proportion employed in fixed-term contracts by sex and age 1990 and 2000, men and women 20-64 years (N in hundreds)

	20-34	35-49	50-49	All 20-64	N
Men					
1990	9.7	2.8	2.0	5.3	1,059
2000	19.3	8.3	5.7	11.5	2,068
Women					
1990	17.1	7.0	4.2	10.0	1,984
2000	29.0	11.5	6.8	15.8	2,867

Source: Labour force survey (AKU).

C. Changes in the Industrial and Occupational Class Structure

Changes were made in the system of industrial classification in the early 1990s, and data from 1980 can therefore not be compared with later years. However, both classifications were used for a few years and a matrix linking the old and new classification schemes has been used to estimate the 1980 figures on an aggregate level (table 4). The 1980 figures should therefore be interpreted with some caution. The greatest change can be found for extractive activities, dominated by agriculture, which have fallen by ½ and now employ merely 2.4% of the population[3]. Another clear trend is the gradual decline of the sector dominated by manufacturing, which has been reduced in size by ¼. In 2000, only ¼ of the labour force were employed in transformative activities, while a total of 73% were employed in services. Trade and communications, the last link in the chain extraction-transformation-distribution, grew quite substantially between 1980 and 1990 but has been stable since then, with 1/5 of the labour force[4]. Producer services, closely related to industry and of strategic importance in an advanced economy, declined by almost 1/3 between 1980 and 1990. This could be interpreted as the beginning of the 1990s crisis, which started in real estate and banking. By 2000, the sector has grown quite considerably and is now somewhat bigger than in 1980. In Sweden large numbers of people are employed in the social services, and their share of the total employment has remained quite stable at 1/3. However, while employment in education and research has increased between 1990 and 2000, employment in health and social work has declined to some extent. The latter sector is greatly dominated by women, and gender segregation has been accentuated during the study period (not shown). In 2000, less than 5% of men compared with 34% of women are employed in this branch. Transformative activities are on the other hand increasingly male, and in 2000 only 11% of women work in these sectors compared with 37% of men.

The Swedish socio-economic classification (SEI) was constructed by Robert Erikson and closely follows the Erikson-Goldthorpe class schema. Its ambition is to identify homogonous groups regarding relations within production, rather than identifying classes with antagonistic interests (Eriksson & Goldthorpe 1992). The first distinction is made between those who sell and those who buy labour, and the self-employed. Employees are mainly categorised according to types of contract: the labour contract, and the service relationship (Goldthorpe 2000). These are further categorised into different groups based on qualificational demands. Examining the Swedish Survey of Living Conditions (ULF) during the latest twenty years we find that the proportion of unskilled workers has dropped for both men and women but much more so for women (table 5)[5]. The proportion of skilled manual

---

[3] The aggregation level of our data means that mining, normally classified as an extracting activity, has been classified with manufacturing. Also, research and development, normally classified as a producer service, is under the heading education.

[4] Note that the data for 1980 is not supported by Hansen (2001), who found a constant proportion between 1970-87-99.

[5] Everyone has been classified according to their own, current or former, occupation

workers has been stable for men, while it has doubled among women (although from a very low level). Manual workers have decreased from ½ to around 40–45% for both sexes. The proportion of lower non-manual employees has been reduced slightly for women but has been quite stable for men. The two highest non-manual classes have generally grown, but again the difference over time is much greater for women, especially for the highest class, which has more than doubled. Today they represent almost 1/3 of women and 36% of men. Entrepreneurs are more often men than women and this pattern has even been strengthened during the period, as there is an increase only for men during the last ten years. As already shown, a very small proportion of the population are farmers and their numbers have been further diminished during the study period. Women's and men's class structures have converged over time, something that reflects women's move from the secondary to the primary labour market, although significant differences still remain.

Table 4: Proportion working in different branches of industry and total number of employees (N in hundreds) 1980-2000

	1980	1990	2000
Extractive			
A+B	5.0	3.4	2.4
Transformative	32.5	29.2	24.6
C-E	25.6	22.0	19.1
D	-	21.0	18.2
F	-	7.2	5.4
Distributive services			
G+I	14.2	20.0	19.2
G	-	13.0	12.5
Producer services			
J+K – R&D	11.9	8.7	13.3
K – R&D	-	6.6	11.2
Social services	29.8	32.0	32.5
M + R&D	7.2	6.9	8.7
N	18.0	19.7	18.5
L+Q	4.6	5.3	5.4
Personal services			
H+O+P	6.7	6.5	7.9
N	41,578	44,799	41,525

A) Agriculture, hunting and forestry; B) Fishing; C) Mining and quarrying; D) Manufacturing; E) Electricity, gas and water supply; F) Construction; G) Wholesale and retail trade, repairs; H) Hotels and restaurants; I) Transport, storage and communications; J) Financial intermediation; banking, insurance; K) Real estate, renting and business activities; L) Public administration; M) Education; N) Health and social work; O) Other services; P) Private households as employers; Q) International organisations.
Source: Labour force survey (AKU).

Over the last few decades, Sweden has changed from an ethnically relatively homogeneous society to a multicultural society with as many as over a million foreign-born inhabitants. In the 1960s, the labour shortage meant that many came to work in industry, while later immigrant flows have consisted both of refugees and relatives of earlier immigrants (Törnell 2003). The percentage of foreign-born in different occupational classes can be seen in table 6. Among men, the group with the most immigrants has always been those who are not classifiable, and this is also true for women at all years, except for 1979/80 when entrepreneurs had the highest proportion. Apart from a relatively large proportion among entrepreneurs, immigrants are predominantly manual workers. This is a result of the history of immigrant labour, but also reflects the difficulties that later immigrants, many highly educated, have had in becoming established in the labour market. Especially those who came as refugees during the recession of the 1990s have had lasting labour market problems (The Welfare Commission 2002: 32).

Table 5: Socio-economic groups based on current or former occupation by sex and study period, men and women 20-64 years (%)

Period	1979-80	1989-90	2000-2001
Men			
Unskilled manual	25.9	24.2	20.7
Skilled manual	22.8	22.7	22.2
Lower non-manual	9.2	10.2	9.1
Intermediate non-manual	16.9	16.9	18.4
Higher non-manual	12.7	14.7	17.3
Entrepreneurs	9.1	9.4	11.2
Farmers	3.4	2.0	1.2
N	5,893	4,291	3,916
Women			
Unskilled manual	41.4	34.6	26.4
Skilled manual	7.4	11.7	13.3
Lower non-manual	24.2	21.7	18.6
Intermediate non-manual	13.2	18.2	23.1
Higher non-manual	6.3	8.5	13.6
Entrepreneurs	4.3	4.1	4.6
Farmers	3.2	1.2	-
N	5,043	4,084	3,762

Source: Survey of Living Conditions (ULF).

Table 6: Percentage of foreign-born in different social classes and not classifiable by sex and study period, men and women 20-64 years (%)

Period	1979-80	1989-90	2000-2001
Men			
Not classifiable	17.0	25.0	14.4
Unskilled manual	13.2	12.5	14.9
Skilled manual	10.6	11.3	12.9
Lower non-manual	5.5	6.2	8.7
Intermediate non-manual	7.1	8.4	8.3
Higher non-manual	6.4	6.8	6.6
Entrepreneurs	5.2	6.7	12.1
Farmers	1.0	0	4.3
N	6,149	4,498	4,254
Women			
Not classifiable	9.4	15.4	19.2
Unskilled manual	15.1	14.5	15.8
Skilled manual	13.2	8.8	12.2
Lower non-manual	6.1	8.0	7.7
Intermediate non-manual	7.4	7.5	7.6
Higher non-manual	7.9	8.0	7.0
Entrepreneurs	10.2	13.3	13.8
Farmers	2.5	6.0	6.7
N	6,415	4,519	4,339

Source: Survey of Living Conditions (ULF).

D. Summary of Labour Market Changes

After very high and stable employment rates in the 1980s, the labour force participation rate declined for both men and women between 1990 and 2000, especially in the youngest age group. This reflects the high and rising proportion of students in this group, as well as difficulties in entering the labour market. Among older people, the proportion on disability benefits has risen, while the group of early retirees (for other than health reasons) has declined. The decline in employment is especially pronounced for female manual workers and lower non-manual employees. For women, part-time employment decreased by 13 percentage points, while for men it rose slightly. During the 1990s there was a marked growth of fixed-term employment in all age groups and for both men and women. There has been a gradual decline of the sector dominated by manufacturing, while the social services have been quite stable. Trade and communications grew quite substantially between 1980 and 1990. In 2000, only ¼ of the labour force were employed in transformative activities, while a total of 73% were employed in services. There has been a change in the occupational structure from unskilled jobs to more qualified non-manual jobs. Overall, the changes for women have been much more pronounced, whereas for men it is only the opposite ends of the occupational structure that have seen any substantial changes.

E. Degree of Unionisation

Along with the other Nordic countries, Sweden has traditionally had a strong union movement, and still enjoys a high membership rate in all occupational groups. A high unionisation has been supported by a union-run unemployment insurance system (also known as the Ghent system); a socially highly segregated union movement, with three major unions for workers, non-manual employees and non-manual employees with tertiary degrees, respectively; a tradition of collective agreements instead of legal regulations (90-95% of all Swedish employees are covered by collective agreements); and a strong union presence at plant as well as peak level (Kjellberg 2003, Blom-Hansen 2000). However, there have been some fluctuations during the last 20 years. Membership numbers increased during the early 1980s, declined during the boom years, only to rise again in the early 1990s (Kjellberg 2000). Since 1993 they have decreased continuously and are now lower than in 1980. This decline can primarily be seen among people under the age of 25. In 1990, overall unionisation was 81% compared with 80% in 2002, having peaked at 85% in 1993. In the age group 16-24 years, rates among employees have declined from 69% in 1993 to 50%. This reflects a shift from public to private sector employment (where unionisation has always been lower) and a large proportion of temporary employees, who have especially low membership rates. Temporary employees may feel that their interests are not well represented by unions, and that their current occupation is a mere transitory state. Women and men have similar degrees of unionisation, women being slightly more likely to be union members, mostly due to the higher unionisation level among public sector employees. The changing class structure is also reflected in the size of major unions. While in 1950, 78% of all members belonged to LO, the workers' union, this decreased to 52% in 2002. TCO, the biggest white-collar union, has increased its share from 17% to 33% during the same period.

F. Income Differentials

Internationally, income differentials have generally been growing since the early 1980s, but not to the same extent in different countries (Le Grand *et al.* 2001b). An overview of the research to date concludes that changes in the demand for labour, as well as institutional and regulational factors, help explain changes over time and between countries (Katz & Autor 1999). Relative to most other countries, Sweden has

a very small income dispersal (Le Grand *et al.* 2001b). The Gini coefficient, which takes into account the total income dispersal in the population, has however increased steadily over the last two decades (SCB
2000). A study using data from the Level of Living Survey (LNU) has
shown that the increasing differentials are due to changes in the upper
part of the income structure, especially for managers (le Grand *et al.*
2001b). During 2000-2003 there has been a small decrease (SCB 2005).

Data from the Income Distribution Survey (HEK) on median income
from work in different socio-economic classes reveal a different picture
(tables 7 & 8)[6]. For men, the differences have been relatively stable
during the study period. If we instead examine disposable income per
family unit, which includes income from capital, taxes and transfers, as
well as the income of other household members, the difference between
classes is reduced. The reduction rests mostly on the class with the
highest income. Here we find an increase in differentials over time,
which is especially influenced by changes among higher non-manual
employees. In 1980, the disposable income was only around 25% higher
in this class compared with unskilled workers. This increased to 35% in
1990 and to 45% in 2000. Taking changes in part-time work as shown
in ULF into account, differentials in income from work seem rather
stable over time also for women[7]. If we turn to the data on disposable
income, income differentials have increased between manual and non-
manual groups. Especially the two highest non-manual classes have
increased their income relative to other groups. Thus, the trends are
roughly equal for men and women. These results emphasise the growing
importance of capital gains in explaining overall income differentials
and the decreasing weight of income from work. However, the situation
in 2000 might be quite unique, as the stock market peaked much due to

---

[6]   There was a tax reform in 1990-1991 which entailed a broadening of the tax base
(extension of the VAT system and changes in the taxation of capital income, real
estate and housing as well as fringe benefits) and cuts in marginal tax rates (Willner
& Granqvist 2002). For 1990 there are two calculations to make possible comparisons over time. As we can see, taxable income as well as disposable income increased, while class differences remained roughly the same. There are however some
tendencies for a larger increase for the two highest non-manual classes.

[7]   For women, the proportion working part-time has an impact on the median income
from work and will also affect differences between classes and over time if the proportion differs. If we are interested in the actual income level among women, it
would be biased to only consider those in full-time employment. In some branches
and sectors this would exclude a majority of employees as positions are normally
part-time. Also part-time and full-time positions within a certain class may be quali-
tatively different, thus distorting class differences. It would be preferable to recalcu-
late part-time wages into full-time equivalents but unfortunately the data quality (according to Statistics Sweden) does not permit this. Therefore the data must be
interpreted with caution.

the 'IT bubble'; the importance of capital gains is likely to have clearly diminished in the following years.

Table 7: Median income from work and total disposable income (work + capital) per family unit in different socio-economic groups by study period, men 20-64 years. Thousand SEK standardised to price level year 2000

	Unskilled manual	Skilled manual	Lower non-manual	Intermediate non-manual	Higher non-manual
Income from work					
1980	172	185	199	230	282
1990	184	206	210	241	313
% difference	+7.0	+11.4	+5.5	+4.8	+11.0
1990*	187	210	213	245	320
2000	213	228	248	269	348
% difference	+13.9	+8.6	+16.4	+9.8	+8.8
Disposable income/ family unit					
1980	95	96	102	111	120
1990	105	110	114	122	141
% difference	+10.5	+14.6	+11.8	+9.9	+17.5
1990*	108	115	118	126	146
2000	112	117	129	135	164
% difference	+3.7	+1.7	+9.3	+7.1	+12.3

* *After the tax reform. Source: Income Distribution Survey (HEK).*

Table 8: Median income from work and total disposable income (work + capital) per family unit in different socio-economic groups by study period, women 20-64 years. Thousand SEK standardised to price level year 2000

	Unskilled manual	Skilled manual	Lower non-manual	Intermediate non-manual	Higher non-manual
Income from work					
1980	118	134	148	163	198
1990	135	147	156	182	231
% difference	+14.4	+9.7	+5.4	+11.7	+16.7
1990*	137	149	157	188	237
2000	158	166	191	213	254
% difference	+15.3	+11.4	+21.7	+13.3	+7.2
Disposable income/ family unit					
1980	94	97	104	107	121
1990	103	102	114	119	137
% difference	+9.6	+5.2	+9.6	+11.2	+13.2
1990*	106	105	118	123	143
2000	108	110	130	134	153
% difference	+1.9	+4.8	+9.1	+9.2	+9.3

* *After the tax reform. Source: Income Distribution Survey (HEK).*

2. Changes in the Work Environment

Since 1989, it has been possible to follow work environment trends in the bi-annual Work Environment Survey (WES). The sample consists of 10,000-15,000 respondents. In 2001, 66.7% of those included in the survey responded to the questionnaire. Here, we have chosen to focus on psychosocial factors at work that in a number of previous studies have been shown to be associated with ill health: demands, control and social support, as well as some indicators of physical strain that may lead to musculoskeletal problems and some other physical work environment factors associated with ill health (Theorell & Karasek 1996, Van der Doef & Maes 1998, Van der Doef & Maes 1999, Bongers *et al.* 1993, Hales *et al.* 1996, Viikari-Juntura 1997).

A. Psychosocial Factors at Work

Studies examining the period before 1990 show that there was an increase in the proportion reporting high job strain during the 1980s (Szulkin & Thålin 1994) in all classes. The increase was dependent on a rise in demands, while job control did not change during this period. The trend was especially strong for female-dominated jobs and sectors. During the 1990s, there was also a general reduction of job control, leading to further increases in high strain (le Grand *et al.* 2001a) across all classes except for unskilled workers. The most noticeable change can be seen for jobs in health care and nursing, education and retail, and the rise in high strain has continued at a faster rate among female-dominated jobs. ULF data also show an increase in high-strain jobs between the late 1980s and mid 1990s, while there was a slight improvement between 1994/95 and 1997/98 (SOU 2000: 37). This analysis confirms an increasing polarisation between men and women in terms of demands but not for high-strain jobs.

Previous studies on the Work Environment Survey confirm an increase in stress and mental strain related to work during the 1990s. As already mentioned, there is a tendency towards increased polarisation between men and women and between the private and public sector in working conditions (AMV/SCB 2001). It is clear that employees in the municipalities and county councils have had a particularly negative trend regarding high-strain jobs. The occupations with the highest proportion reporting high strain are female-dominated jobs such as schoolteachers and employees in health care. For women, other high-strain jobs are lower-level service occupations that involve direct customer contact, and for men, motor vehicle drivers. The general picture is that especially those jobs that involve a great degree of contact with other people – whether as students, patients or customers – are most exposed to poor psychosocial conditions. These jobs are also those that, according to Maslach's original formulation, are at risk of burnout (Maslach *et al.* 2001).

For our psychosocial variables we have used those proposed by Fredlund *et al.* (2000), with one exception (see appendix 1 for variables and index construction). The variables constituting skill discretion in the WES are quite 'ergonomic' (with questions on bending and turning) and do not include questions on opportunities for acquiring skills or participating in on-the-job training – skill acquisition being an integral part of the concept. Thus, we are rather cautious of the specific operationalisation of skill discretion in WES and have excluded it. As skill discretion is lacking, we have not calculated any high-strain variable. Our analysis starts in 1991 as there was a large (30%) internal non-response for the psychosocial work environment questions in 1989.

The general picture concerning psychosocial factors is that the exposure to adverse conditions has increased, while overall class differences have been stable (figures 1-6). This is true for high demands and low decision authority, while levels of low social support have decreased slightly for men. The detrimental changes are more pronounced for women, as previously mentioned.

B. Psychological Demands

The proportion reporting high demands shows a steep class gradient, with the highest non-manual class 2.5-3 times more likely to be in the exposed group compared with unskilled workers (figures 1-2). For men, the level has increased for all groups between 1991 and 1995, significantly for manual workers. Between 1995 and 2001, the proportion was stable for all classes except the highest, where it was reduced to the 1991 level. However, for those in the public sector (not shown), demands remain on a higher level. For women, the highest non-manual group has been stable at around 50%. For all other groups, there has been a significant increase. Thus, there is a tendency for diminishing class differentials between 1991 and 2001 for both men and women.

Figure 1: Proportion of men in high-demand jobs

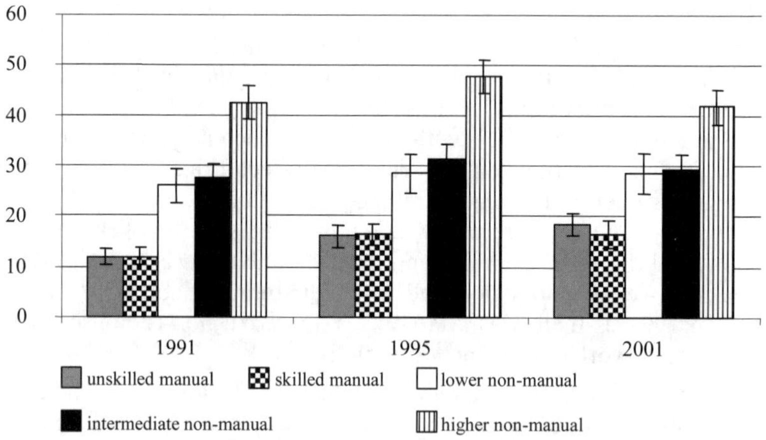

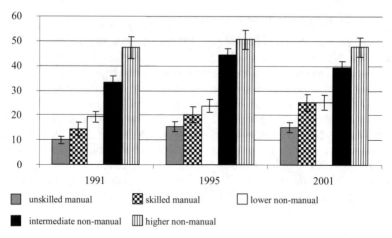

Source: WES.

Figure 2: Proportion of women in high-demand jobs

Source: WES.

C. Decision Authority

Among men, low decision authority has increased for all classes except for the highest non-manual class, where there has been no change (figure 3). Significant changes can again be found for manual workers.

For women, class differences are not as pronounced as among men, and the proportion with low decision authority is higher than for men (figure 4). This reflects that the type of jobs that women hold tend to be more controlled by the demands of others, which implies less individual autonomy for the worker. The proportion reporting low decision authority has generally increased significantly. However, there has been no change in the highest non-manual class.

D. Social Support at Work

The proportion experiencing low social support at work fell for men between 1991 and 1995, but since then it has increased slightly (figure 5). This tendency can also be seen for women (figure 6). Social support tends to be lower in the highest non-manual class for both men and women, and for women there is a slight gradient. An analysis of individual questions shows that it is more common not to receive support and encouragement from fellow workers, and not to have access to advice or help when tasks feel difficult in the highest class, while there are no differences concerning support from supervisors or expressed appreciation from supervisors, colleagues or others.

E. Physical Working Conditions

Previous analyses of LNU show that between 1968 and 1991 the prevalence of heavy lifting fell considerably, while hazardous working conditions (being exposed to gas, dust, smoke or toxic substances) increased slightly (Fritzell & Lundberg 1994). Class differentials were large but decreased for heavy lifting and dangerous working conditions between 1968 and 1981 (Vågerö & Lundberg 1995) Physically demanding work, including heavy lifting as well as monotonous and unsuitable working postures, was as common in 1981 as in 1991 (Fritzell & Lundberg 1993). Women had a negative development relative to men for all physical working conditions, while hazardous working conditions continued to be more prevalent among men.

Figure 3: Proportion of men with low decision authority

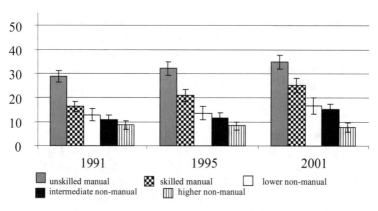

Source: WES.

Figure 4: Proportion of women with low decision authority

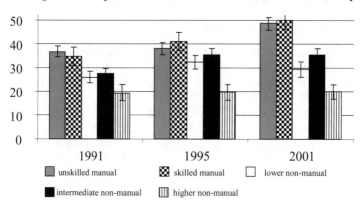

Source: WES.

Figure 5: Proportion of men with low social support at work

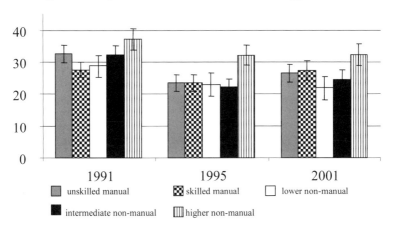

Source: WES.

Figure 6: Proportion of women with low social support at work

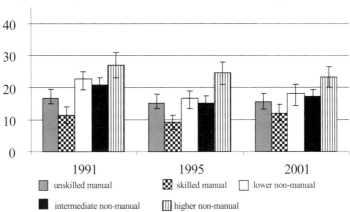

Source: WES.

F. Ergonomic Load

Our analyses of the WES show that for men generally there has been no change in the proportion who are exposed to ergonomically strenuous working conditions (heavy lifting several times a day *or* working bent forward without support *or* working above shoulder height *or* working in a bent position *or* whole-body vibration *or* hand-arm vibration, ¾ of the time or more), nor has there been any change in overall class differentials over time (figure 7). Skilled manual workers, where the exposed group increased from 48 to 55% between 1995 and 2001, are the one group showing a significant change over time. The class distribution is heavily skewed, with the highest non-manual class having less than 5% exposed. For women, there has been an increase in the proportion reporting these conditions over time, but only between 1991 and 1995 (figure 8). The development rests mostly on skilled manual workers, where there has been a rise from 39 to 48%, and they are now the most exposed class.

Figure 7: Proportion of men in ergonomically exposed jobs

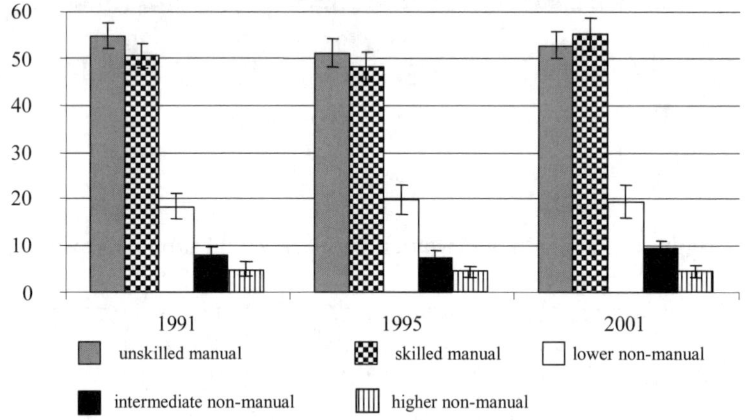

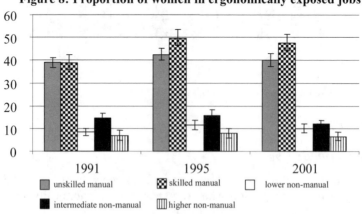

Source: WES.

Figure 8: Proportion of women in ergonomically exposed jobs

Source: WES.

G. *Physical and Chemical Hazards*

The prevalence of exposure to certain physical/chemical hazards (tobacco smoke *or* chemical vapours *or* dust *or* noise *or* skin contact with cleaning agents/disinfectants *or* oil/cutting fluids, ¾ of the time or more) has much the same distribution as ergonomic working conditions, and there has likewise been no overall change for men, either in levels or class differences (figure 9). The most exposed group is skilled manual workers: 43% compared with 36% for unskilled manual workers. Intermediate non-manual employees decreased their exposure between 1991 and 1995. For women, there has been an increase in exposure for skilled manual workers who are now on the same level as unskilled workers (figure 10).

Figure 9: Proportion of men with physical/chemical exposure

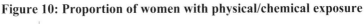

Source: WES.

Figure 10: Proportion of women with physical/chemical exposure

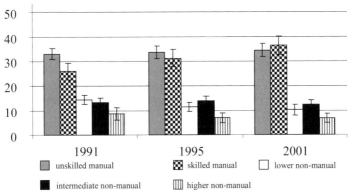

Source: WES.

353

H. Conclusion

In conclusion, psychosocial working conditions have gradually become worse. Results suggest that during the 1980s there was an increase in demands while job control stayed the same. The increase in demands continued during the early 1990s but has been stable since then. While class differences in demands are large, they tend to become smaller due to, for men, large increases among manual workers and, for women, increases for all classes except the highest non-manual one. Low decision authority is much more common in lower classes and increases have also been clearer for these groups, while proportions in the higher non-manual class have been stable. Throughout the period, female-dominated jobs have had the worst development, and the occupations most exposed to high strain are those in health care, education and retail. It is interesting to note that despite the continuing decline of the industrial sector, according to the available questionnaire data, physical working conditions have not been improved. Exposure to heavy physical work has been stable during the period, while results suggest that hazardous working conditions increased slightly up until 1991. During the 1990s, the most exposed group, skilled manual workers, had a negative development for both men and women, and for both ergonomic working conditions and for physical/chemical exposure. What we might expect from the general development of working conditions in terms of health could be a gradual increase in class differentials as well as gender differences, at least during the 1990s. As inequalities have increased regarding psychosocial variables it is probable that the health indicators most affected would be stress-related health measures such as mental health, but possibly also CVD. It is also possible that the increase in detrimental physical working conditions alongside growing demands and decreasing decision authority implies a particularly high burden for skilled manual workers, and thus increasing health problems for this group.

3. Health Inequalities

In 1979 a group of researchers commissioned by the Swedish government concluded that 'social class, income or socio-economic status has a fairly limited explanatory value (...) as a basis for studying the correlation between environment and health' (Carlsson *et al.* 1979). The differences that did exist were considered minor and did not warrant further inquiry. However, the debate following the Black report (published first in 1980), as well as a renewed political interest, inspired an increased activity in the field (Lundberg 1990). A trickle of papers in the late 1980s was followed by a growing number of publications and international collaborations during the 1990s, as well as regional public health reports moulded on the national report first published in 1987. The foundation of CHESS (Centre for Health Equity Studies) in 2000 may be seen as the chief example of the institutionalisation of the academic field. In this section, some of those previous studies on mortality and health differentials between social classes will be reviewed, and data on health differentials for 1980-2000 are presented.

A. Mortality

In a large cross-country comparison of mortality differentials between occupational classes Kunst *et al.* (1998) stated that '... comparisons both over time and across countries underline the persistent nature of socio-economic differences in premature mortality' (age 30-64 years). However, extending the period of inquiry back in time reveals changes in mortality differentials over time. Census data covering the period 1961-1990 show that among Swedish middle-aged men (45-69 years) there has been a shift in total mortality rate ratios between occupations in industry (92% manual workers) and professional/managerial occupations (79% high or intermediate non-manual) between the early 1960s to the late 1980s (Diderichsen & Hallqvist 1997). When controlling for deaths among the not employed, the absolute rates in the two groups were equal in 1966-1979. Between 1966 and 1980 those in industry experienced an increase in absolute mortality, while those in professional/managerial positions saw a sharp decline during the entire period up until 1990, resulting in the inequalities we see today. Underlying the trend is mainly CVD mortality.

Vågerö (1991) also demonstrates a shift in (IHD) mortality differentials among middle-aged men between the 1960s and 1970s, and discusses this finding as a shift from 'material to 'behavioural' factors as the most salient in explaining class patterns in mortality. However, for women there is no corresponding change, as women in manual occupations had higher total and CVD mortality also in the 1960s. A comparison of all-cause mortality between 1961-5 and 1981-6 in different socio-economic groups (age 35-69 years) confirms the relatively negative development for men in manual classes during a period when there were large reductions in mortality for all other groups (Vågerö & Lundberg 1995). For women, there were considerable improvements in all groups at this time but also a slight widening of inequalities due to a slower decline for manual workers.

Calculations made by the Epidemiological Centre (EpC) at the National Board of Health and Welfare based on census data with a follow-up period of five years, show that during the late 1980s and early 1990s there was declining total mortality in all classes (table 9). Although they experienced falling mortality rates, unskilled male manual workers and lower non-manual employees increased their relative difference to the reference group, while absolute differences stayed the same. The group of unclassifiable (mainly economically inactive) have decreased their absolute as well as their relative mortality considerably during the time period, which implies a decreasing importance of health-related selection (although this group has the highest mortality by far). For women this group has had stable absolute mortality while relative and absolute differences have risen, reflecting the disappearance of the housewife and a growing importance of health-related selection to the group. For women, unskilled workers and, to a lesser extent, lower non-manual employees saw rising relative, but also absolute, differences in total mortality compared with the reference group. If we examine IHD especially we find large absolute reductions for men in the periods 1986-1990 and 1991-1995 in all groups; but the group with the most favourable development is that of high and intermediate non-manual employees, resulting in increased differences between them and unskilled manual workers and lower non-manual employees (table 10) (Persson G. *et al.* 2001). Also for women, the reductions are large (in relative if not absolute terms). However, unskilled manual workers have hardly decreased their absolute mortality, and both the relative and absolute rate between unskilled workers and higher and intermediate non-manual employees has increased.

To sum up, what we can see for (middle-aged) men is insignificant or even small reversed class differences in the 1960s, followed by an increase up until 1980 due to a negative development for men in manual classes, and since then rather stable differences, while the highest non-manual group and skilled workers have had the highest reduction in total and IHD mortality. Since 1980 all groups have had a favourable development. For women, there is less data but we can note that differences seem to be stable over a long time. Whereas female manual workers experienced reduced mortality rates almost on a par with other groups between the 1960s and early 1980s, unskilled workers have clearly been lagging behind since the late 1980s. This has resulted in a gradual increase of mortality differentials.

Table 9: Age-standardised total mortality (deaths/100,000 person years) relative rates and absolute differences in different socio-economic groups, men and women 20-64 years

		Men			Women		
		Mortality	RR	Absolute difference	Mortality	RR	Absolute difference
Unskilled	1986-90	338.7	1.56	120.9	157.8	1.20	26.8
manual	1991-95	309.4	1.63	119.1	155.5	1.25	30.8
Skilled manual	1986-90	295.1	1.35	77.3	156.1	1.19	25.1
	1991-95	261.8	1.38	71.5	139.3	1.12	14.6
Lower	1986-90	274.0	1.26	56.2	151.9	1.16	20.9
non-manual	1991-95	252.6	1.33	62.3	148.3	1.19	23.6
Higher and intermediate non-manual	1986-90	217.8	1	-	131.0	1	-
	1991-95	190.3	1	-	124.7	1	-
Not classifiable	1986-90	849.9	3.90	632.1	353.6	2.70	222.6
	1991-95	679.8	3.57	489.5	354.9	2.85	230.2

Source: Calculations made by the Epidemiological Centre, census data.

Table 10: Age-standardised IHD mortality (deaths/100,000 person years) relative rates and absolute differences in different socio-economic groups, men and women 20-64 years

		Men			Women		
		Mortality	RR	Absolute difference	Mortality	RR	Absolute difference
Unskilled	1986-90	91.6	1.55	32.5	14.9	1.82	6.7
manual	1991-95	72.5	1.74	30.9	13.9	2.17	7.5
Skilled manual	1986-90	76.9	1.30	17.8	15.5	1.89	7.3
	1991-95	56.7	1.36	15.1	12.4	1.94	6
Lower	1986-90	76.1	1.29	17	13.8	1.68	5.6
non-manual	1991-95	59.8	1.44	18.2	10.5	1.64	4.1
Higher and intermediate non-manual	1986-90	59.1	1	-	8.2	1	-
	1991-95	41.6	1	-	6.4	1	-
Not classifiable	1986-90	201.8	3.41	142.7	43.2	2.92	35
	1991-95	145.6	3.50	104	42.5	3.06	36.1

Source: Persson et al. (2001).

B. Morbidity

Analyses of LNU data 1968-1981 show stable class differences in health (measured as an index of physical and mental ailments) (Vågerö & Lundberg 1995). This runs contrary to the reported increase in mortality differentials for that period. Lundberg *et al.* (2001) studied changes in health (self-rated health and limiting long-standing illness) and health inequalities between 1986-1987 and 1994-1995. Their conclusion is that overall prevalence rates were almost identical across the two periods, and that there were few if any changes in health inequalities, regardless of whether social class or education are considered. These results are not influenced by including or excluding those not economically active in the analysis. That no change has occurred despite the economic crisis would suggest that the welfare state has had a buffering effect through unemployment benefits, social assistance and expansion of the educational system. However, cuts in public expenditure were implemented primarily in 1995 and 1996, which means that the potential consequences of these are still to be analysed (*ibid.*). Also work environment changed most drastically in the early 1990s, the results of which may not be immediate.

Looking at the development during our study period, the ULF study shows stable inequalities in self-rated health, as well as for long-standing illness with serious complaints (figures 11-14). For both men and women, the proportion reporting less than good health has been rather stable, although overall levels have decreased slightly for men (figures 11-12). Only those not classifiable among men have had a significant change. For long-standing illness with serious complaints, there is a clear trend of growing levels of ill health during the 1990s for both sexes (figures 13-14). Significant increases can be found for unskilled manual workers (bordering on significance for men) and male intermediate non-manual employees. Logistic regressions with age, social class and period were performed, including an interaction term class*period to take into account changes in overall health, as well as any change in health inequalities over time (table 11). These confirm that overall class differentials have been stable, as the interaction term is not significant (not shown). Class differences are steeper for men than for women, and for women there is no significant difference between higher and intermediate non-manual employees. For men, class differentials are very similar for the two outcomes, but for women there are much smaller differences concerning long-standing illness with serious complaints. Looking at overall changes, there has been a significant decrease in the proportion of men reporting less than good health between the first and second period, whereas for women there has been no change over time. For serious long-standing illness, there is instead a substantial increase in the third period for both men and women, and for women also during the 1980s.

As we can see, class differences in health seem to have been stable for a long time, with no increase in health inequalities in the period leading up to 1980. Self-rated health has been quite stable in all classes also after 1980. In contrast, long-standing illness with serious complaints has increased for both men and women in the 1990s, while inequalities have been stable. Unskilled workers remain the most affected social class, and women are more affected than men.

Figure 11: Self-rated health less than good, men 20-64 years. Age-standardised

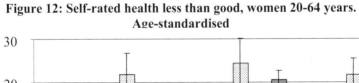

Source: ULF.

Figure 12: Self-rated health less than good, women 20-64 years. Age-standardised

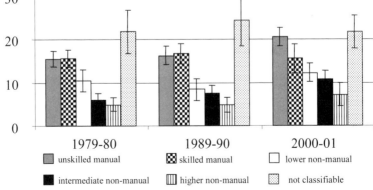

Source: ULF.

359

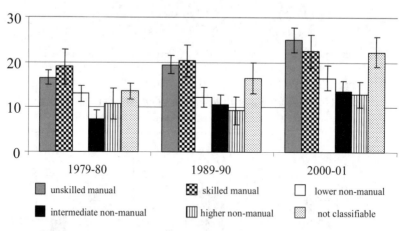

Figure 13: Long-standing illness with serious complaints, men 20-64 years. Age-standardised

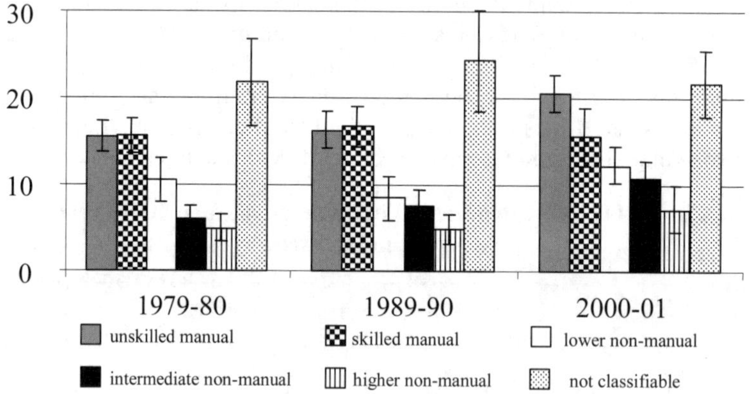

Source: ULF.

Figure 14: Long-standing illness with serious complaints, women 20-64 years. Age-standardised

Source: ULF.

C. Conclusion

As Diderichsen *et al.* (Diderichsen & Hallqvist 1997) mention, the period 1961-1985 was distinguished by narrowing income differentials and low unemployment. The two main causes of mortality to increase at this time were CVD and injuries. For both smoking and alcohol consumption, those in higher socio-economic groups used to have the highest consumption, and groups lower in the social hierarchy have followed them (SCB 1986, Sos/EpC 2001), changes consistent with Bourdieu's notion of hierarchical diffusion (Leifman 1998, Bourdieu 1987, Sulkunen 1989). This would all point to a growing importance of behavioural factors in explaining the increase in differentials, which is due to increasing mortality among male manual workers and a positive trend for other groups up until 1980. Class differences in both smoking and alcohol are smaller for women, and they have not had the same bearing on class differentials in mortality. Thus, a shift from 'material' to 'behavioural' factors as an explanation for class differentials is much less clear for women[8]. After 1980, we have witnessed growing differentials in disposable income for both men and women, due to a relatively better development for above all the highest social class. This class is also the least affected by the negative developments in the psychosocial work environment. Class differences in both smoking and physical activity have been stable, while there has been a positive trend with decreased smoking and increased activity in all groups (SpC/SCB 2001). Taken together, these factors might imply an increasing importance of economic and working conditions for social class differences in health since 1980, and a decreasing importance of behavioural factors. The pattern for alcohol consumption is more worrying as there has been an overall increase in consumption, and in the late 1990s male manual workers had the highest proportion of heavy consumers (Leifman 1998).

As Vågerö & Lundberg (1995) indicate, the relative importance of work environment and behavioural factors may be different for mortality and morbidity. For morbidity, factors causing impaired musculoskeletal function may be more important, whereas for mortality, factors causing cardiovascular problems should be given more weight. The fact that class differences in self-reported health have been so stable may therefore not be inconsistent with an increase in mortality differentials. The shifting patterns of smoking and alcohol consumption that occurred in earlier decades may take their full toll on mortality differentials only now; we are experiencing a 'lagged effect'. It is interesting to note that class inequalities continue to be stable also in the aftermath of the crisis for both health measures. The fact that no change in overall self-rated health has occurred would seem to indicate that even major welfare restructuring, as well as increased psychosocial stress at work and higher unemployment figures, have had little impact on the health

---

[8]   We acknowledge that health-related behaviours are more than an aggregate of individual lifestyles, and that cultural explanations are no less structural than materialist explanations (Vågerö & Illsley 1995).

361

of the population. It is not necessarily a contradiction that long-standing illness has increased and self-rated health has remained stable. Long-standing illness with serious complaints is a health measure close to diagnosed illness, and conditions such as high blood pressure and diabetes properly managed do not necessarily impair the subjective feeling of health. This may also be true for other long-standing conditions such as musculoskeletal complaints and allergies. The fact that women have had a more negative development than men could partly be due to an effect of accumulated exposure to paid work (reflecting a development from the 1960s onwards), which should not be the case for men. From the available data, it is difficult to conclude why increases in long-standing illness have as yet not been accompanied by increasing class inequalities.

Table 11 a: Odds ratios, 95% confidence intervals and significance level for less than good health and long-standing illness with serious complaints, controlled for age. Men 20-64 years

Men	Odds ratio	95% C.I	p		Odds ratio	95% C.I	p
SRH				LSIS			
Higher non-manual	1.00				1.00		
Intermediate non-manual	1.42	1.18-1.71	0.000		1.43	1.13-1.81	0.003
Lower non-manual	1.89	1.54-2.33	0.000		2.01	1.55-2.59	0.000
Skilled workers	3.11	2.62-3.67	0.000		3.34	2.71-4.12	0.000
Unskilled workers	3.73	3.16-4.40	0.000		3.75	3.05-4.61	0.000
Not classifiable	5.06	4.00-6.39	0.000		4.31	3.26-5.71	0.000
1979-80	1.00				1.00		
1989-90	0.87	0.78-0.98	0.016		1.05	0.92-1.20	0.475
2000-01	0.88	0.79-0.98	0.021		1.31	1.16-1.49	0.000

Source: ULF.

Table 11 b: Odds ratios, 95% confidence intervals and significance level for less than good health and long-standing illness with serious complaints, controlled for age. Women 20-64 years

Women	Odds ratio	95% C.I	p		Odds ratio	95% C.I	p
SRH				LSIS			
Higher non-manual	1.00				1.00		
Intermediate non-manual	1.24	1.00-1.54	0.045		1.03	0.82-1.29	0.812
Lower non-manual	1.85	1.51-2.27	0.000		1.41	1.14-1.76	0.002
Skilled workers	2.62	2.10-3.26	0.000		2.18	1.73-2.76	0.000
Unskilled workers	3.24	2.68-3.92	0.000		2.32	1.89-2.84	0.000
Not classifiable	2.74	2.23-3.36	0.000		1.94	1.56-2.42	0.000
1979-80	1.00				1.00		
1989-90	0.93	0.85-1.05	0.184		1.20	1.07-1.35	0.002
2000-01	1.08	0.96-1.21	0.124		1.67	1.49-1.86	0.000

Source: ULF.

4. How much of Inequality in Health May Be Explained by Work Environment Factors?

The changes in working conditions in Sweden in recent years would imply a gradual increase in class differentials, at least during the 1990s. Skilled manual workers seems to be the group with the most unfavourable development, especially concerning physical working conditions, and consequently could be experiencing increasing health problems. However, self-rated health has been quite stable in all classes except for a slight improvement among men between the first and second period. On the other hand, long-standing illness with serious complaints increased for both men and women in the 1990s, and for women more so than men. This is consistent with the deterioration in working conditions that took place in the early 1990s. What may seem surprising here is the fact that skilled manual workers as a group have been little affected, which is a striking contrast to the trend for unskilled workers. It is not impossible that health-related mobility out of the group contributes to this finding, even though we have included those who are early retired or currently unemployed. Earlier studies show that there is health-related mobility from physically heavy to light occupations (Östlin 1988). Of course, there could also be a case of health-related mobility into the group – only those who are exceptionally fit are recruited to these physically heavy jobs. Unskilled workers may also be comparatively more vulnerable due to experienced detrimental conditions in other areas.

In this section, we will try to quantify the contribution of different health-related factors to the current class inequalities in health. The analysis has been inspired by Lundberg's previous work on LNU data (Lundberg 1991, 1992). The results of Lundberg's studies indicate that for physical illness, physical working conditions (heavy and dangerous work) was the most important explanation for existing class differences in 1981, followed by economic hardship during childhood and then health-related behaviours. The impact of work factors (physical and psychosocial) on class inequalities in physical illness was twice as large in 1991 as it was in 1981. All factors had a greater impact on class differences in 1991 than in 1981, and all differences became insignificant in the full model. For psychological distress, class inequalities were generally smaller, and also seem to have decreased between 1981 and 1991. In 1991, controlling for any set of factors individually made differences become insignificant. In 1981, the most important factor seemed to be economic hardship during childhood.

We have chosen ULF 1996/97, as this survey is unique in containing a number of questions on both the physical and psychosocial work environment, as well as several measures of health-related behaviours. Included are those currently employed aged 20-64 (N=5982, 49.2% males, 50.8% females)[9]. Explanatory variables are physical and psychosocial working conditions, behavioural factors including physical activity, alcohol consumption and smoking, obesity, measures of economic hardship and indicators of social isolation (lacking a close friend) and living in a single household (see appendix for variable definitions and categorisation). The only factor in ULF that might be directly related to adverse childhood conditions is achieved height, and this variable was included in an earlier analysis. However, as short stature failed to show any relationship to health it was excluded, and the same is true for lacking a close friend. A measure of high strain was first included in the model. When all psychosocial working conditions are included in the model, high strain is no longer significant for either sex for any of the outcomes. This variable was therefore excluded.

---

[9] Those who are economically inactive are systematically found to experience worse health, and as a bigger proportion in lower social classes are economically inactive, excluding them will lead to class differentials being underestimated. However, including them here might underestimate the importance of working conditions as they lack a current exposure, although present ill health may in many cases be related to previous work exposure.

A. *Results*

First, the relationship between each independent variable and the two health outcomes was tested in a series of logistic regression including only that variable and controlling for age (not shown). As mentioned, all included variables were shown to have a significant effect on health. For our work environment variables, psychological demands are only related to health for women, and social support at work also shows a much stronger association for women than it does for men.

The prevalence of each independent variable in different classes was also assessed (not shown). High demands and low control showed the expected association with class. Low social support at work was prevalent among unskilled manual workers for both sexes, and for women also skilled manual workers had a higher proportion. Both behavioural factors and economic difficulties showed the expected association with social class. For women, there was no difference between classes in the proportion living alone, while there was a noticeable class gradient for men, reflecting gender norms in partner choice.

Turning now to the explanatory analyses, we can note that compared with our previous analyses of ULF that included those not currently employed (see table 11), class differentials are generally reduced (tables 12 a + b). Another difference is that skilled workers have as bad or worse health as unskilled workers. Smaller differences could partly be explained by the exclusion of those not employed, as these are most prevalent in the unskilled group. Again, class inequalities are more pronounced for men, especially for self-rated health. Examining the models in figures 15-18, we can get an understanding of the weight that work environment factors have in explaining class differentials in health. Explained fraction, i.e. how much each set of factors has reduced the odds ratio between a group and the reference group has been calculated net (when added to the base model) and gross (when added to the full model). Overall, included factors explain more of the class differences in women; this is partly due to smaller differences in the base model. For women, differences between the higher and intermediate non-manual class are small and always insignificant. The intermediate non-manual class has therefore been excluded from the figure.

Table 12 a: Class differences in self-rated health and long-standing illness with serious complaints among employed men 20-64 years. Odds ratios adjusted for age and adjusted for the full model (age, working conditions, behavioural factors, measures of economic hardship and living in a single household)

		Base model	Model VII		Base model	Model VII
		Age adjusted	Full model		Age adjusted	Full model
Men	SRH			LSIS		
Unskilled manual		3.30 (2.26-4.82)	1.89 (1.15-3.09)		2.66 (1.69-4.17)	1.53 (0.86-2.72)
Skilled manual		3.63 (2.50-5.26)	2.53 (1.56-4.09)		2.86 (1.84-4.44)	2.05 (1.17-3.58)
Lower non-manual		2.51 (1.61-3.91)	2.05 (1.25-3.35)		2.88 (1.75-4.75)	2.39 (1.37-4.16)
Intermediate non-manual		1.68 (1.12-2.52)	1.5 (0.97-2.32)		1.89 (1.18-3.01)	1.63 (0.98-2.71)
Higher non-manual		1	1		1	1

Source: ULF.

Table 12 b: Class differences in self-rated health and long-standing illness with serious complaints among employed women 20-64 years. Odds ratios adjusted for age and adjusted for the full model (age, working conditions, behavioural factors, measures of economic hardship and living in a single household)

		Base model	Model VII		Base model	Model VII
		Age adjusted	Full model		Age adjusted	Full model
Women	SRH			LSIS		
Unskilled manual		2.39 (1.64-3.48)	1.33 (0.83-2.12)		2.11 (1.38-3.23)	1.19 (0.71-1.99)
Skilled manual		2.41 (1.57-3.70)	1.51 (0.91-2.51)		2.62 (1.63-4.19)	1.62 (0.94-2.77)
Lower non-manual		1.71 (1.14-2.56)	1.43 (0.92-2.22)		1.64 (1.04-2.59)	1.26 (0.77-2.06)
Intermediate non-manual		1.14 (0.75-1.71)	0.98 (0.63-1.52)		1.24 (0.78-1.96)	1.03 (0.63-1.66)
Higher non-manual		1	1		1	1

Source: ULF.

Looking first at self-rated health, both psychosocial (model II) and physical working conditions (model III) contribute to the increased risk for manual workers (figures 15-16). However, physical working conditions are more important. The gross effect of psychosocial work factors is generally negative, which means that when all other factors have been included, it does not reduce but rather exacerbates differentials. Its initial effect may thus be due to its co-variation with other health-related factors. Total working conditions (model IV) is the most crucial factor for manual workers, with behavioural factors (not shown) coming in second. Adding psychosocial working conditions increases the odds ratio for lower non-manual employees for both men and women, and behavioural factors have the greatest relative weight for this group. Overall, the impact of economic and social factors is relatively small (not shown). In the full model, no significant differences for women remain, while for men there are still rather large differences. For long-standing illness with serious complaints, the impact of working conditions for manual workers is even more pronounced (figures 17-18). Psychosocial working conditions take on a greater significance for women, and they appear to be more important than the physical working environment. Both behavioural factors, economic conditions and social relations are less important in explaining class differentials in long-term illness than they were for self-rated health. In the full model, male lower non-manual and skilled manual workers still have a significantly higher risk of illness.

Figure 15: The effect of work environment factors for class differences in SRH. Employed men 20-64

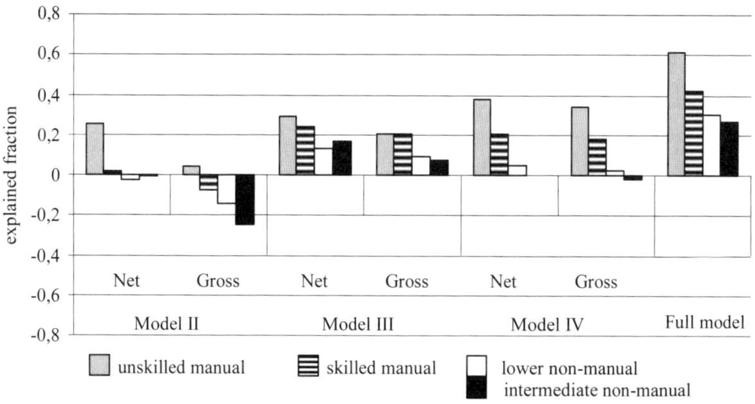

367

Figure 16: The effect of work environment factors for class differences in SRH. Employed women 20-64

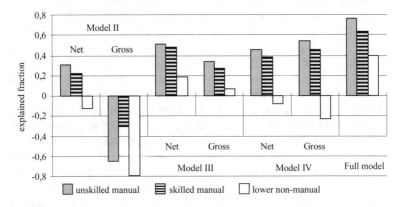

Source: ULF.

Figure 17: The effect of work environment factors for class differences in LSIS. Employed men 20-64

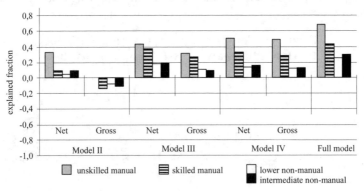

Source: ULF.

Figure 18: The effect of work environment factors for class differences in LSIS. Employed women 20-64

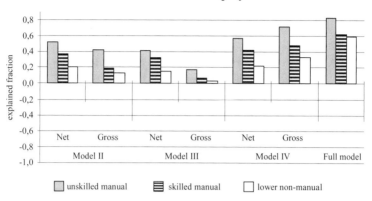

Source: ULF.

B. Trend Analyses

Earlier waves (1979 and 1986/87) of ULF have included the same battery of questions regarding work environment, and thus it is possible to repeat the above analysis for earlier years. However, as health-related behaviours were not included those years the full model cannot be accounted for, only working conditions. In 1986/87 questions on social support at work are missing, and we have therefore also excluded those questions for the other years. The above data for 1996/97 and these analyses will therefore not be entirely comparable. The analyses are presented in figures 19-20. As shown, the effect of total working conditions on class differences in health was at its highest in 1986/87, and it had the least impact in 1996/97. Looking at physical and psychosocial working conditions separately (not shown) for self-rated health, psychosocial factors have become relatively more important and physical factors relatively less so. For long-standing illness, there is no clear pattern for men, whereas for women psychosocial factors have again clearly become more important overall, while physical factors decreased in importance between the mid-1980s and 1990s.

Figure 19: The effect of work environment for class inequalities in health 1979-1997. Employed men 20-64 years

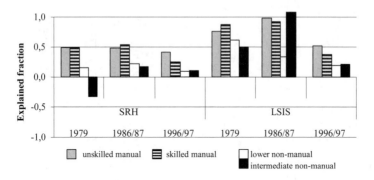

Source: ULF.

Figure 20:The effect of work environment for class inequalities in health 1979-1997. Employed women 20-64 years

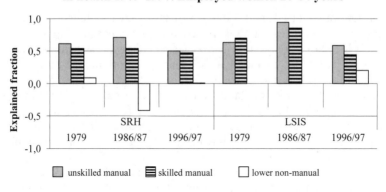

Source: ULF.

C. Discussion

These analyses confirm the continuing role that working conditions play in explaining class inequalities in health, especially for those groups who experience the highest level of ill health. Behavioural factors seem in their turn to be relatively more important for non-manual employees. The biggest difference between men and women is the impact of psychosocial conditions on long-standing illness. This is consistent with deteriorating psychosocial working conditions in fe-male-dominated occupations and sectors.

A major shortcoming of this study is its cross-sectional design. This means that we cannot control for health-related mobility. One example where this might contribute to the findings is for long-standing illness, where male lower non-manual employees have as poor health as manual workers. Further, their high risk is poorly explained by any of the included factors. This might reflect the character of 'retreat position' that these jobs may have for former manual workers. The most common occupations in this category are those of salesmen (wholesale and retail), caretakers, and secretarial positions. Health-related mobility out of exposed groups and out of the labour market may also lead to a depreciation in the effect of working conditions, just as previous health-related behaviours which have led to current ill health are not accounted for. One may note here that when Lundberg repeated his analysis with a longitudinal design, previous findings were generally confirmed, including the relative size of different factors (1990). Another aspect that has not been taken into account is the complex interaction effect of concurrent variables. The analysis presented here is rather crude and could be developed. However, for the sake of clarity the number of models has been kept to a minimum. What has been demonstrated is that poor working conditions are indeed related to health and that they contribute strongly to existing class differentials in health.

Among employees, the weight of working conditions for overall class differences seems to have decreased somewhat between the mid-1980s and 1990s. Given what was shown about the development during the early 1990s, how can this be explained? One obvious candidate is the employment rate, which was at its highest in 1990 and decreased considerably up until 1997. It is quite possible that health-related mobility out of the labour force during this time has meant that deteriorating working conditions have not had the expected effect, due to a generally healthier workforce. Also, it is only after 1997 that sickness absence has increased, and it is quite possible that we are now witnessing a lagged effect of earlier changes. In 1996/97, these might not have been observable. Unlike what was shown in the WES, according to our analyses of ULF, high psychological demands have not generally increased among manual workers, and low control has been rather stable. Thus we cannot find the same trends as in the WES. As noted, demands have been measured using only two questions (see appendix 2), which is likely to be less valid.

D. Research on the Relationship between Work Environment and Class Inequalities in Health

A recent overview of all public health research in Sweden has shown that out of all international scientific publications from Jan 2000 to June

2003, 21% dealt with working life and health (Carsjö 2005). Out of fifteen different research areas, working life was in fourth place and inequality in health came eighth when institutions were asked to state the four most prominent areas for their own research. Much of the research in occupational medicine is of course directly related to social inequalities in health, but this broader perspective is rarely applied. This is for instance true of much research at the National Institute for Working Life. Institutes or departments that explicitly focus both on working life and social inequalities are Social Medicine at Karolinska Institutet, the Sociological Department at Umeå University and Social Medicine at Lund University. At those institutions especially concerned with equity in health, such as the Centre for Health Equity Studies (CHESS) at Karolinska Institutet/Stockholm University and the Department for Public Health and Clinical Medicine at Umeå University, working conditions are seldom a special focus, although CHESS has projects dealing with labour market position and health. However, there is a wealth of research on working conditions, work organisation and health at a number of institutions, and this research is helpful regarding both the causation and prevention of work-related social inequalities, even in cases when these are not explicitly addressed. The problem lies more in systematising and using this knowledge – a formidable task which has not been within the scope of this chapter.

5. Concluding Discussion

The effect of working conditions on health differentials between classes is dependent on two things: the size and composition of the labour force, and working conditions as such. During the last decade the labour force has diminished, which should mean that selection processes in and/or out of work have been strengthened. In such a situation, we can have the paradoxical effect of deteriorating working conditions alongside no increase in health problems (at least among the economically active population) and no increase in health differentials, due to a 'healthy worker' effect. Trend analyses of ULF seem to indicate that this might be the case, at least up until 1997.

A. In-/Outflow from the Labour Force

As we have seen, the major change in labour force participation has been in the lower age range rather than the higher ages, contrary to what has been found in many other European countries (European Commission 2003). Between 1990 and 2000, labour force participation fell most for men and women aged 20-34, while the oldest age group saw the least change. The 'establishment age', when 75% are in the labour force, has increased from 20 years to 26 years for men and 28 years for women (SCB 2002). At the other end of the age range, the corresponding threshold has decreased by less than a year. Thus it would seem that changing demand has led to a decrease in labour supply primarily through a higher proportion of young people entering higher education, rather than an increased selection out of the labour force. However, the threefold increase in long-term sickness absence might very well change that picture, as more and more of those currently off sick become early retired due to disability. As shown earlier, the employment rate has declined especially for manual workers, and those most affected are female unskilled manual workers and lower non-manual employees. Also the proportion who have retired before 65 (for any reason) in the ULF study has increased most for female unskilled manual workers and lower non-manual employees. Small average changes in exit age might therefore hide large class differentials, and a healthy worker effect might therefore be evident.

Thus it is clear that there are increasing labour market problems for those with low education and low skills, but also what seems to be a growing health selection out of the labour force. While the growing non-participation of lower classes might entail a diminished effect of working conditions (and a growing importance of labour market status), the increase in sickness absence and disability benefits since 1997 suggest that working conditions may have become more important. These forces are at work simultaneously and it is not obvious what the net effect might be.

B. Labour Market Policy as a Means of Maintaining Full Employment

In Sweden, labour market policy has been part of the general economic policy and its main goals are to promote growth and full employment while restricting inflation (Bergeskog 1999). The fundamentals of the Rehn-Meidner model (so called after its inventors) have been in force since the 1950s (Olsen 1999). Active labour market policies have been a particularly salient part of the Swedish policy, and consist of policies which increase labour mobility between markets and regions (through retraining programmes, job placement and mobility grants) and stimulate growth in weak markets and regions, as well as helping those who have particular difficulties in finding employment, especially those with functional disabilities. Apart from active measures, the basic elements are a generally restrictive economic policy and a wage policy of solidarity which means 'the same wage for similar work' in both strong and weak parts of the economy (Wadensjö 1998). Both of these might lead to unemployment, and this is where the active measures come in. In the 42 years between 1950 and 1991, Sweden's share of open unemployment exceeded 3% for short periods on only three occasions (Olsen 1999). This would point to an extremely successful labour market policy in the pre-recession era. However, the policy came under increasing attack for giving rise to substitution and displacement effects (Wadensjö 1998), and it is clear that on its own it could not prevent the rise in unemployment in the 1990s. Studies point to a developed wage bargaining framework, a high level of demand through welfare state policies, and the use of devaluation as more important for full employment than active labour market policies. Evaluations suggest that the most effective aspect of the active policy was its job placement service, which reduces mismatch and increases mobility (Fraser 1999).

The labour market model developed by Rehn & Meidner was part of a coherent economic policy grounded in the theories of Keynes. Today, labour market policy operates in an environment of decentralised wage bargaining and with no scope for public sector expansion, and it has failed to establish a new theoretical base (Wadensjö 1998). Policies are increasingly being targeted to specific groups such as young people and newly arrived immigrants, and the range of measures has increased. It is difficult to tell what impact these measures will have by themselves, but for disadvantaged groups, targeted active labour market measures together with adult secondary education has at least the potential to remedy some of the current problems. Earlier research has shown that differences in employment rates between people with and without chronic illness have been less pronounced in Sweden than in Britain, also in the 1990s (Burström *et al.* 2000, 2003). Country differences were especially large among unskilled manual workers. This suggests that policies such as strong employment protection which makes it illegal to dismiss someone on the grounds of illness, as well as state-subsidised jobs for people with functional impairments, has had a real impact on employment opportunities for this group. However, high employment rates may sometimes mask long-term sickness absences, as sickness benefits can be claimed for an indefinite time in Sweden without loss of employment. It is to the increase in sickness absence that we now turn.

C. *Sickness and Disability Benefits as Exit Routes*

We have already touched upon the rise in sickness absence and disability benefits, an issue which has been hotly debated in Sweden and is the subject of several governmental reports. Since 1997, when sickness absence (total number of spells) was at a historically very low level, the rate has doubled (source: www.rfv.se). The total number of cases has long followed the economic cycle, so this is nothing new. What is perhaps more alarming is the rise in long-term sickness absence: the number of cases with a sick leave period of 90 days or more increased by 100% for men and 130% for women between 1997 and 2001. With the rise in sickness absence, the number of people on disability benefit has also increased. The number of newly granted disability benefits increased by 85% between 1998 and 2002, and it is now at the highest level recorded.

A comparison between Sweden and seven other European countries (Norway, the Netherlands, Denmark, Finland, France, the UK and Germany) shows that sickness absence has been considerably higher in Sweden, Norway and the Netherlands since the 1980s (RFV 2002). These countries have all experienced a sharp increase during the latter part of the 1990s, for all ages and among both men and women. For the countries with the highest rates, sickness absence clearly varies with the economic cycle, so that in times of high unemployment, rates go down, and when the unemployment decreases, sickness absence rises. The report comes to the conclusion that the high employment rate among people over 60, especially older women, is a strong causal factor underlying Sweden's (and Norway's) higher sickness absence – as women and older people generally have the highest rates. A dubious downside to the high employment rate in older age groups is thus a high rate of sickness absence overall, and especially in that age group.

Another contributing factor is of course differences in the social security system, which were not specifically examined in this study. The authors state that the rules regarding sickness absence were most generous in the three countries with the highest rates. Another Swedish study of long-term trends in sickness absence came to the conclusion that changes during the last 20 years could primarily be attributed to the combined effect of expansive or restrictive changes in the regulations in the sickness insurance and the economic development (Lidwall & Skogman Thoursie 2000). As expansions in the system have often taken place in an economic upturn and vice versa, the effects tend to be mutually reinforcing. In Sweden, the benefit level is 80% of the previous income. Since 1993 there is a qualifying period of one day before any benefits are paid, which has a deterrent effect against using the insurance at all. The main explanations for the rise in long-term sickness absence are, according to Lidwall & Skogman Thoursie an ageing workforce, combined with deteriorating working conditions. Also, class differentials in sickness absence can mainly be attributed to the working environment, especially physically strenuous work (Hemmingsson 2001).

D. *Working Conditions*

As concluded earlier there has been a gradual and general deterioration of psychosocial working conditions, especially in the 1990s. There is a tendency towards increased polarisation between men and women, and between the private and public sector, while overall class differences have been stable. However, the highest non-manual class has seen the least change. Physical working conditions are, not unexpectedly, much more arduous among manual workers, and they seem not to have improved over the period. During the 1990s, both men and women in the most exposed group, skilled manual workers, experienced a negative development.

The fact that there have been no overall changes in self-reported physical working conditions for decades does seem puzzling. One possible interpretation is that expectations of what is a reasonable working environment have changed over time. The official statistics regarding work accidents and diseases up until 1999 shows that occupational accidents fell from 40 cases per 1,000 employees per year to 10 cases for men between 1980 and 1999, the biggest drop being in the period between 1988 and 1993 (Nordin & Bengtsson 2001). For women, the number of cases peaked at below 15 in the late 1980s and is now around 6 cases per year. Also fatal accidents, which are reliably reported, have decreased, and dropped by half between the late 1980s and today (figure 21[10]). This indicates that hazardous work situations have indeed become less common.

---

[10] Estonia capsised and foundered in the Baltic in 1994, with the death toll exceeding 800 people.

**Figure 21: Fatal accidents at work and to/from work,
N and number per 10,000 employees**

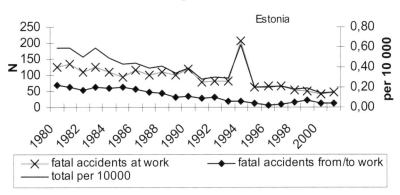

Source: SWEA.

E. Impact of Work Environment Policy

The Work Environment Act, which was passed in 1977, states that its purpose is to prevent ill health and accidents at work, and to achieve a good work environment (SWEA 2001). The Act also says that working conditions should be adapted to people's different physical and mental aptitudes, and that the employee should be given the opportunity to participate in the design of his/her own work situation. It is thus concerned with not simply physical aspects of the job but also job content and work organisation. Further, the employer is required to document the work environment and set up action plans for measures to improve it (systematic work environment management) and is responsible for training employees to avoid risks at work. The responsibility for implementing the policy rests mainly with the Swedish Work Environment Authority (SWEA). The wording of the Act is quite general, and defines the frame of the regulatory activities of SWEA, who lay down more detailed Provisions. There are at present about 140 Provisions and General Recommendations in force. Inspections at worksites are central to SWEA's enforcement of the policy, and employers who do not rectify deficiencies within a set time may be prohibited to carry on a certain activity and/or required to pay a fine. Some breaches of the act are also directly penalised.

There is evidence that inspections can increase compliance and also workplace safety (Lindblom & Hansson 2003). However, it might in practice be impossible to know the total effects of the Authority's activities, as many other conditions influence trends. Examples of single measures that have most likely had an effect include regulations concerning use of certain chemicals in cement, inspections resulting in a written notice regarding ergonomic conditions, and inspections to increase safety against violence and threats in the retail trade (Eriksson 2003). Evaluations of regulations concerning ergonomic working conditions and of a special campaign to decrease negative stress are underway. What might be concluded so far is that actions to prevent accidents have been more successful than those to prevent ill health or to achieve a good working environment. This could point to a priority of 'worst things first' – problems which may also be more easily dealt with. This focus also has a built-in equity perspective, as the jobs with the most dangerous working conditions are manual jobs.

Safety delegates, appointed by the local union in worksites with five or more employees (SWEA 2001), supervise the safeguards against ill health and accidents, and take part in the planning of new or altered facilities, work processes and work organisation. They also participate in the preparation of action plans and monitor the employer's fulfilment of systematic work environment management. It is within the powers of a safety delegate to suspend work if there is imminent danger to life or health, and also if the employer does not comply with a prohibition issued by SWEA. Safety delegates may also turn to SWEA if the employer fails to take remedial action in an area requested by the delegate. Workplaces with at least 50 employees are required to have a safety committee consisting of representatives of both employer and employees, including at least one safety delegate. One of the basic ideas of the act is therefore an emphasis on local cooperation between the parties. This should ensure a continuous monitoring of the work environment and hopefully a preventive effect. An on-site agent might also be more sensitive to the effects of psychosocial working conditions than irregular inspection activities. SWEA consider systematic work environment management to be important enough to be selected as an indicator of how well the authority is fulfilling the Government's national goal for decreasing ill health at work (by which is meant sickness absence) (Arbetsmiljöverket 2003). According to its own survey, 41% of employers say they have introduced systematic work environment management, compared with 29% of safety delegates (Eriksson 2003). Of those who said they had documented the work environment, 70% of employers and 60% of safety delegates say identified risks have been attended to. These figures show that there is still a long way to go before the Act is fully implemented. Important policy changes that may have contributed to the negative development during the 1990s are the dismantling of the occupational health services after state subsidies were abolished, as well as reduced state contributions to regional safety delegates for smaller workplaces without local delegates. There was a marked decline in the number of safety delegates between 1997 and 1999-2000, but the recent resurgence in interest for work environment issues has paid off, and in 2003 the number had risen again to the 1997 level (Kjellberg 2003).

F. *Impact of Unions*

While unions may have been weakened at peak level due to decentralisation of bargaining, they continue to play an important role at the plant level, and some even argue that decentralisation may promote workplace participation and grass-roots activity (Thörnqvist 1999). Through the appointment of safety delegates, union participation is an integral part in the day-to-day monitoring of working conditions. However, many unions report a rise in the number of workplaces without local union representation (Kjellberg 2003). As many as 70% of union members rated work environment as a 'very important' issue for the union in a recent survey. However, the high unemployment in the 1990s gave employers less incentive to attract employees by creating a good work environment, and unions were forced to primarily deal with personnel reductions and efforts to increase productivity and employment opportunities (Kjellberg 2000). For example, in the late 1990s almost half of all local metal workers' unions did not work with issues pertaining to work organisation. Through its long history of cooperation between the parties in the labour market and its well-organised unions Sweden still provides better opportunities for unions to influence work environment policy than most European countries. Today, none of the three peak level unions have formulated policies on social inequalities in health. They all mention the importance of a good work environment, but while the Swedish Confederation of Professional Employees, TCO (which organises non-manual employees) and the Swedish Trade Union Confederation, LO (the workers' union) want to strengthen existing institutions like occupational health services and safety delegates, the Swedish Confederation of Professional Associations, SACO (which organises employees with tertiary-level degrees) focuses on the right to continuing competence-building, and opportunities for occupational and social mobility (SACO 2001, TCO 2005, LO 2000). TCO and LO have highlighted work environment issues that are important for their own members in reports, and LO has published reports on health with a clear class perspective (Nelander & Lönnroos 2004). While work environment is an area where all unions work actively, health at work tends to be primarily associated with sickness absence, and health inequalities *per se* have so far attracted little attention – unions are above all concerned with the working conditions of their own members.

6. A Look at the Future

According to Statistics Sweden (SCB) the labour market situation will improve and the number of adults in secondary education, which expanded considerably due to special measures during the crisis, will decrease, while the expansion of higher education that took place during the 1990s should be permanent (SCB 2002). This means that there will be some increase in labour market participation for those who are 20-34 years old. For the age group 35-54, Statistics Sweden forecast a marked rise in participation rates – for women back to the pre-crisis level in 1990, while for men it will not quite reach the unprecedented high level of the boom years but still increase substantially. This is primarily due to the effect of the new pension system that was introduced in 1999, but also an effect of demand in the wake of the 'baby-boomers' gradually leaving the labour force. The new pension system differs from the old in several crucial ways: the final pension is determined by the income during the entire working life rather than the best 15 years. Also, while the old pension consisted of two tiers – a basic flat-rate universally provided income support, and a supplementary pension determined by previous earnings – in the new system the earnings-related benefits will form the first tier, with pension supplements only for those with little or no supplementary pension (Olsen 1999). The principle of universality has thus been abandoned in the Swedish pension system. Moreover, while earlier everyone was entitled to a full pension after 30 years of working, now there is no guaranteed level of income replacement; rather this is determined entirely by previous contributions. The effects of this system will be to encourage people to work for longer – especially as each year will increase the level of their pension, also after the normal retirement age. This will affect both those who enter paid labour late due to higher education, and those who can expect a low pension due to periods of part-time work or unemployment. As an effect of the pension system, Statistics Sweden predict no further decline in labour force participation in the age group 55-64 up until 2020. These predictions all point to an increasing role of working conditions on health, as more people will be in employment, and the 'disciplining effect' of the pension system might mean increasing health inequalities if labour market exit is less of an option.

The National Labour Market Board (AMS) forecast that the trends we have witnessed during the last few decades will continue, as industry can expect a continued increase in production, coupled with a decrease in demand for labour (Johnreden & Wallin 2002). The private service sector is expected to experience the largest increase in labour demand, but there will also be a serious shortage in the public sector, as a large part of its workforce will have to be replaced. Although this is a rather crude categorisation, it points to the fact that expanding sectors are those where psychosocial working conditions have been an increasing problem. The shortage might however lead to an upgrading of the work environment as a necessary means to attract labour. An improvement might also make it possible for those with some functional impairment to stay on for longer. This would also entail living up to the Work Environment Act, which states that working conditions must be adapted to people's differing physical and mental abilities. The low economic rewards for 'women's work' combined with the continued importance of part-time work – voluntary and involuntary – makes early retirement a costly alternative. However, deteriorating working conditions and a weak labour market have pushed these older and less educated workers out of the labour market through the means available: long-term sick leave and disability benefits, as they can seldom find other employment. (Health problems may not always be caused by the work environment – but an intensified working life may make it impossible to stay in employment with reduced health) In the worst-case scenario, these would be forced to stay on despite no improvements, through a combined effect of the sharpening of sick insurance regulations and a decrease in benefit levels, and the demands of the new pension system.

7. National Goals for Health

In Sweden, reducing inequality in health was established as a political goal with the adoption of the WHO strategy "health for all, 2000" in 1984. The first Swedish public health report in 1987 pointed out that despite increased longevity and health in the population, certain groups lagged behind (Boman 2002). This is a declaration which is echoed in the latest report's statement that social differences in health are still marked and have not diminished during the last twenty years, despite a general positive trend (SoS/EpC 2005). Following the 1987 report, a national public health group with experts and politicians was commissioned to devise a strategy for reducing observed inequalities. The recommendations were presented to the right-wing government in 1991. The group proposed measures directed both at the structural and the individual level, from economic policy to health education. The Government, however, demanded more knowledge on what caused health inequalities. One result of the group's work was the establishment of the Swedish National Institute of Public Health (SNIPH) in 1992. In 1997, a national public health committee was formed, with the aim of proposing national goals with a "health for all" perspective. These goals were made public in 2000 (Boman 2002).

In late 2002, the social democratic government finally proposed 11 domains of objectives, with the overarching aim to "create social conditions that will ensure good health on equal terms for the entire population" and with a particular focus on those groups who are worst off (Hogstedt *et al.* 2005). The bill was passed by Parliament in April 2003. It is an example of a comprehensive policy, with objectives ranging from upstream to downstream approaches. Rather than focusing on health *per se*, the domains all deal with health determinants on different levels. The first six concern structural causes of social ine-qualities and are formulated as: participation and influence in society; economic and social security; secure and favourable conditions during childhood and adolescence; healthier working life; healthy and safe environments and products; and health and medical care that more actively promotes good health. More detailed objectives for the different areas and indicators for measuring them have been proposed by SNIPH, based on, if possible, existing objectives within the different policy areas involved. For goal 4, healthier working life, the main indicators proposed are the proportion of employees with work-related ill health or specific complaints, and an index of job demand/control/support. The last five target areas are directed at health-related behaviours and in-clude protection from communicable diseases, reproductive health, physical activity and nutrition, tobacco, alcohol and illicit drugs. While much of the concrete work will take place on the local and regional level – over which the Government have no right of determination – the role of the State will be to set up targets, undertake regular follow-ups and report on the results. In the area of working life, nine national agencies are directly involved. All involved agencies and authorities must report on their efforts to achieve the national public health target, and SNIPH is responsible for supporting and coordinating this work. What the public health objectives provide is a framework to employ in existing policy areas, and a call for health impact assessments by re-sponsible agencies.

Burström *et al.* assess that within the action spectrum described by Whitehead (1998) Sweden is in the stage where 'more structured devel-opments' have taken place (2002). The political will has been and continues to be strong, but as Boman rhetorically asks: Why does the government persist in bringing attention to class differences in health when no obvious measures have been implemented to reduce them (Boman 2002)? How public health issues will be prioritised along with other pressing concerns in a world of limited resources is as yet an open question. It is worth noting that the bill does not contain any extra means to support the new focus, nor does it entail any new commit-ments for municipalities or county councils.

Acknowledgment

We would like to extend our gratitude to Ingvar Lundberg for extensive discussions and detailed comments during different parts of the manuscript preparation. We also thank the Swedish reference group for helpful comments and suggestions; Bo Burström, Olle Lundberg, Tomas Hemmingsson, Christer Hogstedt and Töres Theorell, and referees from the international group for comments on an earlier version of the manuscript.

References

ARBETSMILJÖVERKET. 2003. *Indikatorer för att följa arbetsmiljön och AV:s bidrag till ohälsomålets uppfyllelse*. Stockholm: Arbetsmiljöverket (the Swedish Work Environment Authority), 15 p.

ARONSSON G., GUSTAFSSON K., DALLNER M. 2000. *Anställningsformer, arbetsmiljö och hälsa i ett centrum-periferiperspektiv*. Arbete och hälsa: Stockholm: Arbetslivsinstitutet (National Institute for Working Life): 9, 25 p.

ARONSSON G. 1999. "Contingent workers and health and safety at work". *Work Employ Soc* 13: 439-459.

BERGESKOG A. . *Arbetsmarknadspolitisk översikt 1999*. Uppsala: Institutet för arbetsmarknadspolitisk utvärdering (The Institute for Labour Market Policy Evaluation, IFAU). 44 p.

BERGQVIST C. 2001. "Jämställdhetspolitiska idéer och strategier". *Arbetsmarknad och arbetsliv* 7(1): 15-29.

BLOM-HANSEN J. 2000. "Still Corporatism in Scandinavia? A Survey of Recent Empirical Findings". *Scand Polit Stud* 23(2): 157-181.

BOMAN J. 2002. *Viljans vägar och villovägar. Den politiska diskussionen om klasskillnader i hälsa under 1980- och 1990-talet*. Linköping: Linköping University: 23-45, 98.

BONGERS PM., DE WINTER CR., KOMPIER MA., HILDEBRANDT VH. 1993. "Psychosocial factors at work and musculoskeletal disease". *Scand J Work Environ Health* 19(5): 297-312.

BOURDIEU P. 1987. "What makes a social class? On the theoretical and practical existence of groups". *Berkeley J Sociol* 32: 1–17.

BURSTRÖM B., DIDERICHSEN F., ÖSTLIN P., ÖSTERGREN P.-O. 2002. "Sweden". In: MACKENBACH JP., BAKKER M. (eds.). *Reducing inequalities in health. A European perspective*. London & New York: Routledge: 274-283.

BURSTRÖM B., HOLLAND P., DIDERICHSEN F., WHITEHEAD M. 2003. "Winners and losers in flexible labour markets: the fate of women with chronic illness in contrasting policy environments – Sweden and Britain". *Int J Health Serv* 33(2): 199-217.

BURSTRÖM B., WHITEHEAD M., LINDHOLM C., DIDERICHSEN F. 2000. "Inequality in the social consequences of illness: how well do people with chronic illness fare in the British and Swedish Labour Markets?". *Int J Health Serv* 30(3): 435-451.

CARLSSON G., ARVIDSSON O., BYGREN L.-O., WERKÖ L. 1979. *Liv och hälsa: en kartläggning av hälsoutvecklingen i Sverige*. Stockholm: LiberFörlag, 228 p.

CARSJÖ K., ERIKSON R., HOGSTEDT C., KAMPER-JÖRGENSEN F., KÄLLESTÅL C. "A status report on Swedish publich health research: History, inventory, and international evaluation". *Scand J Public Health* 33: Suppl 65: 84.

CASTELLS M. 2000. *The information age: economy, society and culture. Vol. 1 The rise of the network society*. Malden: Massachussets: Blackwell, 594 p.

DIDERICHSEN F., HALLQVIST J. 1997. "Trends in occupational mortality among middle-aged men in Sweden 1961-1990". *Int J Epidemiol* 26(4): 782-7.

ERIKSON R., GOLDTHORPE J. 1992. *The constant flux*. New York: Clarendon Press, 429 p.

ERIKSSON O. 2003. *Effektutvärdering inom Arbetsmiljöverket*. Stockholm: Arbetsmiljöverket (the Swedish Work Environment Authority, 33 p.

EUROPEAN COMMISSION D-GFEASA. 2003. *Employment in Europe 2003. Recent Trends and Prospects*. Luxembourg: Office for Official Publications of the European Communities: 159-160.

FELSTEAD A., JEWSON N., (eds.) 1999. *Global trends in flexible labour*. Basingstoke: Macmillan, 213 p.

FRASER N. 1999. "How strong is the case for targeting active labour market policies? A review of efficiency and equity arguments". *Int J Manpower*: 20(3/4): 151-164.

FREDLUND P., HALLQVIST J., DIDERICHSEN F. 2000. *Psykosocial yrkesexponeringsmatris. En uppdatering av ett klassifikationssystem för yrkesrelaterade psykosociala exponeringar*. Stockholm: Arbetslivsinstitutet (National Institute for Working Life): 37 p.

FRITZELL J. (eds.). 2000. *Välfärdens förutsättningar. Arbetsmarknad, demografi och segregation*. Stockholm: Socialdepartementet (Ministry of Health and Social Affairs). *SOU*: 37

FRITZELL J., LUNDBERG O. 1993. *Ett förlorat eller förlovat årtionde? Välfärdsutvecklingen mellan 1981 och 1991*. Stockholm: Institutet för social forskning (SOFI), Stockholms universitet: Report No. 3, 88 p.

FRITZELL J., LUNDBERG O. 1994. "Välfärdsförändringar 1968-91". In: FRITZELL J., LUNDBERG O. (eds.). *Vardagens villkor. Levnadsförhållanden i Sverige under tre decennier*. Stockholm: Brombergs: 235-259.

GOLDTHORPE J. 2000. *On Sociology. Numbers, Narratives, and the Integration of Research and Theory*. Oxford: Oxford University Press, 337 p.

GOUDSWAARD A., ANDRIES F. 2002. *Employment status and working conditions*. Luxemburg: European Foundation for the Improvement of Living and Working Conditions. Office for Official Publications of the European Communities, 80 p.

HÅKANSSON K. 2001. *Språngbräda eller segmentering? En longitudinell studie av tidsbegränsat anställda*. Uppsala: Institutet för arbetsmarknadspolitisk utvärdering (The Institute for Labour Market Policy Evaluation, IFAU): Report No.1, 77 p.

HALES TR., BERNARD BP. 1996. "Epidemiology of work-related musculoskeletal disorders". *Orthop Clin North Am* 27(4): 679-709.

HANSEN LH. 2001. *The division of labour in post-industrial societies.* Gothenburg: University of Gothenburg.

HEMMINGSSON T. 2001. "Sjukskrivning, arbetslöshet och utslagning under 1990-talet". In: HEMMINGSSON T. (ed.). *Hälsa och hållbart arbetsliv i Stockholms län.* Stockholm: Yrkesmedicinska enheten, Samhällsmedicin, Stockholms läns landsting: 57-68.

HOGSTEDT, C. LUNDGREN B., MOBERG H., PETTERSSON B., ÅGREN G., "The Public Health Objective Bill (Govt. Bill 2002/03: 35) – Extended summary". Ch 2. In 'The Swedish Public Health Policy and the National Institute of Public Health'. *Scand J Public Health* 32 (Suppl 64): 18-59.

JOHNREDEN A.-C., WALLIN C. 2002. *Den framtida personalförsörjningen. Tre scenarier till år 2015.* Stockholm: Arbetsmarknadsstyrelsen (the Swedish National Labour Market Board, AMS), 28 p.

KATZ LF., AUTOR DH. 1999. "Changes in the wage structure and earnings inequality". Ch. 26. In: ASHENFELTER O., CARD D. (eds.). *Handbook of Labor Economics* 3. Amsterdam: North-Holland.

KJELLBERG A. 2003. "Arbetsgivarorganisationer och fackföreningar i ett föränderligt arbetsliv". In: VON OTTER C.(ed.). *Ute och inne i svenskt arbetsliv. Forskare analyserar och spekulerar om trender i framtidens arbete.* Stockholm: Arbetslivsinstitutet (National Institute for Working Life): 345-376.

KJELLBERG A. 2000. "Facklig organisering och arbetsmarknad: marginalisering av ungdomar och invandrare?" In: TEGLE S., (ed.). *Har den svenska modellen överlevt krisen? Utvecklingstendenser i arbetslivet inför 2000-talet.* Stockholm: Arbetslivsinstitutet (National Institute for Working Life: 49-75.

KUNST AE., GROENHOF F., MACKENBACH JP. 1998. "Mortality by occupational class among men 30-64 years in 11 European countries. EU Working Group on Socioeconomic Inequalities in Health". *Soc Sci Med* 46(11): 1459-76.

LE GRAND C., SZULKIN R., TÅHLIN M. 2001a. "Lönestrukturens förändring i Sverige". In: FRITZELL J., GÄHLER M., LUNDBERG O., (eds.). *SOU 2001: 53. Välfärd och arbete i arbetslöshetens årtionde.* Stockholm: Kommittén Välfärdsbokslut, Socialdepartementet (Ministry of Health and Social Affairs: 121-174.

LE GRAND C., SZULKIN R., TÅHLIN M. 2001b. "Har jobben blivit bättre? En analys av arbetsinnehållet under tre decennier". In: FRITZELL J., GÄHLER M., LUNDBERG O., (eds.). *SOU 2001: 53. Välfärd och arbete i arbetslöshetens årtionde.* Stockholm: Kommittén Välfärdsbokslut, Socialdepartementet (Ministry of Health and Social Affairs): 79-120.

LEIFMAN H. 1998. *Socialklass och alkoholvanor – en empirisk analys av alkoholvanor i olika sociala skikt och implikationer för alkoholpreventionens utformning*. Stockholm: Folkhälsoinstitutet (the Swedish National Institute of Public Health): 14. 88.

LIDWALL U., SKOGMAN THOURSIE P. 2000. *Sjukfrånvaro och förtidspension. En beskrivning och analys av utvecklingen under de senaste decennierna*. RFV analyserar: 2. Stockholm: Riksförsäkringsverket.

LINDBLOM L., HANSSON S.O. 2003. *The evaluation of inspections*. Stockholm: The Swedish Work Environment Authority: 3, 45 p.

LO. 2000. *Det här vill LO. Fackliga och politiska riktlinjer antagna av Demokratikongressen 2000 2-6 sept*. Landsorganisationen (LO).

LUNDBERG O. 1990. *Den ojämlika ohälsan*. Stockholm: Stockholm University.

LUNDBERG O., DIDERICHSEN F., ÅBERG YNGWE M. 2001. "Changing health inequalities in a changing society? Sweden in the mid-1980s and mid-1990s" *Scand J Public Health* 29: Suppl 55.

LUNDBERG O. 1991. "Causal explanations for class inequality in health – an empirical analysis". *Soc Sci Med* 32(4): 385-93.

LUNDBERG O., *The contribution of structural factors vs health-related behaviours to class inequalities in health*. Conference paper presented at the 2nd International Conference in Behavioral Medicine. Hamburg, Germany: 15-18 July 1992

LUNDBORG P. "Vilka förlorade jobben under 1990-talet?". In: FRITZELL J., (ed.) *SOU 2000: 37 Välfärdens förutsättningar*. Arbetsmarknad, demografi och segregation. Stockholm: Socialdepartementet (Ministry of Health and Social Affairs).

MAGNUSSON L., OTTOSSON J. 2002. "Har den svenska arbetsmarknaden förändrats?". In: *Hela folket i arbete?: Arbetslivsforum 2002 – en mötesplats för forskare och praktiker*. Stockholm: Forskningsrådet för arbetsliv och socialvetenskap (FAS).

MAGNUSSON L. 1999. *Den tredje industriella revolutionen*. Stockholm: Prisma & Arbetslivsinstitutet (National Institute for Working Life), 159 p.

MASLACH C., SCHAUFELI WB., LEITER MP. 2001. "Job burnout". *Annu Rev Psychol* 52: 397-422.

AMV/SCB. 2001. *Negativ stress och ohälsa. Inverkan av höga krav, låg egenkontroll och bristande socialt stöd i arbetet*. Stockholm: Arbetsmiljöverket (The Swedish Work Environment Authority, AV) & Statistiska centralbyrån (Statistics Sweden, SCB), 181 p.

NELANDER S., LÖNNROOS E. 2004. *Ohälsans trappa*. Stockholm: Landsorganisationen, 82 p.

NORDIN H., BENGTSSON B. 2001. *Occupational accidents and work-related diseases in Sweden*. Stockholm: Swedish Work Environment Authority, 49 p.

OLSEN G.M. 1999. "Half empty or half full? The Swedish welfare state in transition". *Can Rev Sociol Anthr* 36(2): 241-267.

ÖSTLIN P. 1988. "Negative health selection into physically light occupations". *J Epidemiol Community Health* 42: 152-156.

PERSSON G., BOSTRÖM G., DIDERICHSEN F., LINDBERG G., PETTERSSON B., ROSÉN M., *et al.* 2001. "Health in Sweden – The National Public Health Report 2001". *Scand J Public Health*: Supplement 58.

RFV. 2002. *Svensk sjukfrånvaro i ett europeiskt perspektiv. RFV analyserar 2002: 11.* Stockholm: Riksförsäkringsverket (RFV), 85 p.

SACO: *Färdriktning för SACO 2002-2005*; Antagen av SACOs kongress 2001. http://www.saco.se/upload/doc_archive/2253.pdf

SCB. 2001. *Utbildning och efterfrågan på arbetskraft. Utsikter till år 2008.* Stockholm: Statistiska centralbyrån (SCB); Information om utbildning och arbetsmarknad: 1, 104 p.

SOS. 1986. *Tobaksvanor i Sverige. En översikt och analys.* Stockholm: Socialstyrelsen (The National Board of Health and Welfare, SoS): 9, 152 p.

SOS/EPC. 2001. *Folkhälsorapport 2001.* Stockholm: Socialstyrelsen (The National Board of Health and Welfare, SoS)/ Epidemiologiskt centrum (EpC): 220-241.

SOS/EPC. 2001. *Folkhälsorapport 2005.* Stockholm: Socialstyrelsen (The National Board of Health and Welfare, SoS)/ Epidemiologiskt centrum (EpC): 14.

SCB. 2000. *Inkomstfördelningsundersökningen 2000.* Stockholm: Statistiska centralbyrån (Statistics Sweden, SCB), 84 p.

SCB. 2005. *Inkomstfördelningsundersökningen 2003. Redovisning på riksnivå.* Stockholm: Statistiska centralbyrån (Statistics Sweden, SCB), 95 p.

SCB. *Arbetskraftsprognos 2002. Utvecklingen till år 2020.* Information om utbildning och arbetsmarknad 2002: 1. Stockholm: Statistiska centralbyrån (Statistics Sweden, SCB): 106 p.

SOCIALDEPARTEMENTET (MINISTRY OF HEALTH AND SOCIAL AFFAIRS). 2002. *Handlingsplan för ökad hälsa i arbetslivet. Mål, ansvar och åtgärder med utgångspunkt från ett övergripande mål för människor i arbete.* Stockholm: *SOU*: 5: 81-131.

SULKUNEN P. 1989. "Drinking in France 1965-79. An analysis of household consumption data". *Br J Addict* 84: 61-72.

SUNDSTRÖM M. 2003. "Part-time work in Sweden: an institutionalist perspective". In: LE GRAND, C. & TSUKAGUCHI, LE GRAND, T. (eds). *Women in Japan and Sweden.* Stockholm: Acta Universitatis Stockholmiensis & Almqvist & Wiksell International: 121-136.

SVENSSON T. 2002. "Globalisation, marketisation and power: the Swedish case of institutional change". *Scand Polit Stud* 25(3): 197-229.

SWEA. 2001. *The Work Environment Act with commentary.* Stockholm: Swedish Work Environment Authority (SWEA).

SZULKIN R., TÅHLIN M. 1994. "Arbetets utveckling". In: FRITZELL J., LUNDBERG O. (eds.). *Vardagens villkor.* Stockholm: Brombergs: 87-118.

TCO. *Inriktning och ekonomi. Verksamhetens inriktning och ekonomi för TCO åren 2004 – 2007.* http://www.tco.se/ArticlePages/200406/30/2004 0630134908_TCO162/20040630134908_TCO162.dbp.asp. June 2005.

THE WELFARE COMMISSION. *Ds 2002: 32. Welfare in Sweden: The Balance sheet for the 1990s.* Stockholm: Ministry of Health and Social Affairs, 216 p.

THE WORKING LIFE DELEGATION. 1999. *Working life and the individual: perspectives on contemporary working life at the turn of the millenium.* Stockholm: Ministry of Labour. *SOU* 69, 28 p.

THEORELL T., KARASEK RA. 1996. "Current issues relating to psychosocial job strain and cardiovascular disease research". *J Occup Health Psychol* 1(1): 9-26.

THÖRNQVIST C. 1999. "The decentralisation of industrial relations: the Swedish case in comparative perspective". *Eur J Ind Relat* 5(1): 71-87.

TÖRNELL B., "Migration, etnicitet och hälsa – begrepp och indikatorer". In: HOGSTEDT C. (ed.). *Välfärd, jämlikhet och folkhälsa – vetenskapligt underlag för begrepp, mått och indikatorer.* Stockholm: Statens folkhälsoinstitut (The Swedish National Institute of Public Health) : 253-296.

VÅGERÖ D., ILLSLEY R. 1995. "Explaining health inequalities: beyond Black and Barker. A discussion of some issues emerging in the decade following the Black report". *Eur Sociol Rev* 11(3): 219-241.

VÅGERÖ D., LUNDBERG O. 1995. "Socio-economic mortality differentials among adults in Sweden". In: LOPEZ AD., CASELLI G., VALKONEN T. (eds.). *Adult mortality in developed countries: from description to explanation.* Oxford: Clarendon Press: 222-242.

VÅGERÖ D. 1991. "Inequality in health – some theoretical and empirical problems". *Soc Sci Med* 32(4): 367-71.

VAN DER DOEF M., MAES S. 1998. "The job demand-control (-support) model and physical health outcomes: a review of the strain and buffer hypotheses". *Psychol Health* 13(5): 909-936.

VAN DER DOEF M., MAES S. 1999. "The job demand-control (-support) model and psychological well-being: a review of 20 years of empirical research". *Work Stress* 13(2): 87-114.

VIIKARI-JUNTURA ER. 1997. "The scientific basis for making guidelines and standards to prevent work-related musculoskeletal disorders". *Ergonomics* 40(10): 1097-117.

WADENSJÖ E. 1998. "Arbetsmarknadspolitiken under AMS första halvsekel". In: MOLIN B., (ed.) *Visioner och vardagar. 50 års aktiv arbetsmarknadspolitik.* Stockholm: Arbetsmarknadsstyrelsen (the National Labour Market Board): 51-76.

WHITEHEAD M. 1998. "Diffusion of ideas on social inequalities in health: a European perspective". *Milbank Q* 76(3): 469-492.

WIKMAN A., ANDERSSON A., BASTIN M. 1998. *Nya relationer i arbetslivet – en rapport om tendenser mot flexibla marknadsrelationer i stället för permanenta anställningsrelationer.* Stockholm: Arbetslivsinstitutet (National Institute for Working Life)/Statistiska centralbyrån (Statistics Sweden), 138 p.

WILLNER J., GRANQVIST L. 2002. "The impact on efficiency and distribution of a base-broadening and rate-reducing tax reform". *Int Tax Public Finan* 9: 273-294.

Appendix 1

1. Psychosocial work environment indices from WES

A. *Job demands*

Do you sometimes have so much to do that you have to skip lunch, work late, or take work home with you?

Is your work sometimes so stressful that you do not have time to talk or even think about anything other than work?

Does your work require your undivided attention and concentration?

Can your tasks feel so difficult that you would like to ask someone for advice or ask for help?/IF SO: How much of your time is devoted to such difficult tasks?

B. *Decision authority*

Is it possible for you to set your own work tempo?

Is it possible for you to decide on your own when various tasks are to be done?

Does it happen that you are involved in planning your work?

In the mains can you take short breaks at any time in order to talk?

C. *Social support*

Can you receive support and encouragement from your superiors when your work becomes heavy?

Can you receive support and encouragement from your fellow workers when your work becomes heavy?

If your tasks feel that difficult, do you have access to advice or help?

Does your superior (boss) ever express appreciation for your work?

Do other persons express appreciation for your work (e.g. fellow workers, patients, customers, clients, passengers, students)?

D. Index construction

All variables were converted to run from 1-6 and added. The indices were dichotomised so that the 25% with the highest or lowest values were considered 'exposed'. All others were included as 'unexposed'.

2. Variables in ULF 1996/97

A. Working conditions

Psychosocial working conditions include questions on demand, control and support. Demand consists of two questions; if the work is hectic or mentally straining. Skill discretion includes questions on monotonous work, repeated and one-sided working movements, possibilities to learn new things on the job, on-the-job training in the previous 12 months and instrumental or expressive attitude towards work. Decision latitude consists of questions regarding the degree of influence on the planning of work, work pace, breaks and vacations, flexible working-hours and possibility to be on compensatory leave. Social support at work is measured by questions on the possibility to talk to fellow workers during breaks, to leave work temporarily to talk to a colleague, and if the subject spends time with work colleagues outside of work. Heavy physical work consists of questions concerning heavy lifting, bent, twisted or other unsuitable working postures, daily perspiration from physical exertion and being exposed to shakings or vibrations.

The indices were constructed by adding the single items, and all were divided in 3 categories with the highest category for control and support and the lowest category for demands and heavy physical work as reference. Indicators for high strain (high demands/low control) and high iso-strain (high demands/low control/low support) were also calculated. Part-time work (<35 h per week) has also been controlled for as it decreases work exposure and therefore also might decrease the association between work environment and health.

B. Health-related behaviours

Included are questions on smoking, alcohol consumption and physical activity. Smoking has been categorised into never smokers (=0), ever smokers (=1) and current daily smokers (=2). Alcohol consumption was calculated using questions on frequency and amount of alcohol consumed during the last seven days and frequency and amount during a normal week for those who have had an atypical week in the last seven days. This was categorised into abstainers (=0), low consumption (=1) and high consumption (=2) (>=20 g alcohol/day for women and >= 30 g/day for men). There was one question on physical activity ranging from no activity at all to strenuous activity several times a week. The variable was dichotomised into no physical activity at all or a couple of times a year (=0) and any activity above that (=1). We have also included obesity as a behavioural factor – properly an outcome measure it does have a close relationship to physical activity and diet. Obesity was dichotomised as BMI<30=0, BMI =>30=1.

C. Economic conditions

We have included two measures. Having access to a certain amount of money (1,500 euros) in case of unforeseen expenses can be seen as an indicator of some economic security. Economic crisis, if there have been difficulties paying rent, food, bills etc. during last 12 months, reflects a more acutely difficult situation. Both were coded so that 1 indicates having economic difficulties as previously defined.

D. Social relations

We have included one question reflecting the existence of close social ties. Family status is dichotomised into married/cohabitating and single households, where single=1.

United Kingdom

Martin HYDE

Introduction

Inequalities in health between and within nations continue to exist despite overall improvements in health and life expectancy throughout most parts of the world (Wilkinson 1997, Mackenback, Kunst, Cavelaars *et al.* 1997, WHO 2004). The psychosocial work environment has long been identified as an important factor in the health of the working population and thus a potential site for the production and reproduction of these inequalities (Marmot, Theorell, & Siegrist, 2002, Marmot *et al.* 1991, Karasek & Theorell 1990). However, the structure of society and the work environment is changing with the introduction of new technologies, work practices and the globalisation of communication, production and services. How, if at all, these changes have affected the distribution of adverse psychosocial working conditions amongst the different social classes in society, and whether these changes have increased or diminished the effects of the psychosocial work environment on the health of the workforce, are key questions for those interested in reducing inequalities in health.

However, such an undertaking would require an entire book or a series of books. Thus the aim of this chapter is rather more modest. After a brief discussion of the political and economic context in Britain since the 1980s, data from the UK[1] are used to describe trends in the composition of the labour market, such as employment, unemployment and non-standard working practices, over the past 20 years. Our aim is to set the context for a review of the trends in socio-economic inequalities in health over the same period. Although it would be impossible to cover all the work that has been done in the UK on this subject, the main message – that those in the lower social classes suffer poorer health – is clear. Following this, data on the contribution of an adverse work environment to socio-economic inequalities in health are presented. Unlike the Scandinavian countries, there are no national work environ-

---

[1]   Where possible data for the whole of the UK have been used. However, in some cases data have only been available for England and Wales.

ment studies in the UK. However, these questions have been at the centre of one of the longest running longitudinal studies of the work environment and health, Whitehall II. Data on the distribution of adverse psychosocial working conditions by social class, from the Health Survey for England, and the changing effects of these conditions on health at work, taken from the Whitehall II study, are presented in this chapter. Finally the social policy response to these inequalities is reviewed in the penultimate section, which is followed by some conclusions.

1. Political and Economic Background

British society has undergone a series of well-publicised and well-researched changes over the final two decades of the 20th century (Ferri, Bynner & Wadsworth 2003, Hutton 1996). The election of the Conservative government under Margaret Thatcher, coupled with the second major OPEC crisis in 1980-1981, resulted in an explicit shift in political ideology within the Government, and changes in accumulation strategy amongst certain sections of capital. However, these trends were also evident under the previous Labour government, which was partly responsible for the economic and social problems which culminated in the 'winter of discontent' in 1979. Conservative governments held uninterrupted power from 1979 to 1997, during which time they aimed to reduce public spending, and although they never achieved reduction in the absolute level of public expenditure, they did slow the growth of spending. They introduced sweeping privatisation and anti-union legislation, and abandoned Keynesian demand-side economics in favour of monetarist supply-side orthodoxy. The impact on the labour market was stark and unemployment rose; union membership fell after several waves of industrial disputes and many public sector industries were privatised.

With the election of New Labour to government in 1997 many hoped that these trends would be reversed. Although it is undeniable that health inequalities, and inequalities in general, have become a focus of the New Labour government (Department of Health 2003), there are still many social and economic problems that affect the health of the population and many wonder if the Government's policies are tackling, or indeed can tackle, the real causes of health inequalities. The Blair government assiduously rejected the social democratic politics of the past in favour of what has now become known as the Third Way. The cornerstone of this new ideology is the notion of a partnership, between government and business, between the public and private sector, and between the citizen and state (Clarke 2004, Giddens 1998).

These political changes have coincided, and are in many ways inter-dependent, with the partial reorganisation of the UK economy. The perceived failure of Fordist mass production techniques to cope with the economic crisis following the OPEC shocks, coupled with the demise of welfarist employment policies, led many large companies to adopt alternative, flexible, methods and organisation (Lash & Urry 1987, Piore and Sabel 1996). But, as many writers are quick to note, both Fordism and post-Fordism ought to be understood as ideal types which co-exist, although invariably in an asymmetrical relation, rather than fully realised systems (Turner 2000, Amin 1996). However, there are many features of the present UK labour market that fit a post-Fordist scenario, such as the increasing numbers of people outside of the labour force and the falling proportions employed in manufacturing, which are described below.

2. Employment Trends since 1980

In the UK, as elsewhere, the nature and organisation of paid work has undergone significant transformations over the past few decades. Although there has been an increase in employment following the decline through the recession of the 1990s there has been a shift from full-time work to increased proportions of the population outside the labour market, as well as an increasing trend towards the casualisation or flexibalisation of certain types of employment. The UK has been characterised as a 40: 30: 30 society, in which 40% of the population are employed in jobs that are, relatively-speaking, stable and secure, 30% are employed in insecure or part-time jobs, and a further 30% are unemployed or otherwise outside the labour market (Hutton 1996).

Figure 1: Numbers of employees and self-employed in 1980, 1990 and 2000: Men

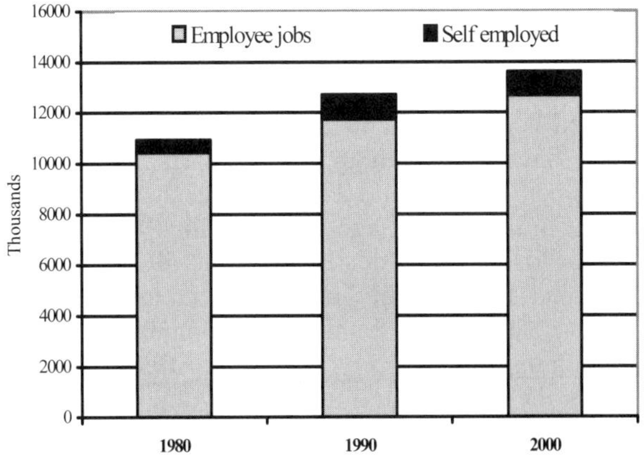

Source: LFS 1981, 1991, 2001.

**Figure 2: Numbers of employees and self-employed in 1980,
1990 and 2000: Women**

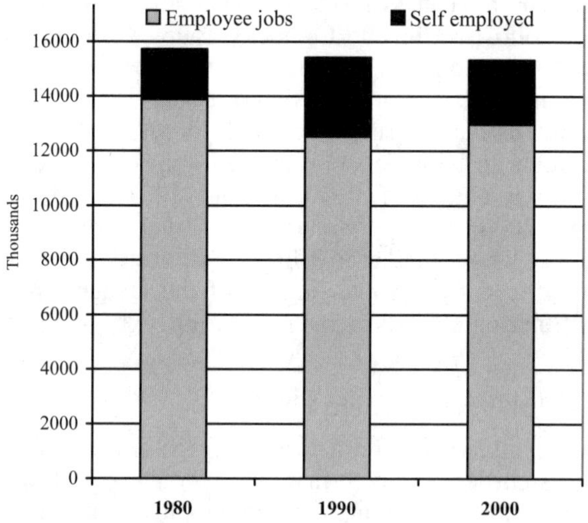

Source: LFS 1981, 1991, 2001.

Figure 1 shows, for men, that there was a drop in the number and proportion of employees, and a rise in the number and proportion of self-employed from 1980 to 1990. This trend had reversed somewhat by 2000, although it did not return to the levels of 1980. For women there has been a steady rise in the numbers of employees from 1980 to 2000 (see figure 2). However, as figure 3 shows, although there has been a general rise in the levels of employment, these are unevenly distributed across the age groups and the sexes. For both men and women, those in the youngest age group, 16-17 years old, have experienced a slight decrease in the proportions employed between 1992 and 2002, and such a decline can also be seen for men in the oldest age group, 65 years and over. Men aged between 25 and 34 years, and those aged between 35 and 49 years, have equally high levels of employment at both time points. For women, in 1992 and 2002, there is a steady increase in rates of employment in subsequent age groups, which reaches its peak in the 35- to 49-year-olds and then decreases in the 50- to 59-year-olds. This reflects the trend towards the increasing feminisation of the labour market. However, when one examines the composition of female labour market participation more closely, it is very different from that of men. Figure 4 shows the percentage of men and women in part-time employment. For men the numbers and proportions in part-time work have successively increased over the past two decades from 4% in 1984 to

8% in 1994, and finally to 10% in 2003. However, the rise from 1984 to 1994 is driven by a slight increase in the numbers working part-time as well as a fall in the numbers in full-time employment, whilst in 2003 the number of full- and part-time workers had both risen, which suggests that part-time work is increasing faster than full-time work for men. For women, despite an overall increase in employment from 1984 to 2004, the proportions of full- and part-time work remain remarkably stable with around 44% in part-time work at all three time points.

Figures 5 and 6 show the reasons that men and women gave for being employed in part-time and temporary jobs respectively, in 1992 and 2002. For both men and women in both years the principle reason given for working part-time was that people did not want a full-time job. However, the extent to which this is the case differs greatly between men and women. Just over 40% of men in 1992 and 2002 said that they did not want a full-time job, compared with around 80% of women who gave the same reason. Conversely, the percentages of men who said that they were working part-time because they could not find a full-time job were two to three times higher than those for women at both time points. In 1992, 22% of men and 9% of women said that they could not find a full-time job. In 2002 this had declined for both sexes but was still higher for men, 16%, than for women, 6%. However, the reasons given for working in temporary employment reveal a somewhat different picture. In 1992 the principle reason given by men for working in temporary jobs, 43%, was that they could not find a permanent job, compared with 19% who did not want a full-time position. The gap had narrowed a little by 2002, when 32% of men said that they could not find a full-time job and 25% said that they did not want a full-time job. For women, at both time points, the situation is reversed. In 1992, 35% of women said that they did not want a full-time job compared with 31% who said that they could not find one. By 2002, 33% said that they did not want a full-time job, whilst the percentage who reported that they could not find a full-time position had fallen to 23%.

Figure 3: Percentages in employment
by age group and sex: 1992 & 2002

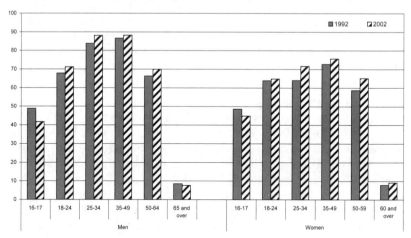

Source: LFS, 1993 &, 2003.

Figure 4: Percentages in part-time employment
by sex: 1984, 1991 & 2000

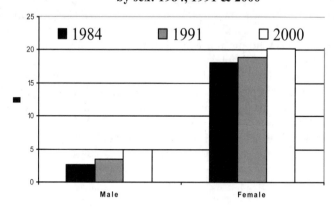

Source: LFS 1985, 1992 & 2001.

Figure 5: Reasons for part time employment:
Men and women 1992 & 2002

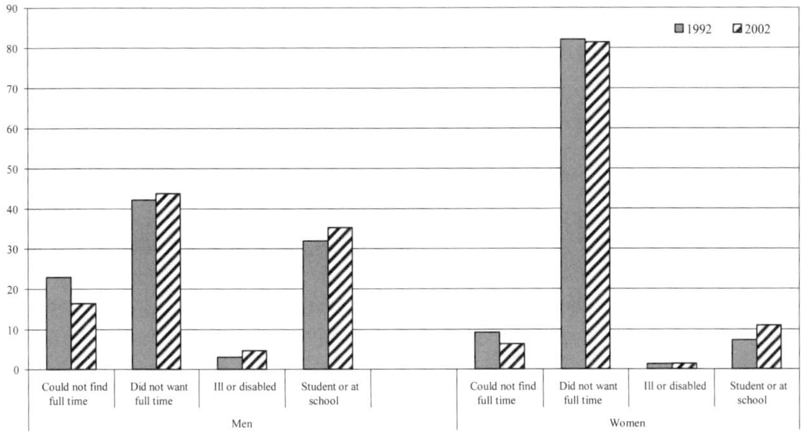

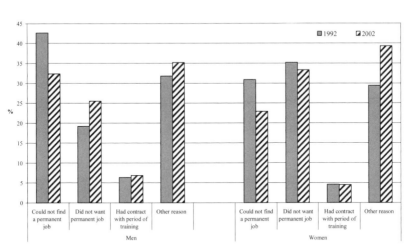

Source: LFS, 1993 &, 2003.

Figure 6: Reasons for being in temporary employment:
Men and women 1992 & 2002

Source: LFS, 1993 &, 2003.

3. Unemployment Trends since 1980

In 1999, over 8 million men in the EU were unemployed, according to the International Labor Organization's definition. One million of these were in the UK (Yeandle 2003). Although, as figure 7 shows, there has been a general decline in unemployment, which is notably sharp after 1991, there remain disparities in the rates of unemployment for different age groups and sexes. For both sexes the actual rates of unemployment and the fall in unemployment have been very similar. For men the rate of unemployment fell from just under 10% in 1981 to around 5% in 2001, and for women the rate fell from 9% to around 4.5%. However, for both sexes in all three years, those aged between 16 and 24 years have the highest rates of unemployment. Amongst men but not women there has also been a high level of unemployment for those approaching state retirement age[2].

Male labour force detachment is becoming an increasingly important feature of the UK labour market. In common with many west European countries, such as France and Italy, the UK has experienced a steady decrease in the labour force participation rates of older men (Guillemard and Rein 1993). The shift to service sector employment, increasing use of technology in the workplace and the need for higher qualifications for employment have all had an effect on employment rates for older men (Taylor, Tillsley, Beausoleil, Wilson and Walker 2000). In conjuncture, successive Tory governments have reconstructed unemployment, through excluding early retirement, the unfit and unemployable. However, male labour force detachment is not explained by any one factor, nor is there any one form that it takes. Indeed the boundaries between different forms of 'economic activity' are becoming increasingly blurred (Yeandle 2003). The data presented in figure 7 give a misleading impression of the change in labour market participation rates at older ages. By aggregating over such large age groups they disguise more complex trends. For men over the age of 55 years there has been a steady fall in employment rates. In 1983, 75% of men aged between 55 and 59 years were employed, and this had fallen to 70% by 1999. For women the trend has been the opposite. In 1983, 47% of women aged between 55 and 59 years were employed and by 1999 this had risen to 54% (see figure 8). However, other data show that the trend for women is mainly the result of women with children returning to work later in life. Labour force participation rates for women without children have

---

[2]   Unlike most European countries the UK has different state retirement ages for men and women. The age of state retirement in the UK for men is 65 years, whereas it is 60 years for women. However, the State Pension age for women is changing and will gradually increase from 60 to 65 between 2010 and 2020.

been relatively stable over the last decade at around 75% (Lindsay 2002).

Figure 7: ILO unemployment rates
by age group and sex: 1981, 1991 & 2001

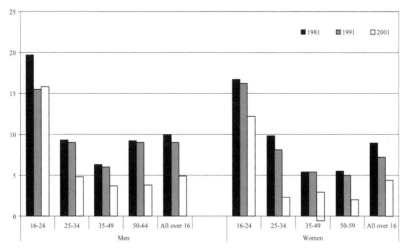

Source: LFS 1981, 1991, 2001.

Figure 8: Percentages of men and women aged 55-59 years
and 60-64 years in employment: 1983, 1990 and 1999

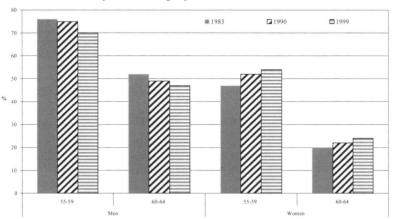

Source: Phillipson 2004.

4. Changes in the Sectoral and Class Composition of the Labour Force

For both sexes there has been a relative decline in the proportions employed in the manufacturing industry, and a corresponding rise in the proportions employed in services. However, as figure 9 shows, the patterns of gender segregation have remained reasonably stable over the past two decades. In 1982 around one third of men were employed in manufacturing compared with 17% of women. By 2002 this had changed to 21% and 8% for men and women respectively. Although there has been little change over time in most of the other industrial sectors, there has been a modest increase in the percentages employed in other services for both sexes. 16% of men and 39% of women were employed in the service sector in 1982, and this had risen to 19% of men and 41% of women by 2002. This increase in service sector employment has come about through the growing numbers employed in the banking and financial services. For both men and women the proportions employed in these sectors and changes over time have been very similar. In 1982, 13% of men and 12% of women were employed in financial and banking services, which grew to 20% and 19% respectively in 2002.

Figure 9: Employee jobs by sex and industry

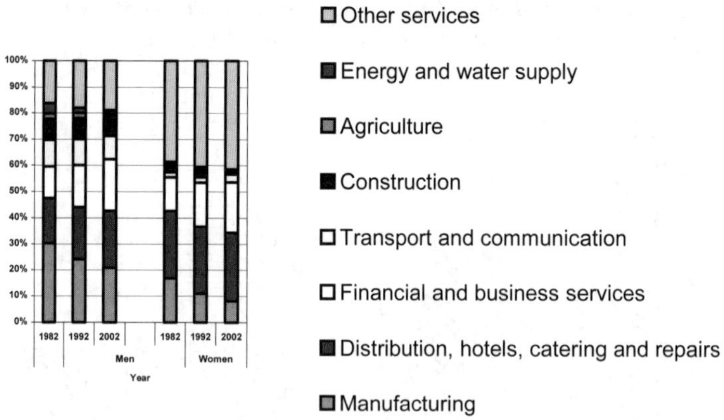

Source: Short-term Turnover and Employment Survey, Office for National Statistics.

The changing sectoral composition of the labour market has been reflected in the changing class structure of British society as measured by the Registrar General's classification system. As figure 10 demonstrates, there has been a general increase in the proportions of the non-manual social classes (I-IIInm) for both sexes. Over the course of the 19 years since 1981, the proportion of men in non-manual classes has risen from around 35% to just below 50%. This has largely been the result of falling proportions of men employed in skilled manual occupations, although this still remains the most common class for men, and slight reductions for the unskilled classes. This was accompanied by a modest increase in the professional and managerial classes of around 5% and 10% respectively. For women, who have traditionally been concentrated in non-manual occupations, the decrease in the proportions of those in the manual classes, from around 50% to around 35%, has been the result of increases in the proportions employed in the upper social classes at the expense of skilled manual and semi-skilled occupations (social class IIInm and IV). However, the proportions working in unskilled occupations (social class V) have remained relatively constant at around 10%.

Figure 10: Percentages in Registrar General's social class by sex; 1981, 1991 & 2000

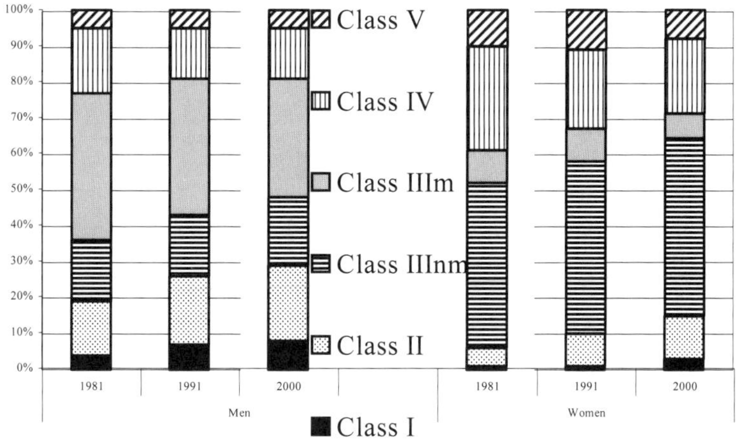

Source: GHS 2001.

5. Changes in Trade Union Membership

These changes in the constitution of the workforce have been accompanied by a reorganisation of industrial relations in the UK. There was a general decline in Trade Union membership throughout the late 1980s and early 1990s, reaching the lowest point in post-war history in 1997. There has been a modest recovery in the late 1990s, although the numbers are still far short of their early 1980s peak. However, as figures 11, 12 and 13 show, there are large differences in Trade Union membership between the sexes and in different industries. In 2001, men were more likely to be in a union than women, and the rates of unionisation were much greater in the public sector than in the private sector (see figure 11).

Figure 11: Percentage of the workforce in Trade Unions by sex and sector: 2001

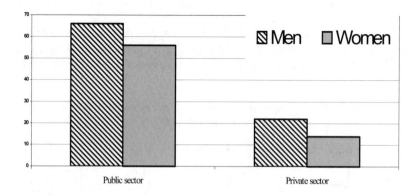

Source: GHS 2001.

Although there was a decline for both sexes in the percentages of workers in trade unions across all occupations, from 1992 to 1998, differences in the gender differences in occupational rates remain. Women in the professional and associated professional sectors are most likely to be in a union, among women, followed by plant and machine operatives, and craft and related occupations. For men, plant and machine operatives and those in the personal and protective services have the highest rates of unionisation, although there is not such differentiation amongst the other occupations, apart from the low rates amongst those in sales and managerial and administrative occupations (see figures 12 and 13).

Figure 12. Percentage of the workforce in Trades Unions by sector: Women, 1992 & 1998

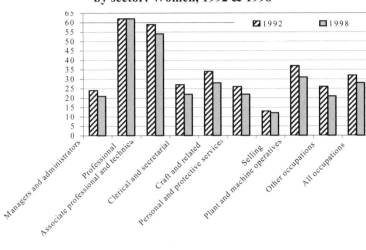

Figure 13: Percentage of the workforce in Trade Unions by sector: Men 1992 & 1998

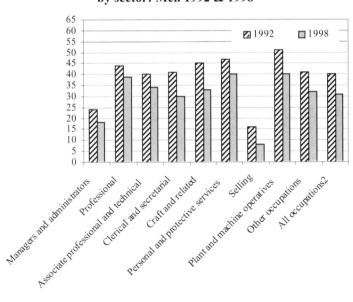

Source: LFS 1992/1998.

6. Social Inequalities and Health

The publication of the Black report, in 1980, was a crucial moment in health inequalities research in the UK. The central message of the report was that those in the lower occupational classes suffered poorer health than those in the upper occupational classes at all points in their lifecourse. Throughout the 1970s and 1980s, class inequalities had widened in many important areas such as low birth weight, inadequate nutrition and poor general health, even though the overall levels in the population had fallen. What was remarkable, however, and what probably provoked the then Conservative government's attempts to diminish the findings from the report, was that the authors firmly placed the blame for the (widening) social inequalities in health on social and economic causes, such as income differentials, experiences at work and unemployment (Macintyre 2002). In summarising their findings later, the authors conclude that:

> Social and economic factors like income, work (or lack of it), environment, education, housing, transportation and what are today called 'lifestyles' all affect health and all favour the better off (Black *et al.* 1982).

Whilst the Black report did not initiate research into health inequalities in the UK, which can be traced back to the 19th century (Goldblatt & Whitehead 2000), it, or the controversy that surrounded it, produced a renewed interest in the field. The study of social inequalities in health is almost by definition interdisciplinary; however, two broad approaches to the study of health inequalities can be identified. One approach, Kwachi and colleagues argue, looks at the distribution of health between different meaningful groups, whilst the other looks at the distribution of health across individuals in a population (such as income). Although the latter avoids political questions and ignores social relations amongst individuals, it allows for comparisons over time; i.e. group definition might change, making comparisons difficult. Furthermore, they note two different approaches to the causes of inequalities in health: the materialist approach which focuses on 'access to tangible material conditions', and the psychosocial one which looks at the 'direct or indirect effects of stress stemming from either being lower on the social hierarchy or conditions of relative socio-economic disadvantage'. However, these approaches are not as opposed as originally thought and many studies incorporate measures of both (Bartley 2003, Kwachi, Subramanian & Almeida-Filho 2002). Hence the data presented below attempt to combine both approaches by looking at the distribution of poor health and psychosocial conditions across socio-economic groups across time.

Over the last two decades or so there has emerged a vast literature devoted to exploring the state and causes of social inequalities in health. The consensus that has emerged from this research is that those who are in the most disadvantaged groups, however measured, generally suffer the worst health, although different outcome measures do not always produce the same picture. The gap in life expectancy between those born into the highest and those born into the lowest social classes has been increasing, despite overall improvements in longevity for all social classes (Donkin, Goldblatt & Lynch 2002). The difference in life expectancy at birth between men from social class I and men from social class V increased from 5.5 years in 1976 to 9.5 years in 1996. Whilst differences in life expectancy for women are less marked, the gap between social class I and social class V grew from 5.3 years in 1976 to 6.4 years in 1996 (Hattersley 1999)[3]. Data from the ONS longitudinal study, presented in figure 14, show that although all-cause mortality fell for men aged between 35 and 64 years of age from the mid-1980s to the end of the century, social class differences in mortality rates persisted amongst both men and women, although they were less pronounced amongst the latter. For men the gap in mortality rates between those at the top of the social classification system, classes I and II, and those at the bottom, classes IV and V, grew from a ratio of 1.69 in 1986-1992 to 1.75 in 1997-1999. As tables 1 and 2 show, this trend is repeated for deaths attributable to ischaemic heart diseases and cerebrovascular diseases (White, van Galen & Chow 2003). Amongst men there is a persistent gradient in mortality due to ishaemic heart diseases over this period, and for cerebrovascular diseases the gap has actually increased. Amongst women a gradient in mortality for both these causes is also clearly visible. However, the difference between those in the upper social classes and those in the lower social classes has decreased slightly over the period.

---

[3] As previously stated, it is important to note that the re-classification of occupations over time can have an effect on mortality rates. For example between 1971 and 1981, 14% of men aged between 16 and 65 years moved occupational classes purely on the basis of reclassification, the net effect of which was to reduce the levels of mortality amongst the non-manual classes. However, changes made between 1981 and 1991 had a negligible impact on mortality rates (Goldbatt & Whitehead 2000).

Figure 14: Trends in all-cause mortality by social class, men and women aged 35-64

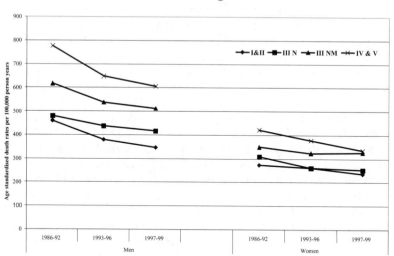

Source: *White, van Galen & Chow 2003.*

This picture is similar for morbidity in later life (Marmot & Nazroo 2001). Those who work in manual occupations are more likely to report poor general health (Chandola, Bartley, Wiggins & Schofield 2003) and having a limiting long-standing illness (White, Nicolaas, Foster, Browne & Carey 1993). When comparing those at the very top of the social class system with those at the very bottom the gap is even more extreme. Scottish data show that unskilled workers are three times more likely than those from the professional class to have a limiting long-standing illness, and also increased likelihood of psychiatric symptoms and poor psychological well-being (Macintyre 1986). Where one puts oneself in the social class system also has an effect on one's health. Data from the Whitehall II study shows that subjective social status is a strong predictor of ill health over and above the effects of education, occupation and income. Even after controlling for these factors, men who put themselves lower in the social order had higher rates of diabetes, respiratory illness and depression (Singh-Manoux, Adler and Marmot 2003).

Table 1: Trends in mortality attributable to ischaemic heart disease (ICD-9 410-414) by Registrar General's social class, 1986-1999, for both sexes aged 35-64. Age-standardised death rates per 100,000 person years

		1986-92	1993-96	1997-99
Men	I & II	160	97	90
	III NM	162	117	117
	III M	228	159	141
	IV & V	270	215	167
	Ratio IV & V:I & II	1.69	2.22	1.86
Women	I & II	31	21	22
	III NM	44	35	30
	III M	58	46	41
	IV & V	74	48	50
	Ratio IV & V:I & II	2.38	2.29	2.27

Source: White, val Galen & Chow, 2003.

Table 2: Trends in mortality attributable to cerebrovascular disease (ICD-9 430-438) by Registrar General's social class, 1986-1999, both sexes aged 35-64. Age-standardised death rates per 100,000 person years

		1986-92	1993-96	1997-99
Men	I & II	29	22	12
	III NM	28	17	13
	III M	33	30	24
	IV & V	39	45	32
	Ratio IV & V:I & II	1.34	2.05	2.67
Women	I & II	14	8	18
	III NM	21	14	9
	III M	17	24	22
	IV & V	33	22	19
	Ratio IV & V:I & II	2.26	2.75	1.06

Source: White, val Galen & Chow, 2003.

Figures 15 to 18 show data on social class differences in the prevalences of long-standing and limiting long-standing illness for men and women, taken from three waves of the General Household Survey for the UK. For men there is a clear social class gradient in the rates of long-standing illness in 1980. 22% of men in the professional class reported a long-standing illness compared with 36% amongst the un-skilled manual group. In 1990 there was an increase in the rates of long-standing illness for all social classes but, although there was still a clear difference between the unskilled manual group and the professional group, the gradient has flattened considerably. In 2000 there was an increase in rates amongst the manual social classes, and those in non-manual classes almost returned to their 1980 levels. Thus not only was the gradient re-established but there is an ever-widening gap between the manual and non-manual occupational groups. For women, although there are wide differences between the lowest and the highest social classes, there is not a clear gradient in either 1980 or 1990. This is principally due to the fact that women in the intermediate and junior non-manual group have worse health than women in the skilled manual group. This gives the impression of two gradients, one within the non-manual occupations and another within the manual occupations. Like the trends for long-standing illness in men there was a general rise for all classes from 1980 to 1990. Unlike the men, this was followed by an improvement in 2000 for all groups apart from those in the unskilled manual class, whose health continued to deteriorate.

The pattern for limiting long-standing illness is quite similar. Amongst men in 1980 there is a clearly observable gradient, with those in the higher social classes reporting lower rates of limiting long-standing illness. Although by 1990 there had been little change in the reported rates for the highest or lowest social classes, there was a general rise in all the intermediate classes. In 2000 the picture was, how-ever, very different. For those in the non-manual occupations the previ-ous trend was reversed and the rates of illness declined, whilst there was an increase in the rates of illness for all manual classes. The result of these developments was a wider gap between the top and bottom classes than had been present in 1980. For women there was an increase in the rates of reported limiting long-standing illness for all classes between 1980 and 1990, although the increase was greatest for those in the lowest class, up from 18% to 33%, and least for those in the highest class, up from 13% to 15%. By 2000 the rates had fallen for all classes, although again the fall was greatest for those in the higher classes than for those in the lower classes.

Figure 15: Percentages of men with a longstanding illness by socio-economic group of household: 1980, 1990 & 2000

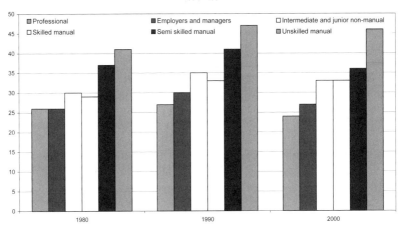

Source: General Household Survey, 1981, 1990 & 2001.

Figure 16: Percentages of women with a longstanding illness by socioeconomic group of household: 1980, 1990 & 2000

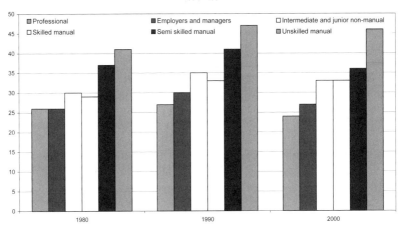

Source: General Household Survey, 1981, 1990 & 2001.

Figure 17: Percentages of men with a limiting longstanding illness by socio-economic group of *household: 1980, 1990 & 2000*

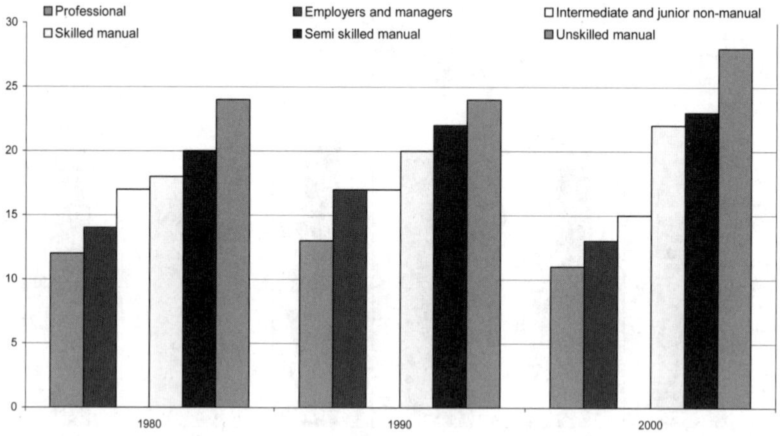

Source: General Household Survey, 1981, 1990 & 2001.

7. The Workplace and Health

A. Accidents and Injury at Work

Data from the Health and Safety Commission (HSC), presented in figure 19 show that there has been a general trend toward a falling incidence of fatal industrial injury rates over the 1980s and 1990s, although there are still wide sectoral differences in risk of injury. Except for the self-employed in the agricultural, forestry and fishing sector, who are at a great and increasing risk of fatal injury, the self-employed are at less risk of injury compared with employees (Health and Safety Commission 2003). Regarding social class differences in the likelihood of suffering from an accident at work the Government notes that although manual workers make up 42% of the workforce in 2003, they account for 72% of reported workplace-related injuries (Tackling Health Inequalities 2003).

Figure 18: Percentage of women with a limiting longstanding ilness by socio-econonis group of household

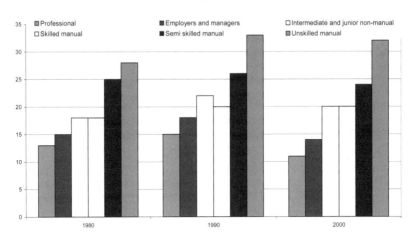

Figure 19: Fatal injury rates

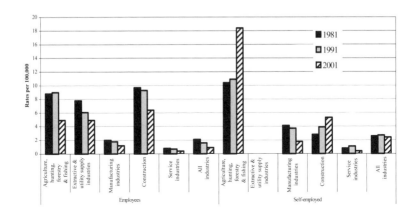

Source: Health and Safety Commission, 2003.

B. Health at Work

Today there are around 2.3 million people in Great Britain who suffer from work-related illnesses. The most common of these are muscoskeletal diseases, followed by stress and depression and then lung disease. Data collected by the HSC show that the prevalence of work-related illness is up from 1998-1999, but muscoskeletal and lung disease are still statistically significantly lower than the rates in either 1990 or

413

1995. However, stress has risen over the decade and is now double the rate it was in 1990. Teachers and nurses are the most likely to suffer from work-related stress. An estimated 32.9 million working days were lost due to ill health in 2001, which works out at an average of 22.9 days off work for each person who is ill. However, those who suffer from stress or depression take more days off work on average, 29.2 days, than those who suffer from other illnesses (Health and Safety Commission 2003).

Increasingly, work environment studies are looking at the effects of stress at work on the health of employees. Unlike the Scandinavian countries there are no national studies of the (psychosocial) working environment in the UK. However, some data on the distribution of adverse psychosocial working conditions for different social groups are available from occasional national studies and some regional studies. A population-based study of around 8,500 people living in Bristol in the South-West of England found that around one fifth of the respondents reported that their occupations were very or extremely stressful. There were no significant differences between the percentages of men and women reporting high levels of stress, although there were differences by age, with middle-aged workers reporting the highest rates of stress. The effects of stress on health and changes in stress were measured at two time points 12 months apart. At both time points respondents who reported high levels of stress were at a significantly increased risk of suffering from physical ill health, such as bronchitis, and psychological symptoms, such as stomach problems or backache, and health-related behaviours, such as reduced sleep (Smith, Johal, Wadsworth, Davey Smith & Peters 2000). The 1994 wave of the Health Survey for England included questions on the work environment derived from the Whitehall II study. The data presented in table 3 show the distribution of psycho-social working conditions for the Registrar General's social classes for men and women. It is apparent from these data that the further one moves down the social class scale, the more monotonous work becomes and the less control one has over one's work. Whilst less than 10% of men in social class I said that they had low variety at work, two thirds of those in social class V reported that this was the case. The situation appears to be more extreme amongst women. Women in social class V were over 10 times more likely than those in social class I to say that their work lacked variety.

Table 3: Percentages reporting adverse psychosocial working conditions by Registrar General's social class; England, 1994

	Registrar General's social class						
Men	I	II	III N/M	III M	IV	V	All
High pace of work	40	40	30	27	24	26	32
Low variety of work	9	18	35	35	62	66	33
Low control at work	6	6	21	22	40	45	20
Low variety and control at work	7	11	29	30	57	68	29
Women	I	II	III N/M	III M	IV	V	All
High pace of work	42	45	30	29	25	20	33
Low variety of work	8	22	56	52	74	92	51
Low control at work	14	10	36	31	50	46	31
Low variety and control at work	7	17	53	49	70	85	47

Source: Talyor 1994.

However, it has been the Whitehall studies which have been at the forefront of work environment research in the UK. The most recent study, Whitehall II, was set up in 1985 (phase 1) and was designed to investigate the degree and causes of health inequalities amongst a working white-collar population. All those working as civil servants, aged between 35 and 55 years, in 20 London-based departments were sent an introductory letter and an initial screening questionnaire. Those who agreed to take part and were eligible (73% response rate) were given a medical examination, at which time a range of baseline health measures were taken such as blood pressure and blood cholesterol. Those who participated in the original survey were sent self-completion questionnaires in 1989 (phase 2), 1995-1996 (phase 4) and 2000 (phase 6). In addition to the questionnaire, phase 3 (1991-1993) and phase 5 (1998-1999) data collection also included a repeat medical examination (Marmot and Shipley 1996).

The effects of employment grade and work environment on general health and chronic illness have been a major focus of the Whitehall II studies. Prospective longitudinal data for several phases of the study have demonstrated a clear association between exposure to adverse psychosocial working conditions, notably low control over work, and an increased risk of CVD incidence, even after controlling for employment grade and health behaviours (Kuper & Marmot 2003). Data from the first wave of the Whitehall II study show that there is an occupational gradient in those reporting low job control, with around 9% of those in the highest grades reporting low job control compared with just over 77% of those in the lowest grades. Furthermore, low job control was a significant factor in predicting the onset of a CHD event at subsequent waves. Data from phases 2 and 3 show a clear occupational gradient in the risk of reporting a CHD event, with those in the lowest occupations around one and a half times more likely to report such an event compared with those in the highest occupations. However, after controlling for low job control the gradient attenuated considerably, with those in the lowest grades only around 18% more likely to report a CHD event (Marmot, Bosma, Hemingway, Brunner & Stansfeld 1997). Conversely, Bosma found that after controlling for employment grade, along with other sociodemographic factors and coronary risk factors, those with low self-reported job control were around one and a half times more likely than those with high job control to report a CHD event (Bosma, Marmot, Hemingway, Nicholson, Brunner & Stansfeld 1997). When Effort-Reward imbalance was controlled for this rose to almost two and half times more likely (Bosma, Peter, Siegrist & Marmot 1998).

The studies have also shown that work and the work environment have an effect on psychological as well as physical health. Longitudinal analysis found that low social support at work and high job demands, at phase one, all predicted poor mental health, at phase three (Stansfeld, Fuhrer, Shipley & Marmot 1999, Stansfeld, Fuhrer, Head, Ferrie and Shipely 1997). Interestingly, when control at home is taken into account gender differences appear. Although for both men and women those who had low control either at work or at home had an increased risk of depression and anxiety, the way in which low control affected psychological health differed by grade and sex. Men in the lowest grade, who had low control, in either sphere, were at increased risk of anxiety, whilst men in the middle grades with low control, in either sphere, were at increased risk of depression. Women in the low or middle grades with low control were at increased risk of both anxiety and depression (Griffin, Fuhrer, Stansfeld and Marmot 2002). The longitudinal nature of the Whitehall II studies has permitted researchers to test for the possible effects of health selection as an explanation for these inequalities in health. Results show that changes in mental and physical health did not have an effect on changes in employment grade, although there was a slight, significant, effect of changes in mental health on change in financial deprivation amongst men (Chandola, Bartley, Sacker, Jenkinson and Marmot 2003).

One study has looked at changes in the social gradient of health and health behaviours between phase 3 and phase 5, using self-reported health, long-standing illness, GHQ 30, cholesterol, diastolic and systolic blood pressure, BMI, alcohol and smoking. It found employment grade differences in most of the health measures at both time points. Apart from GHQ and cholesterol, there was little evidence that these differences had changed over time. However, there was some evidence that the effects of grade had changed over time. At phase 5 men in the lowest grade had a significantly increased risk of having a limiting long-standing illness, where this had neither been the case at baseline nor at phase 3 (Ferrie, Shipely, Davey-Smith *et al.* 2002). For the present chapter we repeated some of the analyses including measures of the psychosocial work environment. Figure 20 shows the percentages in each grade with poor self-rated health in 1995 and 1998. For both the top and middle grades there has been an increase in the percentage who report poor health, whilst in the lowest grade there has been a slight decrease from 1995 to 1998. However, at both time points the social gradient in health is very much in evidence, with the upper grades reporting less poor health than the lower grades. The data also showed that at both time points there was a clear gradient in the percentages reporting high demands and low decision authority, with around 50% of the highest grades reporting high demands and between 60% and 70% of the lowest grades reporting low decision authority. There appears to be a slight decrease over time in the percentages of the middle grades reporting high demands, and a rise in the percentages of the lowest grades reporting low decision authority.

**Figure 20: Percentages of the Whitehall II sample
reporting poor health by grade: 1993 & 1998**

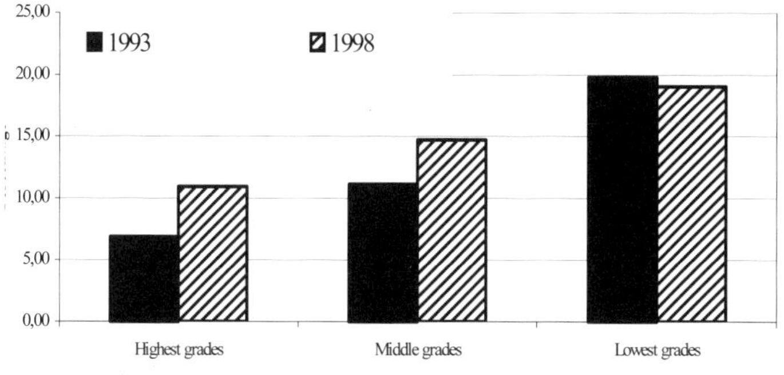

Source: Own calculation.

Tables 4 to 7 show the results of binary logistic regression analyses for the effects of employment grade and psychosocial working condi-tions on the likelihood of reporting poor health or long-standing illness in 1993 and in 1998. The results in table 4 show that in 1993, those in the middle and lowest grades had significantly increased likelihoods of reporting poor health compared with the top grades. Those in the top tertile of decision authority were about half as likely to report poor general health as those in the lowest tertile, whilst those with high job demands were around 30% more likely to report poor general health than those with low job demands. The inclusion of decision authority in the model slightly attenuated the effects of the employment grade, although the job demands did not significantly do so. In the fully adjusted model in the final columns of the table, both employment grade and adverse psychosocial working conditions have an effect on general self-rated health. The results for the same analyses done on the phase 5 data in 1998, presented in table 5, show a similar pattern. With the exception of the fact that those in the middle tertile of decision authority no longer had an advantage over those in the lowest tertile the results are almost exactly the same as in 1993. Conversely, tables 6 and 7 show no significant effects of either employment grade or decision authority on the likelihood of reporting a long-standing illness. Only being in the highest tertile of job demands, in both 1993 and 1998, led to an increased risk of reporting a long-standing illness.

Table 4: The effects of employment grade, decision latitude and job demands on the risk of reporting a poor general health in 1993. Analyses controlled for age and sex

	Odds ratio	95% CI	Odds ratio	95% CI	Odds ratio	95% CI	Odds ratio	95% CI
Top grades	1		1		1		1	
Middle grades	**1.45**	(1.31-1.61)	**1.23**	(1.11-1.37)	**1.51**	(1.36-1.68)	**1.29**	(1.15-1.44)
Low grades	**2.25**	(1.93-2.62)	**1.56**	(1.31-1.85)	**2.50**	(2.12-2.94)	**1.73**	(1.45-2.08)
Decision authority bottom tertile			1				1	
Decision authority middle tertile			**0.73**	(0.64-0.84)			**0.72**	(0.63-0.82)
Decision authority top tertile			**0.55**	(0.48-0.63)			**0.53**	(0.46-0.60)
Job demands bottom tertile					1		1	
Job demands middle tertile					**1.21**	(1.07-1.37)	**1.27**	(1.13-1.44)
Job demands top tertile					**1.30**	(1.14-1.50)	**1.41**	(1.22-1.62)

Figures in bold are significant at the p = .05 level. Source: Own calculation.

Table 5: The effects of employment grade, decision latitude and job demands on the risk of reporting a poor general health in 1998. Analyses controlled for age and sex

	Odds ratio	95% CI	Odds ratio	95% CI	Odds ratio	95% CI	Odds ratio	95% CI
Top grades	1		1		1		1	
Middle grades	**1.41**	(1.23-1.61)	**1.21**	(1.05-1.39)	**1.44**	(1.26-1.65)	**1.24**	(1.07-1.43)
Low grades	**2.08**	(1.70-2.55)	**1.51**	(1.21-1.89)	**2.30**	(1.87-2.83)	**1.62**	(1.29-2.03)
Decision authority bottom tertile			1				1	
Decision authority middle tertile			0.87	(0.74-1.03)			0.85	(0.72-1.01)
Decision authority top tertile			**0.56**	(0.47-0.66)			**0.54**	(0.46-0.64)
Job demands bottom tertile					1		1	
Job demands middle tertile					1.22	(1.04-1.43)	**1.28**	(1.09-1.50)
Job demands top tertile					1.34	(1.13-1.58)	**1.41**	(1.19-1.68)

Figures in bold are significant at the p = .05 level.
Source: Own calculation.

Table 6: The effects of employment grade, decision latitude and job demands on the risk of reporting a long-standing illness in 1993. Analyses controlled for age and sex

	Odds ratio	95% CI	Odds ratio	95% CI	Odds ratio	95% CI	Odds ratio	95% CI
Top grades	1		1		1		1	
Middle grades	1.00	(0.89-1.11)	0.96	(0.86-1.08)	1.05	(0.94-1.18)	1.01	(0.90-1.14)
Low grades	0.98	(0.84-1.15)	0.91	(0.76-1.09)	1.10	(0.93-1.30)	1.00	(0.83-1.21)
Decision authority bottom tertile			1				1	
Decision authority middle tertile			0.93	(0.81-1.07)			0.92	(0.80-1.06)
Decision authority top tertile			0.89	(0.77-1.02)			0.86	(0.75-0.99)
Job demands bottom tertile					1		1	
Job demands middle tertile					1.08	(0.95-1.24)	1.10	(0.96-1.25)
Job demands top tertile					**1.33**	(1.15-1.53)	**1.35**	(1.17-1.56)

Figures in bold are significant at the p = .05 level.
Source: Own calculations.

Table 7: The effects of employment grade, decision latitude and job demands on the risk of reporting a long-standing illness in 1998. Analyses controlled for age and sex

	Odds ratio	95% CI	Odds ratio	95% CI	Odds ratio	95% CI	Odds ratio	95% CI
Top grades	1		1		1		1	
Middle grades	1.10	(0.96-1.26)	1.10	(0.95-1.26)	1.12	(0.98-1.29)	1.12	(0.97-1.29)
Low grades	1.07	(0.88-1.31)	1.07	(0.86-1.33)	1.13	(0.92-1.38)	1.12	(0.90-1.40)
Decision authority bottom tertile			1				1	
Decision authority middle tertile			1.00	(0.84-1.18)			0.99	(0.84-1.17)
Decision authority top tertile			0.99	(0.84-1.17)			0.98	(0.83-1.16)
Job demands bottom tertile					1		1	
Job demands middle tertile					1.04	(0.89-1.22)	1.07	(0.91-1.25)
Job demands top tertile					**1.21**	(1.02-1.43)	**1.24**	(1.04-1.47)

Figures in bold are significant at the p = .05 level.
Source: Own calculation.

8. Social Policies for Addressing Health Inequalities

The Tory government's response to the publication of the Black report in 1980 is now well known and occupies an important place in the story of British social policies towards reducing health inequalities. The Government released the report over the August Bank Holiday, one of the busiest public holidays in the British calendar, and then only 260 copies were made available. Despite – or because of – this, the media championed the importance of the Report's findings about the persistence of social inequalities in health (Berridge 2003). However, the main effect of this was to encourage a renaissance of health inequalities research amongst academics, as the issue largely disappeared from the policy agenda for the duration of Tory rule.

This situation changed somewhat with the election of a Labour government in 1997. One of the first acts of the incoming government was to set up the Independent Inquiry into health inequalities in the UK under the chairmanship of Sir Donald Acheson. Firstly, the Inquiry was charged to provide a review of the latest available information on the state of health inequalities in the country, using data from a range of national sources. Secondly, it was to use this information to identify priority areas for future policy development for cost-effective and affordable interventions to reduce health inequalities. The Acheson Report was published in 1998 and received a much more favourable reception than its predecessor. In all, the report made 39 recommendations (see Box one) covering action for a wide range of determinants of health. However, the Inquiry identified three crucial recommendations:

- All policies that are likely to have an impact on health should be evaluated in terms of their impact on health inequalities.
- A high priority should be given to the health of families with children.
- Further steps should be taken to reduce income inequalities and improve the living standards of poor households (Exworthy 2003).

In response, the Government published its White Paper *Saving lives – Our Healthier Nation* in 1999, in which they set out their programme of policies designed to reduce health inequalities. They identify as one of the key aims of the Government's health strategy for England that of improving the health of the worst-off in society and narrowing the health gap (Department of Health 1999: 1). Seemingly heeding the call from the Acheson Report to broaden the scope of health policy beyond service delivery, the Government has constructed its health policy around the notion of a 'fairer society...that means promoting social inclusion and increasing opportunities for *all* members of society to enjoy the best possible health and general well being' (*ibid.*, p. 5). Their principle vehicle for achieving this has been a combination of New Deal policies, tax and benefit reforms, aimed at alleviating poverty amongst the poorest groups and making work financially viable; reform of the employer's national insurance contribution, to help remove barriers to employment; and policies to improve skills through education and training. Specific focus is given to the health and economic well-being of young families and mothers. In regard to the Acheson Report's recommendations concerning work and working life (Nos. 8 & 9), the Government has enacted a series of employment policies designed to get people back to work, the young, the long-term unemployed and the over-1950s, and has introduced the 'healthy workplace initiative'. This initiative, which is supported by £1 million from the Department of Health, aims to 'strengthen partnerships necessary to improve the overall health of the workforce and help to protect employees from avoidable harm' (p. 20). This is being carried out in conjunction with the new Health and Safety Commission (HSC) goals to improve the safety of the work environment. The aim is to reduce the number of fatal and major injuries by 10% by 2010; to reduce the incidence of rate of new cases of work-related injury by 10% by 2004/5, and by 20% by 2010; and to reduce the number of days lost by 30% by 2010, with an interim goal of a 15% reduction by 2005 (Health and Safety Commission 2003). However, policies aimed at improving the psychosocial work environment are noticeable by their absence in all these documents.

Nevertheless, some argue that there are other policies that have already been implemented which might also have an (indirect) effect on population health and reducing health inequalities. Increases in the national minimum wage and changes in tax credit and welfare payments have had a modest redistributive effect. The Government's *Strategy for Neighbourhood Renewal* (www.odpm.gov.uk) has focused on rebuilding local communities and building strategic partnerships between local government and service providers to ensure that local needs are addressed. The *Sure Start* programme (www.surestart.gov.uk) and the *Fuel Poverty Strategy* (http://dti.gov.uk/energy/fuel/poverty/index.htm) have also focused resources on the poorest sections in society (Nutbeam 2003). A raft of New Deal programmes aimed at assisting various groups, such as young people, the long-term unemployed and the 50+ group, back into work represents a novel approach to unemployment by shifting the focus from benefit cuts and including some provision for personalised job-seeking advice (Alcock, Beatty, Fothergill, Macmillan & Yeandle 2003).

However, serious challenges still exist for the Government. Crucially, their ability to achieve the aims they have proposed to tackle health inequalities relies to a large extent on the wider political and economic climate. Poor economic performance will not only place restrictions on the Government's ability to finance these programmes but could also have a detrimental effect on employment and conditions in the workplace. Furthermore, there is concern that the Government is ill-equipped to deal with such a broad issue as health inequalities that requires the sort of joined-up government that Tony Blair has called for, but which seems far from being realised. Ministerial and civil service careers are still too closely wedded to a single department to be able to provide the necessary policy overview and connections. As such, although most authors welcome the Government's commitment, the actual programmes are falling short of their intended aim (Exworthy, Blane & Marmot 2003). For example, the *Sure Start* programme and *Health Action Zones* only cover around one third of all children in poverty (Exworthy 2003). Although the Government's response to the Acheson inquiry, *Tackling Health Inequalities*, acknowledges that social class differences are important for health, the authors principally focus on lifestyle factors such as smoking, or area effects, as the key areas for policy interventions (see page 29: C21). Where the study does focus on reducing inequalities due to social class is in infant mortality. One of the stated aims is to reduce the gap in mortality in children under one year of age by at least 10% between routine and manual groups, and the population as a whole.

9. Conclusion

As mentioned in the introduction, social inequalities in health continue to be a feature of British society. Countless studies have shown that the most disadvantaged groups, however defined, tend to have the worst health. The aims of this chapter were to ascertain the extent to which the work environment has contributed to the construction and maintenance of these inequalities, and how changes in the structure of the labour market and the organisation of work might have affected this contribution. It is apparent that the work environment continues to be an important dimension in the construction of these disparities in health. The data presented in this chapter show that the likelihood of suffering an injury at work varies considerably between different industrial sectors. Findings from the Whitehall II study have consistently shown that those in the lowest grades and with the worst work environments suffer the worst health (Bosma, Marmot, Hemingway, Nicholson, Brunner & Stansfeld 1997, Marmot, Bosma, Hemingway, Brunner & Stansfeld 1997, Bosma, Peter, Siegrist & Marmot 1998). This was confirmed in the analyses presented here. Both employment grade and work environment had significant effects on poor general health at the beginning and the end of the 1990s. In addition, high job demands had a persistent effect on long-standing illness at both time points. But without the large-scale representative workplace studies available in other countries, it is impossible to draw any definitive conclusions based on these data about the ways in which changing working practices have altered the effects of the work environment on health. Furthermore, two questions remain to be answered. Firstly, why is work organised in the way that it is and, secondly, what will the future hold for health inequalities.

The changing nature of the labour market and work are sure to have an effect on the future state of social inequalities in health. New ways of working, associated with deindustrialisation, may eliminate certain risks (Yeandle 2002) but could introduce new health risks. These changes in the labour market and the nature of work have prompted some to call for a re-theorisation of class relations and health. The Office for National Statistics, the UK's official statistical body, recently introduced a new social classification system the NS-SEC (Donkin, Lee & Toson 2002, Chandola 2000). This is based on a more theoretical conception of class, drawing on the Goldthorpe schema, to replace the old Registrar General's schema, which had originally been constructed using life expectancy as an indicator of social class, thus introducing a potential confounder into any association between class and mortality (Guy 1996). Some studies have found associations between the NS-SEC and mortality or morbidity (Donkin, Lee & Toson 2002, Fitzpatrick and Dollamore 1999, Fitzpatrick *et al.* 1997), whilst others have not (Chandola 2000).

However, such questions are unlikely to be resolved by empirical means alone. Much research into health inequalities in general, and the effects of the work environment in particular, have been criticised for lacking any explicit theory about why class gradients exist (Scambler & Higgs 1999). There is a long tradition of industrial sociology or the sociology of work that has sought to explain the organisation of (control at) work. Possibly the most well-known of these is Braverman's (1976) description of the introduction of 'time and motion' into the production process and latterly into white-collar occupations. For Braverman, Talyorism represented a logical, even necessary, response to the increasing concentration of capital and the socialisation of labour, and its threat of action, under the conditions of monopoly capital. These ideas have been built on by writers such as Friedman (1977) and Edwards (1980). Friedman extended Braverman's original conception of Taylorism as a means of controlling workers, by arguing that managers must deploy a range of strategies in order to achieve the optimal match between control and innovation. He argued that these strategies tend towards either 'relative autonomy', characteristic of core workers, or 'direct control', characteristic of peripheral workers. Managers must negotiate which is the best strategy to maximise productivity, and consequently profit, whilst maintaining loyalty. These two situations, relative autonomy and direct control, bear a clear resemblance to the concepts of job control, job demands and skill discretion used in work environment research. Thus, in order to understand how changes in the work environment will affect the health of future employees, it is necessary to understand why the work environment is changing. These ideas offer a potentially useful theoretical framework.

However, as the data presented above show, the most important feature of the British labour market is possibly not so much the changing nature of work that has been underway since the 1970s or earlier, but the dramatic reconstruction of the labour market relations for certain groups. The increasing numbers of older people, mostly men but increasingly women as well, leaving the labour market before state retirement age creates a new set of questions about how to tackle health inequalities. Firstly, what are the effects of early labour market exit; and secondly, what will these changes mean for work environment research.

Undoubtedly these changes will bring new risks with them but the limited research that exists in the UK at present shows that retirees, of either early or normal age, do not differ significantly in terms of physical health from those who continue in work and actually have improved mental health (Mein *et al.* 2003). Given that work will occupy an increasingly shorter proportion of the lifecourse, based on present projections, it might be tempting to think that the effects of the work environment on health will be diminished in the future. As such it is becoming increasingly important to look at the lack of control in non-work spheres of life, such as the home, and how this contributes to psychological disorders (Griffin, Fuhrer, Stansfeld and Marmot 2002). Longitudinal data from the BHPS show that occupational class and working conditions have relatively strong effects on self-rated health for the economically active population. Those from the lower social classes were 1.7 times more likely to have poor health than those from the managerial and professional classes. Part-time work also had a negative impact on health, independent of sex, but for the economically inactive, household factors had the strongest effect on health (Chandola, Bartley, Wiggins & Schofield 2003). However, work retains a key role within the lifecourse and casts a 'long shadow' into post-working life. A study of the health of retired civil servants from Whitehall II found that pre-retirement circumstances at work continue to exercise an influence on health in retirement (Hyde, Ferrie, Higgs, Mein & Nazroo 2004).

Perhaps one should not be overly concerned with the future so much as the past, or rather the effects of the past. Although we are living through a period of change it is important to remember that those groups which are most likely to suffer poor health lived and worked through different times. Thus, some researchers have been drawing attention to the importance of measuring the effects of stress over the entirety of the working life rather than at single or repeated time points. Pavalko and colleagues have rightly argued that most health inequalities research focuses on the demands and rewards of single jobs and the influence of health, and as such overlooks the broader implications of working life patterns. They found that men who experienced a series of unrelated jobs had the highest morbidity, whilst those men who experienced steady career progress had the lowest risk of premature mortality. As the labour market becomes more flexible they argue that the health effects of career patterns means that work should be conceptualised as a process that evolves, and changes will become more and more relevant (Pavalko, Elder & Clipp 1993). In 1981 the Black report concluded with the statement that, although the social class inequalities in health were real, there was no 'single or simple explanation' for these differences. The ways in which disadvantage affects health are evidently complex. Evidence from the Whitehall II study on the effect of education, occupation and income on psychological health found that although there was a gradient for all three measures of socio-economic position, each had a different effect. The authors argue that as different diseases have different aetiological periods, different influences will act at different points in the lifecourse. Thus, health inequalities research needs to be sensitive to the temporal sequencing of factors that affect health (Singh-Manoux, Clarke and Marmot 2002).

Acknowledgements.

I would like to thank both Ingvar Lundberg and Tomas Hemmingsson from the WINNER group for their helpful comments and guidance through the entire process of writing this chapter. I would also like to extend special thanks to Jane Ferrie and Elisa Diaz-Martinez from UCL (Belgium) for their comments and discussions, and to Jenny Head and Martin Shipley for their assistance in accessing the relevant data.

Appendix 1

A short description of any data sets that would be suitable for international and comparative analyses of work-related inequity in health.

1. The General Household Survey

The General Household Survey (GHS) is a multi-purpose survey carried out by the Social Survey Division of the Office for National Statistics which collects information on a range of topics from people living in private households in Great Britain. The survey started in 1971 and has been carried out continuously since then, except for breaks in 1997-1998 (when the survey was reviewed) and 1999-2000. The main aim of the survey is to collect data on a range of demographic issues, including health and health behaviours. The GHS has documented the major changes in households, families and people which have occurred over the last 30 years. These include the decline in average household size and the growth in the proportion of the population who live alone, the increase in the proportion of families headed by a lone parent and in the percentage of people who are cohabiting. It has also recorded changes in housing, such as the growth of home ownership, and the increasing proportion of homes with household facilities and goods such as central heating, washing machines, microwave ovens and home computers. The survey also monitors trends in the prevalence of smoking and drinking. For more details on the measurement of trends, see measuring changes over time below. Fieldwork for the GHS is conducted on a financial year basis, with interviewing taking place continuously throughout the year. The set sample is approximately 13,000 addresses per year, selected from the Postcode Address File. All adults aged 16 and over are interviewed in each responding household and some information is collected about children in the household. For 2000, the survey response rate was 67%, which produces a sample size of over 19,000 adults.

2. The Health Survey for England

The Health Survey for England (HSE) began in 1991 as a new series of annual surveys commissioned by the Department of Health. Initially, the HSE was carried out by the Social Survey Division of the ONS National Statistics. Since 1994, the survey has been carried out by the Joint Health Surveys Unit of the National Centre for Social Research and the Department of Epidemiology and Public Health at University College, London. The HSE is based on a nationally representative sample of the population living in private households in England. It was designed to provide baseline data from which to monitor health trends, and in particular, to assess progress towards health targets (especially those relating to cardiovascular disease, blood pressure and obesity). The HSE is a continuous survey conducted every year throughout the year, with a new sample issued each month. The survey runs to a five-year plan with a particular focus in some years; for instance, the 1999 survey focused on the health of ethnic minorities, and the 2000 survey on the health of older people and social exclusion. Each year interviews are carried out with around 16,000 adult respondents and 4,000 children, around 80% of whom agree to a follow-up interview by a nurse who makes a number of measurements and takes a blood sample. Fieldwork is carried out throughout the year to minimise seasonal variation.

3. The Labour Force Survey

The Labour Force Survey [LFS], which began in 1973, is the largest survey carried out across the United Kingdom. Since 1992 the survey has been known as the Quarterly Labour Force Survey [QLFS] as statistics are now published for each month on a quarterly basis. Interviews are achieved at around 59,000 addresses with 138,000 individual respondents each quarter. The main purpose of the QLFS is to provide internationally comparable statistics on the levels and changes in employment, unemployment and economic inactivity, but data is also collected on sickness, accidents and health problems or disabilities which affect work. The Labour Force Survey has conducted four surveys of self-reported health and work from 1991 using a sub-sample from the main survey. However, there are some problems of comparability between baseline and the later waves.

4. Whitehall II

Whitehall II was set up in 1985 (phase 1) and was designed to investigate the degree and causes of health inequalities amongst a working white-collar population. All those working as civil servants, aged between 35 and 55 years, in 20 London-based departments were sent an introductory letter and an initial screening questionnaire. Those who agreed to take part and were eligible (73% response rate) were given a medical examination, at which time a range of baseline health measures were taken such as blood pressure and blood cholesterol. Those who participated in the original survey were sent self-completion questionnaires in 1989 (phase 2), 1995-6 (phase 4) and 2000 (phase 6). In addition to the questionnaire, phase 3 (1991-3) and phase 5 (1998-9) data collection also included a repeat medical examination.

5. Useful Websites

Office of National Statistics – http://www.statistics.gov.uk/
Whitehall II – http://www.ucl.ac.uk/whitehallII/
Office of the Deputy Prime Minister – www.odpm.gov.uk
The Sure Start programme – www.surestart.gov.uk
Fuel Poverty Strategy – http://dti.gov.uk/energy/fuel/poverty/index.htm

References

AMIN A. 1996. "Post Fordism: Models, fantasies and phantoms of transition". In: AMIN A. 1996. *Post Fordism: A reader*. Oxford; Blackwell: 1-40.

ACHESON D. 1998. *Independent Inquiry into Inequalities in Health Report*. London : HMSO.

ALCOCK P., BEATTY C., FOTHERGILL S., MACMILLAN R. & YEANDLE S. 2003. "New roles, new deal". In: ALCOCK P., BEATTY C., FOTHERGILL S., MACMILLAN R. & YEANDLE S. (ed.) *Work to welfare. How men became detached from the labour market*. Cambridge: Cambridge University Press.

BLACK D., MORRIS JN., SMITH C. & TOWNSEND P. 1982. *Inequalities in health: The Black report*. London: Pelican.

BOSMA H., MARMOT MG., HEMINGWAY H., NICHOLSON AC., BRUNNER E., STANSFELD SA. 1997. "Low job control and risk of coronary heart disease in Whitehall II (prospective cohort) study". *BMJ* 314: 558-565.

BOSMA H., PETER R., SIEGRIST J. & MARMOT M. 1998. "Two alternative job stress models and the risk of coronary heart disease". *American Journal of Public Health* 88: 68-74.

BRAVERMAN H. 1976. *Labor and Monopoly Capital: The Degradation of Work in the Twentieth Century*. New York: Monthly Review Press.

CAUSER P. & VIRDEE D. 2004. *Regional Trends* 38, London: HMSO.

CHANDOLA, T. 2000. "Social class differences in mortality using the new UK national statistics socio-economic classification". *Social Science and Medicine* 50: 641-9.

CHANDOLA T., BARTLEY M., WIGGINS R. and SCHOFIELD P. 2003. "Social inequalities in health by individual and household measures of social position in a cohort of healthy people". Journal *of Epidemiology and Community Health* 57: 56-62.

CHANDOLA T., BARTLEY M., SACKER A., JENKINSON C. & MARMOT M. 2003. "Health selection in the Whitehall II study, UK". *Social Science and Medicine* 56: 2059-72.

CLARKE J. 2004. *Changing Welfare, Changing States: New Directions in Social Policy*. London: Sage.

DEPARTMENT OF HEALTH. 2003. *Tackling Health Inequalities. A Programme for Action*. London: The Stationary Office.

DEPARTMENT OF HEALTH. 2002. *Reducing Health Inequalities: An action report*. London: The Stationary Office.

DONKIN A., LEE YH. & TOSON B. 2002. "Implications of changes in the UK social and occupational classifications in 2001 for vital statistics". *Population Trends* 107: 23-9.

EDWARDS R. 1980. *Contested Terrain*. London: Ashgate.

ERIKSON HR. & URSIN H. 1999. "Subjective health complaints: is coping more important than control?". *Work and stress* 13: 238-252.

EXWORTHY M., BLANE D. and MARMOT M. 2003. "Tackling health inequalities in the United Kingdom: The progress and pitfalls of policy". *Health Services Research* 38: 1905-21.

FERRI E., BYNNER J. & WADSWORTH M. 2003. *Changing Britain, Changing Lives: Three Generations at the Turn of the Century*. London: Institute of Education.

FERRIE JE., SHIPLEY MJ., DAVEY SMITH G., STANSFELD SA. & MARMOT MG. 2002. "Change in health inequalities among British civil servants: The Whitehall II study". *Journal of Epidemiology and Community Health* 56: 922-926.

FUHRER R., STANSFELD S.A., CHEMALI J. & SHIPLEY M.J. 1999. "Gender, social relations and mental health: prospective findings from an occupational cohort (Whitehall II study)". *Social Science and Medicine* 48: 77-87.

FITZPATRICK R., BARTLEY M., DODGEON B., FIRTH D., LYNCH K. 1997. "Social variations in health: relationship of mortality to the interim revised social classification". In: ROSE D & O'REILY K (ed.). *Constructing classes*. ESRC, Swindon.

FRIEDMAN AL. 1977. *Industry and Labour: Class Struggle at Work and Monopoly Capitalism*. London: Palgrave Macmillan.

FITZPATRICK J. & DOLLAMORE G. 1999. "Examining adult mortality rates using the National Statistics Socio-Economic Classification". *Health Statistics Quarterly* 2: 33-40.

GIDDENS A. 1998. *The Third Way: The Renewal of Social Democracy*. Oxford: Polity Press.

GOLDBLATT P. & WHITEHEAD M. 2000. "Inequalities in health – development and change". *Population Trends* 100: 14-19.

GUILLEMARD A.M. and REIN M. 1993. "Comparative patterns of retirement: recent trends in developed societies". *Annual Review of Sociology* 19: 469-503.

GUY W. 1996. *Health for all? In Levitas R. and Guy W. (ed.). Interpreting official statistics*. London: Routledge, 90-114.

GRIFFIN J.M., FUHRER R., STANSFELD S.A. & MARMOT M. 2002. "The importance of low control at work and home on depression and anxiety: do these effects vary by gender and social class?". *Social Science and Medicine* 54: 783-798.

HUTTON W. 1996. *The State We're in: Why Britain Is in Crisis and How to Overcome It*. London: Vintage.

HEALTH and SAFETY COMMISSION. 2003. *Health and safety. Statistical highlights 2001/2*. London: HMSO.

HEMINGWAY H., SHIPLEY M., MULLEN MJ., BRUNNER E., TAYLOR M., DONALD AE., DEANFIELD JE. & MARMOT M. 2003. "Social and psychosocial influences in inflammatory markers and vascular function in civil servants (the Whitehall II study)". *American Journal of Cardiology* 92: 984-7.

HYDE M., FERRIE J., HIGGS P., MEIN G. and NAZROO J. 2004. "The effects of pre-retirement factors and retirement route on circumstances in retirement: findings from the Whitehall II study". *Ageing and Society* 24: 279-96.

KARASEK RA. & THEORELL T. 1990. *Healthy Work: Stress, Productivity, and the Reconstruction of Working Life*. New York: Basic Books.

KAWACHI I., SUBRAMANIAN SV. & ALMEIDA-FILHO N. 2002. "A glossary for health inequalities". *Journal of Epidemiology and Community Health* 56: 647-52.

KUPER H. & MARMOT M. 2003. "Job strain, job demands, decision latitude, and risk of coronary heart disease within the Whitehall II study". *Journal of epidemiology and community health* 57: 147-153.

LABOUR FORCE SURVEY HISTORICAL QUARTERLY SUPPLEMENT. 2004. London: HMSO.

LASH S. & URRY J. 1987. *The End of Organized Capitalism*. Cambridge: Polity Press.

LINDSAY C. 2002. *State of the labour market 2001*. London: HMSO.

MACINTYRE S. 1986. "The patterning of health by social position in contemporary Britain: directions for sociological research". *Social Science and Medicine* 23: 393-415.

MACINTYRE S. 2002. "The Black report and beyond. What are the issues?". *Social Science and Medicine* 44: 723-45.

MACKENBACH J.P., KUNST Q.E., CAVELAARS A.E.J.M., GROENHOF F., GEURTS J.J.M. and THE EU WORKING GROUP ON SOCIOECONOMIC INEQUALITIES IN HEALTH. 1997. "Socioeconomic inequalities in morbidity and mortality in western Europe". *The Lancet* 349: 1655-1659.

MARMOT MG., THEORELL T. & SIEGRIST J. 2002. "Work and coronary heart disease". In: STANSFELD S.A. and MARMOT M.G. (eds.) *Stress and the heart*. London. BMJ Books, 50–71.

MARMOT MG. and SHIPLEY MJ. 1996. "Do socioeconomic differences in mortality persist after retirement? 25 year follow up of civil servants from the first Whitehall study". *BMJ* 313: 1177-80.

MARMOT MG., BOSMA H., HEMINGWAY H., BRUNNER E. and STANSFELD S. 1997. "Contribution of job control and other risk factors to social variations in coronary heart disease incidence". *The Lancet* 350: 235-9.

MARMOT MG., SMITH GD., STANSFELD S., PATEL C., NORTH F., HEAD J., WHITE I., BRUNNER E & FEENEY A. 1991. "Health inequalities among British civil-servants – the Whitehall-II study". *The Lancet* 337: 1387-1393.

MATHESON J. & SUMMERFIELD C. 2000. *Social Trends* 30: London: HMSO.

MEIN G., MARTIKAINEN P., HEMINGWAY H., STANSFELD S. and MARMOT M. 2003. "Is retirement good or bad for mental and physical health functioning?". *Whitehall II longitudinal study of civil servants. Journal of Epidemiology and Community Health* 57: 40-49.

OFFICE OF THE DEPUTY PRIME MINISTER. 2003. *Factsheet 2: The national strategy for neighbourhood renewal*. Crown Copyright, 2003.

PAVALKO EK., ELDER GH. & CLIPP EC. 1993. "Worklives and longevity: Insights from a life course perspective". *Journal of Health and Social Behaviour* 34: 363-80.

RICKARDS L., FOX K., ROBERTS C., FLETCHER L. & GODDARD E. 2002. *Living in Britain*. Results from the 2002 General Household Survey: 31. London: HMSO.

SABEL CF. 1996. "Flexible specialisation and the re-emergence of regional economies". In: AMIN A (ed.) *Post-Fordism. A reader*. Oxford: Blackwell, 101-156.

SCAMBLER G. and HIGGS P. 1999. "Stratification, class and health. Class relations and health inequalities in high modernity". *Sociology* 33: 275-96.

SINGH-MANOUX A., CLARKE P & MARMOT M. 2002. "Multiple measures of socio-economic position and psychosocial health: proximal and distal measures". *International Journal of Epidemiology* 31: 1192-1199.

SINGH-MANOUX A., ADLER NE. & MARMOT M. 2003. "Subjective social status: its determinants and its association with measures of ill health in the Whitehall II study". *Social Science and Medicine* 56: 1321-33.

SMITH A., JOHAL S., WADSWORTH E., DAVEY SMITH G. & PETERS T. 2000. "The scale of occupational stress. The Bristol stress and health at work study". London: HMSO.

STANSFELD SA., FUHRER R., SHIPLEY MJ. & MARMOT MG. 1999. "Work characteristics predict psychiatric disorder: prospective results from the Whitehall II study". *Occupational and environmental medicine* 56: 302-307.

STANSFELD S., FUHRER R., HEAD J., FERRIE J. and SHIPLEY M. 1997. "Work and psychiatric disorder in the Whitehall II study". *Journal of psychosomatic research* 43: 73-81.

TAYLOR A. 1994. "Psychosocial well-being". In: COLHOUN H. & PRESCOTT-CLARKE P. (eds.). *Health Survey for England 1994*. London: HMSO.

TAYLOR P., TILLSLEY C., BEAUSOLEIL J., WILSON R. and WALKER A. 2000. *Factors Affecting Retirement. Department for Education and Employment*. London: HMSO.

TURNER B. 2000. *Modern conditions, Post modern controversies*. Oxford: Routledge.

TROUP C. & DEWE P. 2002. "Exploring the nature of control and its role in the appraisal of workplace stress". *Work and stress* 16: 335-55.

VAN ROSSUM CTM., SHIPLEY MJ., VAN DE MHEEN H., GROBBEE DE. and MARMOT MG. 2000. "Employment grade differences in cause specific mortality. A 25 year follow up of civil servants from the first Whitehall study". *Journal of Epidemiology and Community Health* 54: 178-184.

WHITE C., VAN GALEN F. & CHOW YH. 2003. "Trends in social class differences in mortality by cause, 1986 to 2000". *Health Statistics Quarterly* 20: 25-37.

WHO. 2004. *World Health Report 2003 – shaping the future*. Geneva: WHO.

WILKINSON R. 1996. *Unhealthy Societies: The Afflictions of Inequality*. Oxford: Routledge.

YEANDLE S. 2003. ALCOCK P., BEATTY C., FOTHERGILL S., MACMILLAN R. & YEANDLE S. (ed.). *Work to welfare. How men became detached from the labour market*. Cambridge: Cambridge University Press, 3-24.

Box One

List of Recommendations

General Recommendations
1. We recommend that as part of health impact assessment, all policies likely to have a direct or indirect effect on health should be evaluated in terms of their impact on health inequalities, and should be formulated in such a way that by favouring the less well off they will, wherever possible, reduce such inequalities.

2. We recommend a high priority is given to policies aimed at improving health and reducing health inequalities in women of childbearing age, expectant mothers and young children.

Poverty, Income, Tax and Benefits
3. We recommend policies which will further reduce income inequalities, and improve the living standards of households in receipt of social security benefits.

Education
4. We recommend the provision of additional resources for schools serving children from less well off groups to enhance their educational achievement. The Revenue Support Grant formula and other funding mechanisms should be more strongly weighted to reflect need and socioeconomic disadvantage.
5. We recommend the further development of high quality pre-school education so that it meets, in particular, the needs of disadvantaged families. We also recommend that the benefits of pre-school education to disadvantaged families are evaluated and, if necessary, additional resources are made available to support further development.
6. We recommend the further development of "health promoting schools", initially focused on, but not limited to, disadvantaged communities.
7. We recommend further measures to improve the nutrition provided at school, including: the promotion of school food policies; the development of budgeting and cooking skills; the preservation of free school meals entitlement; the provision of free school fruit; and the restriction of less healthy food.

Employment
8. We recommend policies which improve the opportunities for work and which ameliorate the health consequences of unemployment.
9. We recommend policies to improve the quality of jobs, and reduce psychosocial work hazards.

Box One cont.

Housing and Environment

10. We recommend policies which improve the availability of social housing for the less well off within a framework of environmental improvement, planning and design which takes into account social networks, and access to goods and services.

11. We recommend policies which improve housing provision and access to health care for both officially and unofficially homeless people.

12. We recommend policies which aim to improve the quality of housing. Specifically:

13. We recommend the development of policies to reduce the fear of crime and violence, and to create a safe environment for people to live in.

Mobility, Transport and Pollution

14. We recommend the further development of a high quality public transport system which is integrated with other forms of transport and is affordable to the user.

15. We recommend further measures to encourage walking and cycling as forms of transport and to ensure the safe separation of pedestrians and cyclists from motor vehicles.

16. We recommend further steps to reduce the usage of motor cars to cut the mortality and morbidity associated with motor vehicle emissions.

17. We recommend further measures to reduce traffic speed, by environmental design and modification of roads, lower speed limits in built up areas, and stricter enforcement of speed limits.

18. We recommend concessionary fares should be available to pensioners and disadvantaged groups throughout the country, and that local schemes should emulate high quality schemes, such as those of London and the West Midlands.

Nutrition and the Common Agricultural Policy

19. We recommend a comprehensive review of the Common Agricultural Policy (CAP)'s impact on health and inequalities in health.

19.1 We recommend strengthening the CAP Surplus Food Scheme to improve the nutritional position of the less well off.

20. We recommend policies which will increase the availability and accessibility of foodstuffs to supply an adequate and affordable diet.

Mothers, Children and Families

21. We recommend policies which reduce poverty in families with children by promoting the material support of parents; by removing barriers to work for parents who wish to combine work with parenting; and by enabling those who wish to devote full-time to parenting to do so, by improving the living standards of households in receipt of social security benefits.

Box One cont.

Young People and Adults of Working Age
24. We recommend measures to prevent suicide among young people, especially among young men and seriously mentally ill people.
25. We recommend policies which promote sexual health in young people and reduce unwanted teenage pregnancy, including access to appropriate contraceptive services.
26. We recommend policies which promote the adoption of healthier lifestyles, particularly in respect of factors which show a strong social gradient in prevalence or consequences.

Older People
27. We recommend policies which will promote the material well being of older people.
28. We recommend the quality of homes in which older people live be improved.
29. We recommend policies which will promote the maintenance of mobility, independence, and social contacts.
30. We recommend the further development of health and social services for older people, so that these services are accessible and distributed according to need.

Ethnicity
31. We recommend that the needs of minority ethnic groups are specifically considered in the development and implementation of policies aimed at reducing socio-economic inequalities.
32. We recommend the further development of services which are sensitive to the needs of minority ethnic people and which promote greater awareness of their health risks.
33. We recommend the needs of minority ethnic groups are specifically considered in needs assessment, resource allocation, health care planning and provision.

Gender
34. We recommend policies which reduce the excess mortality from accidents and suicide in young men (see also: recommendation 24).
35. We recommend policies which reduce psychosocial ill health in young women in disadvantaged circumstances, particularly those caring for young children.
36. We recommend policies which reduce disability and ameliorate its consequences in older women, particularly those living alone.

Box One cont.

The National Health Service

37. We recommend that providing equitable access to effective care in relation to need should be a governing principle of all policies in the NHS. Priority should be given to the achievement of equity in the planning, implementation and delivery of services at every level of the NHS.

38. We recommend giving priority to the achievement of a more equitable allocation of NHS resources. This will require adjustments to the ways in which resources are allocated and the speed with which resource allocation targets are met.

39. We recommend Directors of Public Health, working on behalf of health and local authorities, produce an equity profile for the population they serve, and undertake a triennial audit of progress towards achieving objectives to reduce inequalities in health.

(Acheson *et al.* 1998)

PART II

SPECIAL THEMES

Globalisation, Work Intensity
and Health Inequalities

A Cross-national Comparison[*]

Karin HALLDÉN

1. Globalisation and Health Inequalities
in the Labour Market

The potential influence of globalisation on domestic labour markets has been an issue of great debate during recent years. It is a widely held view that globalisation implies increased inequality in wages and a rise in unemployment in developed countries (Deardorff and Stern 2002, Deardorff 2003). Another prevalent assumption is that weaker groups in the labour market in developed countries, for example individuals with a low level of education and in less skilled work, are especially vulnerable (Wood 1995, Deardorff 2003). Though empirical findings differ to some extent[1], current research on Swedish data indicates that globalisation, defined in economic terms, has not had any impact on the stability of employment or job mobility (Korpi and Stern 2006, Korpi and Tåhlin 2006). Nor do the results confirm the connection between globalisation and an increased risk of unemployment for individuals with a low level of education and in unskilled work, compared with other groups (*ibid.*). These findings support research by Bentivogli and Pagano (1999), studying the effects of globalisation on unemployment in four European countries.

However, it is not reasonable to assume that growing international trade and economic integration leave domestic labour markets unaffected. Increased international integration might influence other areas

---

[*] Earlier versions of this chapter were presented at the LNU seminar at the Swedish Institute for Social Research (SOFI), Stockholm University, January 2004, and at the Swedish Sociological Association Conference 2004, February 2004. I most gratefully acknowledge the help and support of my supervisor Michael Tåhlin. I also would like to thank my colleagues at the LNU project for helpful comments and Martin Hällsten for advice concerning the analyses.

[1] Cf. Strauss-Kahn (2003) indicating an impact (though minor) of globalization on unemployment for unskilled manufacturing workers in France.

than the ones considered above. Such an area could be the relation between working life and health. If increased international competition results in firms changing the production process in such a way that the work pace accelerates and the stress in work increases, this process of change is likely to have implications for health (McCormick and Cooper 1988, Green 2001).

The aim of this chapter is to examine if globalisation can be related to the intensification of work and health inequalities. If globalisation implies increased work intensity and a decline in health, workers in industries that are most exposed to rising international competition would be more at risk. Besides, employees in unskilled work in such industries should be more susceptible than others. The analyses are based on data from two points in time (1995/1996 and 2000). Furthermore, when studying the potential influence of globalisation on work intensity and health, a cross-national approach can help to separate a potential effect of globalisation on health from trends due to institutional factors on domestic labour markets. Hence, the countries within the European Union will be analysed.

The chapter has the following structure. In section 2 the concept of globalisation is discussed and in section 3 the notions of economic globalisation and trade theory are accounted for. Section 4 presents implications of globalisation on health, and support for a link between globalisation, work intensity and a decline in health. Objectives and hypotheses are provided in section 5. Section 6 explains the measure of economic globalisation and section 7 accounts for the development of economic globalisation in the European Union. Section 8 and 9 provide information on the data and indicators used, as well as methodological limitations. The empirical results are presented in section 10 and section 11 concludes the chapter.

2. The Concept of Globalisation

During the last two decades the research and literature on globalisation in disciplines such as sociology, economics and political science has grown rapidly (Guillén 2001). The concept of globalisation has several connotations and the term is defined in diverse ways, not only between disciplines, but also within disciplines. In sociology, globalisation generally has a wide definition, including flows of information and new technology, political interdependencies, cultural interchange and economic aspect[2]. Though a broad definition might be preferable for some purposes, it makes assumptions concerning globalisation that can

---

[2]   Guillén (2001) discusses the concept and summarises current sociological research.

be difficult to test empirically. Thus, globalisation is defined here in economic terms as growing international flows of trade, capital and labour[3].

In the literature the concept of globalisation is often presented as a phenomenon of recent occurrence. One might argue that economic globalisation is nothing new, at least not for small countries (such as Sweden). But the degree of interdependence between countries with regard to trade (i.e. exports and imports) is clearly higher today than in the past (cf. Bordo *et al.* 1999), and other aspects of economic global-isation, such as flows of capital (for example flows of short-term capital and foreign direct investment), have increased during recent years to an even greater extent than trade (Guillén 2001, CEIES 2003, OECD 2003). Moreover, increased establishment of trade agreements and the magnitude of multinational companies distinguish the contemporary era of globalisation (Bordo *et al.* 1999, OECD 2003).

3. Theoretical Connections to Economic Globalisation

As mentioned above, the economic dimension of globalisation gen-erally includes three growth elements: international trade flows, interna-tional flows of capital and international flows of labour. In line with most of the literature in the field, the theoretical connection used is mainly linked to the trade aspect of globalisation; thus trade is empha-sised in the following discussion. This focus does not imply that flows of capital and labour are unimportant, only that they fall outside the scope of the present analysis.

What impact is then to be expected on a country's domestic labour market if trade with other countries increases? Heckscher-Ohlin's economic trade theory discusses this issue (cf. Ohlin 1933). In short, the theory implies that countries which differ regarding factor endowments have different comparative advantages on an international market[4]. A country with a relatively large supply of labour has comparative advan-tages with regard to labour-intensive production, for example mass production in manufacturing. Conversely, countries with an abundant supply of capital and skilled labour specialise in manufacturing products that require large capital investments and human capital, such as ad-vanced technological production for comparative advantages interna-tionally. The theory argues that an increase in trade between developing

---

[3] See section 6 for a precise definition.

[4] The theory of countries' comparative advantages in trade (only regarding labour pro-ductivity though) was developed by Ricardo ([1911] 2004). Adam Smith discussed countries' respective advantages in production already in the 18th century, but with an emphasis on absolute labour productivity costs.

and developed countries causes developed countries to increase their import of labour-intensive goods from developing countries, and raise their export of goods, requiring capital and highly skilled workers in the production process. The opposite applies for the developing countries.

Heckscher-Olin's theory states that increased international competition implies specialisation in production that brings about a change in demand for labour. The demand for skilled workers will then increase in the developed countries, and simultaneously the demand for less skilled workers will decrease[5]. The declining demand for unskilled workers in developed countries should, according to economic theory, be reflected in a growing compensation for education and qualifications, leading to increased inequality in wages between skilled and less skilled workers. The reverse change in demand for labour is expected to occur in developing countries. Thus, a growing international trade would imply decreased wage inequalities between groups with diverse qualifications in the latter countries.

The changed demand for labour implied by theory, that arises when a country's international integration increases, can be seen as an adjustment pressure (WTO 2003). The effect of such an adjustment pressure on domestic labour markets is diverse, depending on the kind of labour market policies applied in the country and the structure of the labour market institutions, so-called adjustment modifiers (*ibid.*). In a country where wage negotiations are centralised to a relatively large extent (for example Sweden), the changed demand for labour should mainly become visible in a higher rate of job mobility, unemployment or exits from the labour market, for individuals with less qualifications compared with other groups. Conversely, the wages for unskilled workers will decrease as a consequence of the reduced demand if a country has a relatively flexible wage-setting system (for example the UK)[6]. Wage flexibility is limited for a majority of the European countries (Bentivogli and Pagano 1999); thus an increased trade with developing countries would imply a higher unemployment rate among unskilled workers for the greater part of the countries within Europe.

Arguments opposing the stated empirical effects of increasing international trade on domestic labour markets claim that trade between developed and developing countries is still a minor part of the former countries' total export and import (Acemoglu 2003). The main part of

---

[5] Multinational companies substituting less skilled workers in developed countries with workers in developing countries has been referred to as a "giant sucking sound" (Ross Perot discussing NAFTA in 1992).

[6] Other labour market characteristics not accounted for might influence the adjustment process as well; cf. WTO (2003).

international trade occurs within the circle of developed countries (Bordo *et al.* 1999), even though trade between developed and developing countries has risen during recent years (Bordo *et al.* 1999, OECD 1997). However, if trade with intermediate goods is taken into account, it makes the share greater. Another argument states that a change in technology (so-called skill-biased technological change), particularly in computer technology, has led firms in developed countries to upgrade their demand for skills. This, rather than globalisation (i.e. increased international trade and competition), would explain changes in the structure of demand towards more skilled workers, and the rising wage inequalities between skilled and less skilled employees (Adams 1997, Acemoglu 2003). The empirical support for such an explanation is however uncertain (Morris and Western 1999, Card and DiNardo 2002). In any case, the effects of trade and the effects of technology might be difficult to separate from each other, since a change in a country's trade policy could also give access to, or require, new technology for domestic firms to remain competitive (Hanson and Harrison 1995, WTO 2003).

4. Globalisation and Implications for Health

A more open market tends to increase competition between firms and countries, and increase domestic growth (Dollar 2001, Garrett 2001, Wacziarg and Horn Welch 2003, WTO 2003)[7]. This might lead to sustained investment in essential public goods and improved public health (Woodward *et al.* 2001). It is commonly held that a reduction of trade barriers increases income, and mostly so in developing countries (Hertzman and Siddiqi 2000, Dollar 2001, Garrett 2001, WTO 2003). It is disputed whether this involves a rising income inequality, whether it benefits the poor or whether it is neutral (cf. Cornia 2001, Dollar 2001, Garrett 2001)[8]. If an income growth does not leave the poor behind distributionally, globalisation would imply improved health for poor people through better nutrition, decreased infant mortality and increased

---

[7] Hallak and Levinsohn (2004) summarising current research on the issue, indicate that the causal relationship between trade policy and growth is ambiguous. Garrett (2001) suggests that globalization implies economic growth primarily in middle-income countries.

[8] It is argued that the positive effects have been limited to some countries, where trade openness has been combined with domestic regulatory institutions (Cornia 2001) or middle-income countries (Garrett 2001). The implication of Heckscher-Ohlin's economic trade theory is an increase in wage inequality for developed countries and a reduced inequality in wages in poor countries.

female education among other things (*ibid.*)[9]. In addition to economic growth and a change in income distribution, the effect of economic globalisation on health could be mediated by economic stability[10], civic affiliation and psychosocial living conditions (Hertzman and Siddiqi 2000, Woodward *et al.* 2001).

Other implications of globalisation for health concern a faster spread of infectious diseases, for example AIDS, due to increased travel and migration (WHO and WTO 2002). On the other hand, access to new technology and knowledge can help prevent and treat diseases. Moreover, as a result of increased international trade, prices of tobacco products are likely to decrease, which might raise the consumption in countries with less efficient production (*ibid.*)[11]. In addition, trade liberalisation can be linked to both positive and negative effects on food quality and nutrition (cf. WHO and WTO 2002).

Also, research has linked globalisation to health through workers' psychological well-being. If employees connect rapid international integration with downsizing and dismissals, workers' might perceive globalisation as a threat, since they are unable to control events taking place on an international arena. This hypothesis is tested on cross-sectional data by Pelfrene *et al.* (2003), using the framework of Karasek's demand-control model (1979). The results suggest that employees perceiving their job as being exposed to high levels of 'world market competition' were more likely to report poor health status (for example sleeping problems and depressive mood). Moreover, perceiving the 'global economic dynamics' as threatening to one's working situation was associated with depressive symptoms as well as sleeping problems (*ibid.*).

Furthermore, research testing the predictions of the Heckscher-Ohlin trade theory using micro data from several countries shows that highly skilled workers in richer (developed) countries have a more positive attitude to globalisation than unskilled workers in the same countries (O'Rourke 2003). In addition, analysis on British panel data shows that employees in industries with a high proportion of FDI (foreign direct investments) are more likely to report economic insecurity (Scheve and

---

[9] As regards income inequalities and inequalities in health, cf. Kawachi *et al.* (1999), Navarro (1999) or Coburn (2004).

[10] Increased international trade could affect economic volatility in two different directions (Garrett 2001). On the one hand, specialization in production would increase vulnerability and raise short-term fluctuation, implying increased volatility. On the other hand, a growth in international trade means a bigger market and more potential buyers, something that would make the fluctuation smaller.

[11] However, it is a common health policy to impose taxes on both domestic and foreign tobacco products (WHO and WTO 2002).

Slaughter 2002). Even though these latter two studies do not focus on the implications of globalisation for workers' health, one might suppose that perceiving economic insecurity and having a negative attitude to globalisation in a situation when international integration increases, could affect employees' mental well-being negatively.

A. The Link between Globalisation, Work Intensity and Health

The trade theory accounted for in the previous section states, in summary, that increased international integration leads to a shift in demand towards skilled workers in developed countries. A skill-biased technological change might have also had some influence on the increased demand for skilled labour. Furthermore, the rise in demand for skilled labour means increased wage inequalities between skilled and unskilled workers, or a rise in job mobility or unemployment for less skilled employees, depending on the wage-setting system applied in the country. The empirical situation is not marked by consensus, neither on the actual effects of globalisation on domestic labour markets, nor on the possible extent of such an impact (Morris and Western 1999). Diverse empirical findings might to some extent be explained by differences in the definition of globalisation, the time period and the country studied.

However, current research indicates no connection between globalisation and increased unemployment (Bentivogli and Pagano 1999, Korpi and Stern 2006, Korpi and Tåhlin 2006). Nonetheless, adjustment pressures of globalisation on domestic labour markets might have appeared elsewhere, for example by firms raising their competitiveness (WTO 2003)[12]. One way for firms to respond to increased international competition might be to reorganise the production process and restructure the work, and it is plausible that this will imply an accelerated work pace and increased work pressure. Yet, few studies have investigated a connection between globalisation and work intensity, even though it is often assumed that a rise in international trade (especially between developing and developed countries) will have such implications on domestic labour markets (Green and McIntosh 2000). If growing international trade increases work pressure, this is likely to affect workers' well-being, since research shows that work intensity leads to impaired psychosocial health among employees (McCormick and Cooper 1988, Green 2001).

Empirical findings on Swedish data indicate a general deterioration in psychosocial working conditions during the 1990s and an increase in work intensity (Bäckman and Edling 2000, Fritzell and Lundberg 2000,

---

[12]   Different strategies of adjustment are however not mutually exclusive (WTO 2003).

le Grand *et al.* 2001). Current research on European data supports the tendency of workers to have experienced a rise in work pressure during the most recent decade (Green and McIntosh 2001, Merllié and Paoli 2001). Though a trend towards work intensity might be evident, there are great differences between the countries within the European Union. Employees in countries in the north of Europe report higher levels of stress, while workers in southern countries to a greater extent report physical symptoms (Eklund *et al.* 2000).

5. Objectives

In the present chapter the crucial assumption is made that a potential impact of economic globalisation should be more visible in the manufacturing industry compared with other industries[13]. If a country increases its international trade, manufacturing becomes exposed to international competition to a greater extent than public service and private service, where a potential effect of globalisation should be more indirect (OECD 2003, WTO 2003). Thus, the basic assumption is that a product is more easily exported and imported than a service[14]. In addition, since increased international integration, according to theory, implies a general decrease in demand for less skilled workers in developed countries, unskilled employees within manufacturing would be most exposed.

By measuring work intensity and health for individuals in different industries at two points in time, possible changes can be observed. If changes differ for workers in manufacturing compared with workers in private and public service, this will indicate that globalisation has implications for work intensity and health. If the development is of a similar kind across industries, this indicates that the impact of globalisation on these factors is not significant. Furthermore, the development in work pressure and health for workers at different skill levels will be compared.

Studying more than one country on the basis of the assumptions made above provides additional knowledge about the potential effect of globalisation on work intensity and health. If globalisation has any

---

[13] This assumption has for example been used by Krugman, *et al.* (1995), Korpi and Stern (2006), Korpi and Tåhlin (2006), Strauss-Kahn (2003) and Edin *et al.* (2004) when empirically testing globalization.

[14] It should however be noted that there has been an increase in firms "outsourcing" or "delocalising" services from developed countries to developing countries in recent years (Bordo *et al.* 1999, CEIES 2003). Examples of such services are support functions and customer services. Nevertheless, the manufacturing industry accounted for 96% of the total Swedish export and 86% of the total import on average during the period 1985 to 1990 (Edin *et al.* 2004).

impact on work pressure and health, countries that have experienced a higher rate of globalisation could also be expected to have a larger variation across industries as regards changes in work effort and health.

It might be argued that manufacturing differs from other industries in that the work is more physically demanding than work in private and public service. Over time, however, the share of manual workers has decreased in manufacturing, so the difference in physical working conditions across industrial sectors has probably diminished. In any case, since the focus in the present study is on reduced mental well-being, variations in physical working conditions between different industries need not be a major concern here. Moreover, one might question to what extent possible effects of globalisation for skilled and unskilled workers within the same firm can be separated. Even though skilled workers might be subjected to some increase in work pressure as well, it is argued that firms within manufacturing will try to increase their competitiveness primarily by raising the work pace of unskilled employees, since the less skilled work can be carried out cheaper somewhere else[15].

A. Hypotheses

On the basis of the discussion above, the following hypotheses may be formulated.

1) If globalisation contributes to increased work intensity and health inequalities, the changes in work intensity and health should differ between workers in manufacturing and workers in private and public service, with a relatively deteriorated situation for workers in manufacturing.

2) The difference in work intensity and health between skilled and unskilled workers should have changed more among employees in manufacturing than among employees in private and public service, and be to the disadvantage of the less skilled workers.

3) The expected differences in the development of work intensity and health for workers in manufacturing compared with workers in public and private service, and skilled versus unskilled workers as accounted for above (i.e. hypotheses 1 and 2), would be greater in countries with a high rate of globalisation compared with countries that have a lower globalisation rate.

---

[15] It is also plausible that an increase in work pace is more easily adjusted for employees in unskilled work. At least it might be simpler to measure. Moreover, less skilled work constitutes the main production process in many manufacturing firms.

6. How to Measure Economic Globalisation

As discussed above, the concept of globalisation is defined here in economic terms. While this approach provides a narrower definition of globalisation than is commonly used in sociology, making estimation easier, there is no generally accepted way of measuring economic globalisation (CEIES 2003). The aggregated trade shares – being a common proxy for openness, are used here to estimate the globalisation rate for the countries within the European Union. Figure 1 shows the change in total trade as a share of GDP for the countries within the European Union between 1990 and 2000[16].

Figure 1: The increase in total trade as a share of GDP 1990-2000 for the countries within the European Union (absolute increase,%)

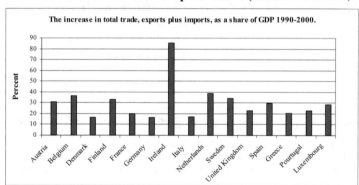

Source: Penn World Tables (Heston et al. 2002), Centre for International Comparisons at the University of Pennsylvania (CICUP).

Ireland, the Netherlands, Belgium, Sweden, Finland, Austria, Spain and Luxembourg are at the top, as countries with a 25% or more increase in total trade during the period 1990-2000, while the United Kingdom, Portugal, Greece, France, Italy, Germany and Denmark have had a slower development as regards openness.

7. The Development of Economic Globalisation for the European Union

The European Union has expanded during the last decades, from six to fifteen member states allowing virtually free movement of goods, individuals, services and capital between them. Trade was one of the

---

[16] Defined as exports plus imports as a share of GDP, constant prices (Penn World Tables, Heston *et al.* 2002).

first agreement areas of the countries. During the 1960s the European Union created a tariff union between the member countries and an external unit tariff was introduced. In 1992 the 'internal market' of the union was initiated, the remaining trade barriers were abandoned and trade was liberalised further (European Commission 2003). The twenty-five member states now negotiate as one unit, both with trade partners and within the World Trade Organisation. The European Union is the world's largest exporter of goods and services, as well as the world's primary source of FDI (foreign direct investments). Furthermore, EU is the second largest receiver of FDI after the United States (*ibid.*).

8. The European Survey on Working Conditions (EFWCS)

The main data set used for the analyses is the European Survey of Working Conditions (EFWCS), a survey based on a standardised questionnaire covering topics on physical and psychosocial working conditions and work environments in the European Union. The survey was carried out by the European Foundation for the Improvement of Living and Working Conditions in association with Eurostat and has been undertaken at three occasions: 1990/1991, 1995/1996 and 2000. The number of countries participating is equivalent to the number of member states[17]. The first and the second survey were conducted with a representative sample of 1000 workers[18] aged fifteen and over in each member state, using a probability sample design (Paoli and Merllié 2001)[19]. In the third survey about 1500 workers in each member state were interviewed[20]. All three surveys were administered using face-to-face interviews.

Though the EFWCS provides a unique opportunity to make cross-national comparisons, since it contains harmonised information from all countries in the European Union for several points in time, the surveys have limitations. One issue is a response rate that differs greatly for

---

[17] Thus, the first survey includes data from twelve countries and the two latter provide data for fifteen countries, i.e. Belgium, Denmark, France, Germany, Greece, Ireland, Italy, Luxembourg, the Netherlands, Portugal, Spain, the United Kingdom, Sweden, Finland and Austria (the three latter countries only provided data for the second and third survey).

[18] Consequently, students, housewives, unemployed or retired individuals etc were excluded. Self-employed people are however included.

[19] In total 12,819 workers were interviewed in the first survey and 15,986 workers in the second survey.

[20] Except for Luxembourg, where approximately 500 workers participated. In total 21,703 workers were interviewed in the third survey.

different countries[21]. For full details, see Paoli (1992, 1997) and Paoli and Merllié (2001). Nevertheless, bearing the objectives of the chapter in mind, EFWCS provides a good opportunity for comparative empirical analyses.

Data from the surveys of 1995/1996 and 2000 are used for the analyses (since Sweden and Finland were not included in 1990/1991). Employed individuals (both full-time and part-time), working 10 or more hours per week, are studied. Self-employed workers and individuals under 18 and over 65 years of age are excluded. The data set after these selections comprises 29,320 employees.

A. Additional Data for Sweden

In addition to the cross-sectional EFWCS data sets, longitudinal data for 1981, 1991 and 2000 from the Swedish Level of Living Survey (Levnadsnivåundersökningen, LNU) are used for panel analyses. These surveys were conducted with national probability samples of individuals between the ages of 18 and 75, and the respondents were interviewed face-to-face (see Gähler 2004 for a further description). The purpose of the panel analyses is to consider a potential health selective mobility related to industry (cf. appendix).

B. Indicators and Methods

The two questions: "Does your job involve working at very high speed?" and "Does your job involve working to tight deadlines?" were used as indicators of work intensity in the EFWCS. The answers to these questions were coded as indexes, taking the value 1 for the answer "Never", and the value 7 for the answer "All of the time"[22]. To create a single indicator of work intensity, the two indexes were added together and then divided by two, forming an index with a range from 1 to 7 with possible half-point values. Green and McIntosh (2001) have used this indicator of work pressure when studying work intensity on the same data set (EFWCS 1990/1991 and 1995/1996).

Mental well-being is measured with an additive index, based on the question: "Does your work affect your health, or not? (IF YES) how does it affect your health? "Yes, stress", "Yes, overall fatigue", "Yes, sleeping problems", "Yes, anxiety", "Yes, irritability". The question has further response options than the five accounted for and they are not

---

[21] Due to such methodologicall restrictions of the EFWCS data, the analyses should be interpreted with caution.

[22] Responses between 1 and 7 take the following values: 2 for *"Almost never"*, 3 for *"Around one quarter of the time"*, 4 for *"Around half of the time"*, 5 for *"Around three quarters of the time"* and 6 for *"Almost all of the time"*.

mutually exclusive. This variable is dichotomised, taking the value 1 if the respondent reports three or more problems related to mental well-being.

With regard to industries, workers are classified in three categories according to NACE codes (Statistical Classification of Economic Activities)[23]:

– *manufacturing* (NACE codes C, D and E): 'mining and quarrying', 'manufacturing' and 'electricity, gas and water supply,

– *private service* (NACE codes F, G, H, I, J and K): 'construction, 'wholesale and retail trade, repair of motor vehicles, motorcycles and personal household goods', 'hotels and restaurants', "transport, storage, and communication', 'financial intermediation and 'real estate, renting and business activities,

– *public service* (NACE codes L, M, N, O, P and Q): 'public admini-stration and defence; compulsory social security', 'education', 'health and social work', 'other community, social and personal service activi-ties and private households with employed persons; extra-territorial organisations and bodies'.

The division of firms into manufacturing, public and private service according to their business activity, as accounted for above, needs to be clarified. First, the 1995 EFWCS data set only comprises the NACE classification codes in combined categories. As a result *'mining and quarrying'* and *'manufacturing'* are treated as one unit (NACE codes C and D). Second, *'Electricity, gas and water supply'* are included in the manufacturing category. It might be questioned whether these latter industries are more exposed to international competition than are public and private service. However, the total share of employees in the EFWCS data set working in *'Electricity, gas and water supply'* are 1.2%, and it is not likely that the inclusion of these industries is of any central importance as regards the analyses. Finally, *'Private households with employed persons; extra-territorial organisations and bodies'* (NACE codes P and Q) are merged with *'education', 'health and social work', 'other community, social and personal service activities'* (NACE codes M, N and O) in the original data set. Thus, these categories cannot be separated, even though exclusion might have been preferable. So, for that reason workers in this category that do not report working in the public sector are sorted to the private service category[24].

---

[23] Individuals working in *'agriculture, hunting, forestry and fishing'* (NACE codes A and B) are excluded.

[24] In the 1995 EFWCS the question was posed: *"Are you working in the public or the private sector?"* For the EFWCS in 2000 the question was put in a different way: *"Are you working in national or local government services/a state-owned com-*

In addition, the countries within the European Union are divided into two categories with regard to the countries' development in terms of economic globalisation (i.e. total trade) 1990-2000:

– Countries with a relatively high rate of globalisation during the period 1990-2000 (an increase in total trade of 25% or more) are: Ireland, the Netherlands, Belgium, Sweden, Finland, Austria, Spain and Luxembourg.

– Countries with a relatively low rate of globalisation in 1990-2000 (less than a 25% increase in total trade) are: the United Kingdom, Portugal, Greece, France, Italy, Germany and Denmark.

This dichotomous variable takes the value 1 for countries with a greater rate of globalisation, and 0 for countries with a lesser rate of globalisation[25].

Finally, a dichotomised variable is constructed to indicate workers' level of qualifications. Employees are classified into two categories[26] according to ISCO-88 codes (International Standard Classification of Occupations):

– *More skilled work* (ISCO-88 codes 1, 2, 3, 4 and 5): 'legislators and senior officials and managers', 'professionals' and 'technicians and associate professionals', 'clerks' and 'service workers and shop and market sales workers'.

– *Less skilled work* (ISCO-88 codes 7, 8 and 9): 'craft-related workers', 'plant and machine operators and assemblers' and 'elementary occupations'.

– *'Skilled agricultural and fishery workers'* or individuals working in *'the armed forces'* (ISCO-88 codes 6 and 10) are excluded.

The variable takes the value 1 for less skilled work and 0 for more skilled work.

The methods used for analyses are OLS regression and logistic regression.

---

pany/another company, another business/other. Employees that are working in the public sector or national/local government services/a state-owned company are counted as being employed in public services.

[25] The measure of economic globalization used is aggregated trade share, defined as import + export as a share of GDP, see section 6: figure 1.

[26] The EFWCS data from 1995/1996 only provides first-digit ISCO-88 codes, making more advanced divisions difficult.

9. Limitations and Methodological Problems

It is possible that individual perceptions in a specific area (in this case regarding work intensity and the impact of work on health) could change over time, due to for example increased media coverage, changes in legislation or individual experience (Wikman 1991). If this were the case, the estimates of change in working conditions as reported by individual workers would be biased. It is reasonable to assume, however, that variations of attitude generally change in a similar way across industries. Since the objective is to study changes in manufacturing compared with changes in other industries, the potential bias due to changing attitudes and perceptions may therefore be considered as minor.

Another potential source of bias in the interpretation of cross-national data is cultural differences in response patterns. When the intention is to compare trends using analyses based on two or more observations across time, cultural differences between countries are very unlikely to affect estimates, since changes and not absolute levels are observed. Even if the European countries differ with respect to levels, it is not likely that cultural differences in response patterns across countries have changed during the time period studied. Hence, no further attention will be paid to this issue.

Moreover, if a specific country makes changes in employment protection legislation and if, for example, the level of unionisation varies, this is likely to have some influence on a potential effect of globalisation on work intensity and mental well-being. This should not be a problem here, however. When studying trends for many countries, it is not reasonable to assume that domestic labour markets institutions have changed in such a way that the main tendencies regarding the plausible connection between globalisation, work intensity and health are affected.

A. Considering a Potential Health-related Selection – 'The Healthy Worker Effect'

A limitation of the EFWC surveys is that they do not provide panel data, hindering the possibility to carry out longitudinal analyses. This is of concern, since a potential health-related selection regarding industry should be taken into account. It is possible that workers in manufacturing with a relative decline in health compared with other employees might decide, or be forced, to leave a job in this industry if the firm becomes exposed to increased international competition and therefore raises work pressure in order to remain competitive. Such possible effects might bias the estimates when analysing cross-sectional data from two points in time, since the average health for workers in manufacturing in this case would be relatively improved compared with employees in other industries, i.e. 'the healthy worker effect'[27] (Östlin 1989). Since a potential underestimation of a possible influence of globalisation on health must be considered, panel data from the Swedish Level of Living Survey (Levnadsnivåundersökningen, LNU) from three points in time (1981, 1991 and 2000) have been analysed. Results from the 1991-2000 panel analyses are presented in the appendix. Similar analyses were conducted on panel data for the period 1981-1991 (results not shown). The results suggest no apparent support for a healthy worker effect, i.e. there are no tendencies for health-related selection as regards mobility between industries or labour market exits that can be connected to a particular industry. Obviously, the analyses only account for the Swedish setting and the results cannot be generalised to other European countries in a straightforward manner. Moreover, the results must be interpreted with caution, since possibly important events taking place between the two interviews are not considered.

Nevertheless, since no health-related selection effect in the manufacturing industry has appeared for this time period, one might argue that it is unlikely that a healthy worker effect would distort the analyses on European data.

10. Empirical Findings on Work Intensity and Health in Europe

As explained in sections 3 and 4.2, a rise in international trade might result in firms changing the work process and increasing work pressure, in order to achieve higher productivity and thus meet increased international competition. A crucial assumption is that this potential effect of economic globalisation on domestic labour markets would be most observable in manufacturing. Since globalisation, defined according to economic terms, has increased during the 1990s (CEIES 2003, OECD 2003), an increased work effort as well as a decline in mental well-being, for workers in manufacturing compared with other industries, is then to be expected for all the EU countries analysed (hypothesis 1). Furthermore, unskilled workers in this industry would be most exposed to increased international competition and, accordingly, the development for unskilled and skilled employees as regards work intensity and health should differ more for workers in manufacturing compared with workers in other industries (hypothesis 2). Finally, these changes in work pressure and mental well-being for employees in manufacturing

---

[27] The expression was first used in a study of rubber workers by McMichael *et al.* (1974).

compared with workers in other industries, and for less skilled workers compared with more skilled employees, would be more visible for countries that have experienced a relatively high rate of economic globalisation (hypothesis 3).

Work intensity is analysed in section A, moving on to workers' mental well-being in section B. In section C a possible connection between increased work pressure and reduced mental well-being is examined.

A. Has Work Become More Intensive in the European Union?

In this section work pressure is analysed. The descriptive statistics (table 1) show a very limited but on average significant rise in work intensity during the period 1995/1996 – 2000, when the EU countries are studied pooled.

Table 1: Work intensity average score
1995/1996 and 2000, all EU countries pooled

Work intensity scale 1-7	1995/1996	2000
Average score:	3,48	3,56**
Manufacturing	3,79	3,85
Private service	3,53	3,56
Public service	3,13	3,25*

Significance levels: **$p \leq 0,01$, *$p \leq 0.05$.

Table 2a (cf. model 1) confirms that the rise in work intensity for all countries between 1995/1996 and 2000 is significant though small (with control for industry, skill level and globalisation rate). Employees in manufacturing and in private service experience more work pressure than workers in public service. However, work intensification has not been greater for individuals employed in manufacturing compared with workers in other industries during the 1990s (cf. table 2a, model 2). Hence, there is no support for hypothesis 1 as regards work intensity.

Work pressure is somewhat higher for employees in less skilled work compared with individuals in more skilled work (cf. table 2a, model 1). But since there has not been any increase in work intensity for unskilled workers in manufacturing compared with less skilled employees in other industries between 1995 and 2000 (cf. the interaction term unskilled*2000, table 2a, model 3), hypothesis 2 is not confirmed regarding work intensity.

Table 2a: Work intensity, employees aged 18-65, EU countries 1995/1996 and 2000. OLS, unstandardised coefficients. Standard errors in brackets

	Model 1	Model 2			Model 3			Model 4		
	Pooled	M.	Pr.	Pu.	M.	Pr.	Pu.	M.	Pr.	Pu.
2000	0.065** (0.022)	0.046 (0.049)	0.048 (0.030)	0.087 (0.046)	-0.044 (0.081)	0.006 (0.037)	0.090 (0.049)	0.081 (0.155)	0.188*c (0.095)	-0.315*c (0.150)
Manufacturing	0.542** (0.036)									
Private service	0.311** (0.028)									
Unskilled work	0.158** (0.025)	0.271** B (0.051)	0.194** C (0.031)	-0.280** BC (0.070)	0.194** B (0.075)	0.123*C (0.049)	0.269** BC (0.096)	0.271** B (0.051)	0.195** C (0.031)	-0.280** BC (0.070)
Countries with faster globalisation rate 1990–2000	0.166** (0.022)	0.108* b (0.049)	0.157* * (0.029)	0.260** b (0.046)	0.109* b (0.049)	0.157** (0.029)	0.260* *b (0.046)	0.121 (0.073)	0.215** (0.047)	0.131* (0.065)
Unskilled work * 2000					0.141 (0.102)	0.121 (0.063)	-0.024 (0.140)			
Countries with faster globalisation rate 1990–2000 * 2000								-0.024 b (0.098)	-0.093 c (0.060)	0.261 **b c (0.093)
Constant	2.895** (0.043)	3.462** (0.088)	3.218** (0.051)	2.788** (0.077)	3.507** (0.094)	3.246** (0.053)	2.786** (0.078)	3.443** (0.120)	3.132** (0.076)	2.980** (0.103)
R-squared [d]	0.02	0.01	0.00	0.01	0.01	0.00	0.01	0.01	0.00	0.01
Observations	28,147	5,902	16,010	6,063	5,902	16,010	6,063	5,902	16,010	6,063

*M. = manufacturing. Pr. = private service. Pu. = public service. Reference categories are: 1995/1996, public service, skilled work and countries with slower globalisation rate. Significance levels: ** p≤ = 0.01, * p≤ = 0.05. [d] The R-square value, not being high in model 1, becomes even smaller in model 2, 3 and 4. This is because the analyses in the latter models are conducted separately for manufacturing, private and public service and thus, industry is omitted as an explanatory variable.*

Significance tests between industries in table 2a:
[a] = a significant difference between the manufacturing industry and private service (* p≤ = 0.05).
[b] = a significant difference between the manufacturing industry and public service (* p≤ = 0.05).
[c] = a significant difference between private service and public service (* p≤ = 0.05).
Bold capital letters indicate that the difference is significant at a level of 99% (** p≤ = 0.01).

Furthermore, the work is more intensive for employees in countries with a relatively faster development of globali*sation*, compared with workers in countries that have a lower rate of globali*sation* (cf. table 2a, model 1).

Even so, work pressure has only increased for workers in public service in countries with a relatively higher globalisation rate during the last years (cf. table 2a, model 4), and employees doing unskilled work in such countries have not had any relative increase in work intensity between 1995 and 2000 compared with employees in more skilled work, irrespective of industry (cf. table 2b). Thus, these results do not provide support for hypothesis 3 regarding work intensity.

Table 2b: Work intensity, employees aged 18-65, EU countries 1995/1996 and 2000. OLS, unstandardised coefficients. Standard errors in brackets

	Countries with faster globalisation rate 1990-2000			Countries with slower globalisation rate 1990-2000		
	M.	Pr.	Pu.	M.	Pr.	Pu.
2000	-0.054^b	-0.038^C	0.200**^{bC}	-0.035	0.052	-0.039
	(0.112)	(0.052)	(0.067)	(0.119)	(0.054)	(0.074)
Unskilled work	0.170^b	0.052^c	-0.282*^{bc}	0.218*^{B}	0.193**^{C}	-0.270*^{BC}
	(0.106)	(0.070)	(0.143)	(0.107)	(0.068)	(0.131)
Unskilled work * 2000	0.144	0.104	0.071	0.140	0.137	-0.106
	(0.142)	(0.090)	(0.197)	(0.147)	(0.089)	(0.200)
Constant	3.746**	3.612**	3.242**	3.597**	3.347**	3.110**
	(0.083)	(0.042)	(0.050)	(0.085)	(0.043)	(0.050)
R-squared	0.00	0.00	0.01	0.01	0.01	0.00
Observations	2,897	8,046	3,258	3,005	7,964	2,805

M. = manufacturing. Pr. = private service. Pu. = public service.
*Reference categories are: 1995/1996 and skilled work. Significance levels: ** $p \leq = 0.01$, * $p \leq = 0.05$.*
Significance tests between industries in table 2b:
[a] *= a significant difference between the manufacturing industry and private service (* $p \leq = 0.05$).*
[b] *= a significant difference between the manufacturing industry and public service (* $p \leq = 0.05$).*
[c] *= a significant difference between private service and public service (* $p \leq = 0.05$).*
Bold capital letters indicate that the difference is significant at a level of 99% (** $p \leq = 0.01$).

Consequently, the analyses of work intensity during recent years in the EU countries do not support hypothesis 1 or 2. Neither is there any clear support for hypothesis 3.

B. Has There Been a Decline in Workers' Mental Well-being?

Secondly, mental well-being is studied. There has been a very slight increase in all symptoms of reduced mental well-being except irritability between 1995/1996 and 2000, when data for all countries are merged (cf. table 3, table 4a, model 1).

Table 3: The change in the distribution of responses to the questions measuring mental well-being (%). All EU countries pooled

Symptoms of reduced mental well-being	1995/1996	2000
Employees that report three or more symptoms of reduced mental well-being (presented in the categories below).	8.7	9.4
Stress	28.0	28.7
Overall fatigue	18.3	20.5**
Sleeping problems	6,8	8.2**
Anxiety	6.3	6.6
Irritability	11.0	9.8

Significance levels; $**p \leq 0.01$, $*p \leq 0.05$.

The measure of reduced mental well-being used in the analyses is a dichotomous variable taking the value 1 if a person reports three or more of the symptoms presented in table 3 above (cf. section 8.B). In table 4a and 4b the baseline is 1 since logistic regression is used. Hence, a coefficient value that exceeds the value of 1 indicates an increase, and simultaneously, a coefficient value below 1 points to a decrease (if it is significant). The regression analyses show that the risk of experiencing reduced mental well-being is relatively lower for manufacturing workers and employees in private service than employees in public service (cf. table 4a, model 1). However, the most interesting result as concerns hypothesis 1 is that mental well-being has decreased for workers in private service during the late 1990s. There is no significant decrease in mental well-being within the manufacturing industry or in public service (cf. table 4a, model 2). Consequently, hypothesis 1 regarding health decline is not confirmed, as it predicted a decline in health for workers in manufacturing that is not matched by a similar trend in the other industries.

Table 4a: Reduced mental well-being among employees aged 18-65, EU countries 1995/1996 and 2000. Logistic regression, odds ratios. Standard errors in brackets

	Model 1	Model 2			Model 3			Model 4		
	Pooled	M.	Pr.	Pu.	M.	Pr.	Pu.	M.	Pr.	Pu.
2000	1.100* (0.046)	1.062 (0.102)	1.174** (0.070)	1.029 (0.079)	0.948 (0.146)	1.265** (0.093)	1.027 (0.082)	0.745 (0.217)	0.825 (0.152)	0.707 (0.177)
Manufacturing	0.705** (0.046)									
Private service	0.669** (0.033)									
Unskilled work	0.798** (0.040)	0.922[b] (0.091)	0.789** (0.052)	0.603**[b] (0.083)	0.833 (0.121)	0.910 (0.092)	0.596** (0.114)	0.924[b] (0.092)	0.788** (0.052)	0.602**[b] (0.083)
Countries with fasterr globalisation rate 1990–2000	0.826** (0.034)	0.730**[b] (0.070)	0.769**[C] (0.044)	1.004[bc] (0.077)	0.731**[b] (0.070)	0.770**[c] (0.044)	1.003[bc] (0.077)	0.633** (0.093)	0.655**[c] (0.064)	0.888[c] (0.097)
Female	1.081 (0.047)	1.161 (0.119)	0.950 (0.057)	1.299** (0.107)	1.162 (0.119)	0.945 (0.057)	1.299** (0.107)	1.158 (0.118)	0.948 (0.057)	1.297** (0.107)
Age	1.011** (0.002)	1.011* (0.004)	1.010** (0.003)	1.012** (0.004)	1.011* (0.004)	1.010** (0.003)	1.012** (0.004)	1.011* (0.004)	1.010** (0.003)	1.012** (0.004)
Unskilled work * 2000					1.204 (0.237)	0.790 (0.102)	1.023 (0.280)			
Countries with faster globalisation rate 1990–2000 * 2000								1.283 (0.249)	1.277* (0.155)	1.275 (0.197)
Pseudo-R2	0.01	0.01	0.01	0.01	0.01	0.01	0.01	0.01	0.01	0.01
Observations	28,730	6,037	16,338	6,178	6,037	16,338	6,178	6,037	16,338	6,178

M. = manufacturing. Pr. = private service. Pu. = public service. Reference categories are: 1995/1996, public service, skilled work, countries with slower globalisation rate and men. Significance levels: **p≤=0.01, *p≤=0.05.
Significance tests between industries in table 4a:
[a] *= a significant difference between the manufacturing industry and private service (* p≤ = 0.05).* [b] *= a significant difference between the manufacturing industry and public service (* p≤ = 0.05).* [c] *= a significant difference between private service and public service (* p≤ = 0.05).*
Bold capital letters indicate that the difference is significant at a level of 99% (** p≤ = 0.01).

The findings in table 4a (cf. model 1) suggest that the risk of experiencing reduced mental well-being is smaller for unskilled workers than for more skilled employees. More importantly in the present context, the interaction term (unskilled*2000, cf. table 4a, model 3) shows there has been no different development in mental well-being for unskilled workers in manufacturing, compared with less skilled workers in private and public service. Thus, the results do not provide support for hypothesis 2 as regards symptoms of mental well-being.

The risk of experiencing reduced mental well-being is smaller for workers in countries with a relatively high rate of globalisation compared with workers in countries that have a slower rate of globalisation (cf. table 4a, model 1). Manufacturing workers have not experienced a decrease in mental well-being, compared with workers in other industries in countries that have a high globalisation rate (this is the situation for employees in private service) (cf. table 4b, Countries with a faster globalisation rate 1990-2000).

Table 4b: Reduced mental well-being among employees aged 18-65, EU countries 1995/1996 and 2000. Logistic regression, odds ratios. Standard errors in brackets

	Countries with faster globalisation rate 1990-2000			Countries with slower globalisation rate 1990-2000		
	M.	Pr.	Pu.	M.	Pr.	Pu.
2000	1.138	1.395**	1.163	0.843	1.160	0.888
	(0.275)	(0.152)	(0.128)	(0.171)	(0.115)	(0.106)
Unskilled work	1.026	0.826	0.799	0.726	0.954c	0.453**c
	(0.242)	(0.135)	(0.216)	(0.135)	(0.124)	(0.123)
Female	1.235	1.034	1.553**	1.114	0.875	1.061
	(0.197)	(0.092)	(0.179)	(0.149)	(0.071)	(0.126)
Age	1.007	1.014**	1.013**	1.014*	1.008*	1.012*
	(0.007)	(0.004)	(0.005)	(0.006)	(0.003)	(0.006)
Unskilled work * 2000	1.121	0.855	0.807	1.247	0.766	1.263
	(0.344)	(0.174)	(0.301)	(0.323)	(0.130)	(0.513)
Pseudo-R2	0.00	0.01	0.01	0.01	0.00	0.01
Observations	2,964	8,209	3,323	3,073	8,129	2,855

M. = manufacturing. Pr. = private service. Pu. = public service.
Reference categories are: 1995/1996, skilled work and men.
*Significance levels: ** $p \leq 0.01$, * $p \leq 0.05$.*
Significance tests between industries in table 4b:
[a] *= a significant difference between the manufacturing industry and private service (* $p \leq 0.05$).*
[b] *= a significant difference between the manufacturing industry and public service (* $p \leq 0.05$).*
[c] *= a significant difference between private service and public service (* $p \leq 0.05$).*
*Bold capital letters indicate that the difference is significant at a level of 99% (** $p \leq 0.01$).*

Moreover, less skilled manufacturing workers in countries with a high globalisation rate have not had any significant decrease in mental well-being during recent years (cf. table 4b). Accordingly, the empirical findings do not support hypothesis 3.

So, the change in the rate of symptoms of reduced mental well-being in the EU countries does not indicate a divergent development in health status for workers in manufacturing compared with other industries. Hence, the analyses provide no support for hypothesis 1. Moreover, since health development for unskilled manufacturing workers has not been more negative than for unskilled workers in other industries, hypothesis 2 is not supported. Lastly, the analyses do not sustain hypothesis 3, given that the health of less skilled manufacturing workers in countries with a faster globalisation rate has not declined relative to similar workers in other industries.

C. Is There a Connection Between Increased Globalisation, Work Intensity and Reduced Mental Well-being?

Finally, the link between work effort and reduced mental well-being is examined. The result shows clearly that work intensity is of importance for mental well-being (cf. table 5a).

Table 5a: Reduced mental well-being among employees aged 18-65, EU countries 1995/1996 and 2000, work intensity included. Logistic regression, odds ratios. Standard errors in brackets

	Model 1	Model 2			Model 3			Model 4		
	Pooled	M.	Pr.	Pu.	M.	Pr.	Pu.	M.	Pr.	Pu.
2000	1.104* (0.048)	1.069 (0.105)	1.190** (0.073)	1.022 (0.081)	0.967 (0.153)	1.296** (0.097)	1.018 (0.084)	0.707 (0.212)	0.815 (0.153)	0.754 (0.193)
Manufacturing	0.602** (0.041)									
Private service	0.608** (0.031)									
Unskilled work	0.747** (0.038)	0.812* (0.083)	0.745** (0.050)	0.603** (0.086)	0.742* (0.111)	0.876 (0.091)	0.590** (0.118)	0.813* (0.083)	0.742** (0.050)	0.602** (0.086)
Countries with a faster globalisation rate 1990–2000	0.770** (0.033)	0.678** (0.067)	0.725** (0.043)	0.922 (0.073)	0.680** (0.067)	0.726** (0.043)	0.921 (0.073)	0.574** (0.087)	0.610** (0.062)	0.834 (0.094)
Female	1.077 (0.048)	1.044 (0.109)	0.995 (0.061)	1.240* (0.105)	1.046 (0.110)	0.989 (0.061)	1.240* (0.105)	1.039 (0.109)	0.991 (0.061)	1.239* (0.105)
Age	1.013** (0.002)	1.015** (0.005)	1.013** (0.003)	1.013** (0.004)	1.015** (0.005)	1.014** (0.003)	1.013** (0.004)	1.015** (0.005)	1.013** (0.003)	1.013** (0.004)
Work intensity	1.345** (0.015)	1.423** (0.039)	1.333** (0.021)	1.313** (0.028)	1.422** (0.039)	1.334** (0.021)	1.313** (0.028)	1.424** (0.039)	1.334** (0.021)	1.312** (0.028)
Unskilled work * 2000					1.178 (0.238)	0.765* (0.101)	1.046 (0.296)			
Countries with a faster globalisation rate 1990-2000 * 2000								1.339 (0.268)	1.301* (0.161)	1.219 (0.194)
Pseudo-R2	0.05	0.06	0.04	0.04	0.06	0.04	0.04	0.06	0.04	0.05
Observations	28,193	5,910	16,039	6,072	5,910	16,039	6,072	5,910	16,039	6,072

*M = manufacturing. Pr. = private service. Pu. = public service. Reference categories are: 1995/1996, public service, skilled work, countries with lesser globalisation rate and men. Significance levels: **p<=0.01, *p<=0.05. Significance tests between industries not conducted.*

Table 5b: Reduced mental well-being among employees aged 18-65, EU countries 1995/1996 and 2000, work intensity included. Logistic regression, odds ratios. Standard errors in brackets

	Countries with faster globalisation rate 1990-2000			Countries with slower globalisation rate 1990-2000		
	M.	Pr.	Pu.	M.	Pr.	Pu.
2000	1.145	1.441**	1.136	0.870	1.179	0.894
	(0.285)	(0.161)	(0.129)	(0.181)	(0.120)	(0.109)
Unskilled work	0.919	0.801	0.789	0.642*	0.911	0.451**
	(0.223)	(0.134)	(0.222)	(0.123)	(0.122)	(0.128)
Female	1.059	1.060	1.440**	1.040	0.929	1.049
	(0.175)	(0.096)	(0.170)	(0.142)	(0.078)	(0.127)
Age	1.013	1.016**	1.012*	1.016**	1.011**	1.014*
	(0.007)	(0.004)	(0.005)	(0.006)	(0.004)	(0.006)
Work intensity	1.342**	1.310**	1.316**	1.482**	1.352**	1.305**
	(0.057)	(0.031)	(0.038)	(0.053)	(0.029)	(0.040)
Unskilled work * 2000	1.156	0.826	0.772	1.173	0.742	1.388
	(0.365)	(0.171)	(0.300)	(0.312)	(0.128)	(0.578)
Psedo-R2	0.04	0.04	0.05	0.08	0.05	0.05
Observations	2,903	8,072	3,267	3,007	7,967	2,805

M. = manufacturing. Pr. = private service. Pu. = public service.
Reference categories are: 1995/1996, skilled work and men. Significance levels:
$**p<=0.01$, $*p<=0.05$. Significance tests between industries not conducted.

Even so, the effect of year does not change significant when controlling for work intensity, neither when analysing all countries pooled or divided by industry (compare table 4a and 5a). The pattern is similar for the interaction term unskilled work*2000 in table 5b, where countries with different globalisation rates are analysed separately (compare table 4b and 5b). Thus, it is not likely that the increase in work intensity between 1995 and 2000 is an important cause of the small increase in symptoms of reduced mental well-being during the same period.

11. Conclusions

The intention of this chapter is to examine whether globalisation has contributed to increased work intensity and health inequalities for the countries within the European Union between 1995 and 2000. A central assumption is that a potential impact of globalisation on a domestic labour market should be more visible in manufacturing compared with other industries, and that less skilled workers within this industry would be in an especially vulnerable position. Furthermore, countries have been compared, based on the logic that the potential influence of globalisation on work pressure and health should be greater in countries with the most rapid change in international integration during recent years.

So, has globalisation contributed to increased work effort and health inequalities in the labour market? The empirical results hardly support the hypotheses accounted for in section 5a. There is no change for workers in manufacturing towards more intensive work, compared with employees in other industries. Furthermore, work pressure has not increased for less skilled workers in manufacturing between 1995 and 2000, and there is no significant difference compared with other industries. Work intensity is higher in countries with a faster globalisation rate, but there has only been an increase in work pressure for workers in public service.

The result that there has been an increase in work pressure in countries with a faster globalisation rate, for employees in public service relative to employees in private service and manufacturing, is of interest. Even though it is assumed here that the manufacturing industry would be most at risk as regards effects of globalisation, public service might have been affected as well. Globalisation could for example imply increased diffusion of New Public Management ideas. The concept refers to the use of market practices in the public sector, meaning that competition and privatisation are seen as strategies for increasing efficiency and keeping expenditures down (Balle Hansen and Lauridsen 2004).

It is important to keep in mind that there are other factors that could affect a possible impact of globalisation on health mediated by work intensity that are not considered in the present chapter. Data from the Swedish Level of Living Surveys were used to examine a possible health-selective mobility related to industry that might bias the results from analyses on cross-sectional data. These analyses do not indicate any great risk of mobility between industries or labour market exits for workers with poor health status employed in manufacturing, compared with similar workers employed in private or public service. Yet, data from other countries and time periods might have provided a different result. A different division of countries according to the rate of globalisation might also affect the conclusion.

In sum, the empirical findings do not support the view that globalisation has had a considerable impact on domestic labour markets in Europe regarding increased work intensity and decline in mental well-being. Accordingly, the findings suggest that economic globalisation, i.e. growing international flows of trade, capital and labour, has not contributed very much to health inequalities in the labour market.

Acknowledgement

The European Foundation for the Improvement of Living and Working Conditions has kindly provided data used in this chapter.

References

ACEMOGLU, D. 2003. "Technology and Inequality". Cambridge: National Bureau of Economic Research.

ADAMS, J. D. 1997. "Technology, Trade and Wages". *Working Paper 5940.* Cambridge: National Bureau of Economic Research.

BALLE HANSEN, M. B. & LAURIDSEN, J. 2004. "The Institutional Context of Markets Ideology: a Comparative Analysis of the Values and Perceptions of Local Government CEOs in 14 OECD Countries". *Public Administration* 82: No. 2 : 491-524.

BENTIVOLGI, C. & PAGANO, P. 1999. "Trade, Job Destruction and Job Creation in European Manufacturing". *Open Economies Review* 10: 165–184.

BORDO, M. D., EICHENGREEN, B. & IRWIN, D. A. 1999. "Is Globalization Today Really Different Than Globalization a Hundred Years ago?". *Working Paper 7195*. Cambridge: National Bureau of Economic Research.

BÄCKMAN, O. & EDLING, C. 2000. "Arbetsmiljö och Arbetsrelaterade Besvär under 1990-talet" (Working Environmentand Work-Related Health Problems in the 1990s). In S. MARKLUND (ed.). *Arbetsliv och Hälsa 2000 Working Life and Health in Sweden 2000.* Stockholm: Arbetarsskyddsstyrelsen and Arbetslivsinstitutet.

CARD, D. & DINARDO, J. E. 2002. "Skill-biased Technological Change and Rising Wage Inequality: some Problems and Puzzles". *Journal of Labor Economic* 20: 733–783.

CEIES. 2003. *Statistics and Economic Globalization.* Eurostat News: 22 and CEIES seminar: Copenhagen: 2 and 3 June.

COBURN, D. 2004. "Beyond the Income Inequality Hypothesis: Class, Neo-liberalism, and Health Inequalities". *Social Science & Medicine* 58: 41–56.

CORNIA, G. A. 2001. "Globalization and Health: Results and Options". *Bulletin of the World Health Organization* 79: 834–841.

DEARDORFF, A. V. 2003. "What might Globalization's Critics Believe?". *The World Economy* 26: 639–658.

DEARDORFF, A. V. & Stern, R. M. 2002. "What you should Know about Globalization and the World Trade Organization". *Review of International Economics* 10: 404–423.

DOLLAR, D. 2001. "Is Globalization Good for your Health?". *Bulletin of the World Health Organization* 79: 827–833.

EDIN, P.-A., FREDRIKSSON, P. & LUNDBORG, P. 2004. "The Effect of Trade on Earnings – Evidence from Swedish Micro Data". *Oxford Economic Papers* 56: 231–241. Oxford University Press.

Karin Halldén

EKLUND, I., ENGLUND, A. & WIKMAN, A. 2000. "Arbetsförhållanden i Sverige och Europa" Working Conditions in Sweden and Europé. In S. MARKLUND (ed.). *Arbetsliv och Hälsa 2000 Working Life and Health in Sweden 2000.* Stockholm: Arbetarsskyddsstyrelsen and Arbetslivsinstitutet.

EUROPEAN COMMISSION. 2003. Publication from the Department of the Commission of the European Communities: Brussels.

FRITZELL, J. & LUNDBERG, O. 2000. *Välfärd, Ofärd och Ojämlikhet Welfare, Disadvantage and Inequalityy,* Kommittén Välfärdsbokslut Reports of the Government Commission (*SOU* 41). Stockholm: Frizes.

GARETT, G. 2001. "The Distributive Consequences of Globalization". Yale University.
http://www.International.ucla.edu/profile/garrett/papers/docs/conseall.pdf

LE GRAND, C., SZULKIN, R. & TÅHLIN, M. 2001. "Har Jobben Blivit Bättre? En Analys av Arbetsinnehållet under Tre Decennier" (Have the Jobs Become Better? An Analysis of the Content of Work During Three Decades). In J. FRITZELL, M. GÄHLER and O. LUNDBERG (eds.). *Välfärd och Arbete i Arbetslöshetens Årtionde Welfare and Work in a Decade of Unempoyment. SOU:* 53.

GREEN, F. 2001. "It's Been a Hard Day's Night: the Concentration and Intensification of Work in Late 20th Century Britain". *British Journal of Industrial relations* 39: 53–80.

GREEN, F. & MCINTOSH, S. 2000. "Working on the Chain Gang? An Examination of Rising Effort Levels in Europe in the 1990s". *Discussion Paper 465.* Centre for Economic Performance: London School of Economics.

GREEN, F. & MCINTOSH, S. 2001. "The Intensification of Work in Europe". *Labour Economics* 8: 291–308.

GUILLÉN, M. F. 2001. "Is Globalization Civilizing, Destructive or Feeble? A Critique of Five Key Debates in the Social Science Literature". *Annual Review of Sociology* 27: 235–260.

GÄHLER, M. 2004. "Levnadsnivåundersökningen (LNU)" (The Swedish Level of Living Survey). In M. BYGREN, M. GÄHLER and M. NERMO (eds.), *Familj och Arbete – Vardagsliv i Förändring Family and work – Everyday Life in Transition.* Stockholm: SNS Förlag.

HALLAK, J. C. & LEVINSOHN, J. 2004. "Fooling Ourselves: Evaluating the Globalization and Growth Debate". *Working Paper 10244.* Cambridge: National Bureau of Economic Research.

HANSON, G. & HARRISON, A. 1995. "Trade, Technology, and Wage Inequality". *Working paper 5110.* Cambridge: National Bureau of Economic Research.

HERTZMAN, C. & SIDDIQI, A. 2000. "Health and Rapid Economic Change in the Twentieth Century". *Social Science & Medicine* 51: 809–819.

HESTON, A., SUMMERS, R. & ATEN, B. October 2002. *Penn World Tables Version 6.1.* Center for International Comparisons at the University of Pennsylvania (CICUP). www.pwt.econ.upenn.edu

KARASEK, R. 1979. "Job Demands, Job Decision Latitude, and Mental Strain: Implications for Job Redesign". *Administrative Science Quarterly* 24: 285–308.

KAWACHI, I., KENNEDY, B. P. & WILKINSON, R. G. (eds.) 1999. *Income Inequality and Health: A Reader*. New York: The New Press.

KORPI, T. & STERN, C. 2006. "Globalization, Deindustrialization, and the Labor Market Experiences of Swedish Women 1950 to 2000". In H. P. BLOSSFELD and H. HOFMEISTER (eds.). *Globalization, Uncertainty, and Women's Careers: An International Comparison*. Cheltenham, UK and Northampton, MA., USA: Edward Elgar.

KORPI, T. & TÅHLIN, M. 2006. "The Impact of Globalization on Men's Labor Market Mobility in Sweden". In H.-P. BLOSSFELD, M. MILLS and F. BERNARDI (eds.), *Globalization, Uncertainty and Men's Careers: An International Comparison*. Cheltenham: UK and Northampton: MA., USA: Edward Elgar.

KRUGMAN, P., COOPER, R. N. & SRINIVASAN, T. N. 1995. "Growing World Trade: Causes and Consequences", *Brooking Papers on Economic Activity* 1, 25th Anniversary Issue: 327–377.

LUNDBERG, O. 1990. "*Den Ojämlika Ohälsan. Om Klass- och Könsskillnader i Sjuklighet*" (Inequality in ill Health. On Class and Sex Differences in Illnes). Swedish Institute for Social Research Dissertation Series 11, Stockholm University.

LUNDBERG, O. 1991A. "Causal Explanations for Class Inequality in Health – An Empirical Analysis". *Social Science & Medicine* 32: 385–393.

LUNDBERG, O. 1991B. "Childhood Living Conditions, Health Status, and Social Mobility: A Contribution to the Health Selection Debate". *European Sociological Review* 7: 149–161.

MCCORMICK, I. A. & COOPER, C. L. 1988. "Executive Stress: Extending the International Comparison", *Human Relations* 41: 65–72.

MCMICHAEL, A. J., SPIRTAS, R. & KUPPER, L. L. 1974. "An Epidemiologic Study of Mortality within a Cohort of Rubber Workers, 1964–72". *Journal of Occupational Medicine* 16: 458–464.

MERLLIÉ, D., & PAOLI, P. 2001. *Ten Years of Working Conditions in the European Union*. Dublin: European Foundation for the Improvement of Living and Working Conditions.

MORRIS, M. & WESTERN, B. 1999. "Inequality in Earnings at the Close of the Twentieth Century". *Annual Review of Sociology* 25: 623–657.

NAVARRO, V. 1999. "Health and Equity in the World in the Era of Globalization", *International Journal of Health Services*. 29: 215–226.

OECD. 1997. *Employment Outlook*. Paris: OECD.

OECD. 2003. *Indicators of Economic Globalization*. Directorate for Science, Technology and Industry: Committee on Industry and Business Environment. Paris: OECD.

OHLIN, B. 1933. *Interregional and International Trade*. Cambridge: Harvard University Press.

O'ROURKE, K. H. 2003. "Heckscher-Ohlin Theory and Individual Attitudes Towards Globalization". *Working paper 9872*. Cambridge: National Bureau of Economic Research.

PAOLI, P. 1992. *First European Survey on the Working Environment 1991–1992*. Dublin: European Foundation for the Improvement of Living and Working Conditions.

PAOLI, P. 1997. *Second European Survey on the Working Environment 1995–1996*, Dublin: European Foundation for the Improvement of Living and Working Conditions.

PAOLI, P., & MERLLIÉ, D. 2001. *Third European Survey on Working Conditions 2000*. Dublin: European Foundation for the Improvement of Living and Working Conditions.

PELFRENE, E., VLERICK, P., MOREAU, M., MAK, R. P., KORNITZER, M. & DE BACKER, G. 2003. "Perceptions of Job Insecurity and the Impact of World Market Competition as Health Risks: Results from Belstress". *Journal of Occupational and Organizational Psychology* 76: 411–425.

RICARDO, D. [1911] 2004. *The Principles of Political Economy and Taxation*. New York: Dover Publications.

SCHEVE, K. & SLAUGHTER, M. J. 2002. "Economic Insecurity and the Globalization of Production", *Working paper 9339*. Cambridge: National Bureau of Economic Research.

STRAUSS-KAHN, V. 2003. "The Role of Globalization in the Within-industry Shift Away from Unskilled Workers in France", *Working paper 9716*. Cambridge: National Bureau of Economic Research.

WACZIARG, R. & HORN WELCH, K. H. 2003. "Trade Liberalization and Growth: New Evidence", *Working paper 10152*. Cambridge: National Bureau of Economic Research.

WIKMAN, A. 1991. "*Att Utveckla Sociala Indikatorer – en Surveyansats Belyst med Exemplet Arbetsmiljö*" (Developing Social Indicators – an efffort with the Survey Method, Illustrated with Example of Working Environment). *Urval* 21. Stockholm: Statistiska Centralbyrån.

WOOD, A. 1995. "How Trade Hurt Unskilled Workers". *Journal of Economic Perspectives* 9: 57–80.

WOODWARD, D., DRAGER, N., BEAGLEHOLE, R. & LIPSON, D. 2001. "Globalization and Health: a Framework for Analysis and Action". *Bulletin of the World Health Organization* 79: 875–880.

WORLD HEALTH ORGANIZATION (WHO) & WORLD TRADE ORGANIZATION (WTO). 2002. *WTO Agreements and Public Health. A Joint Study by the WHO and the WTO Secretariat*. Geneva: WTO Secretariat.

WORLD TRADE ORGANIZATION (WTO). 2003. "Adjusting to Trade Liberalization, The Role of Policy, Institutions and WTO Disciplines". In BACCHETTA, M. and JANSEN, M., *Studies Special 7*. Geneva: WTO publications.

ÖSTLIN, P. 1989. "Occupational Career and Health. Methodological Considerations on the Healthy Worker Effect", Dissertation from the Faculty of Medicine 224: Uppsala University.

Appendix

The Healthy Worker Effect –
Analyses on Swedish Panel Data

Introduction

In this section, a possible impact of declined health on sectoral mobility will be analysed. If the influence of health on labour market mobility is greater for employees in manufacturing compared with workers in private service and public service, the results support a healthy worker effect, implying that workers in manufacturing might change industry due to declining health more often than workers in other industries. Furthermore, the relation between health and labour market exits is studied. If poor health status affects labour market exits in manufacturing more than such exits in other industries, this indicates that workers' health has different implications in different industries and thus supports a healthy worker effect.

A. Indicators and Methods

The data consist of information from 2517 employees[1] in the panel of the Swedish Level of Living Survey (LNU) 1991 and 2000, i.e. individuals included in both surveys[2] (see section 8A for a description of the data used). The industries are categorised according to the Swedish Standard Industrial Classification (Svensk Näringsgrensindelning, SNI), classifying activities of firms in accordance with the NACE codes (standard for the European Union). Thus, manufacturing, private service and public service were distinguished in a similar way as for the analyses on EFWCS data (see section 8B).

---

[1] The selection of individuals was made in a similar way as for the analyses on EFWCS data: full-time or part-time working employees (1991), not over 65 years of age at the time of the second interview (i.e. 2000). Employees working less than 10 hours per week (1991) were excluded.

[2] Employment status between the two interviews is not ascertained in the analyses. This means that sectoral mobility or a labour market exit that takes place after the first interview and that does not last until the time of the next interview is not considered.

Two dichotomised variables have been constructed as indicators of health, one measuring mental well-being and the other indicating physical health. The indicator of mental well-being is partly based on an additive index including the five items [*"Have you during the past twelve months experienced:*] *"overall tiredness", "sleeplessness", "nervous troubles", "depression", "overstrain"*[3], and partly based on a question about mental illness. Individuals that score three or more on the index or answered *"Yes, minor"* or *"Yes, severe"* to the question about mental illness are classified as having reduced mental well-being and are thus coded 1.

The measure for physical health is partly created out of three additive indexes covering *"Aches"*[4], *"Stomach problems"*[5] and *"Circulatory problems"*[6]. A person with three points or more on any of these indexes is considered as having poor physical health. Moreover, if an individual who has myocardial infarction or organic nerve disease, has answered *"Yes, severe"* to questions about serious health problems such as cancer, diabetes, asthma, struma, tuberculosis, gall problems, gastric ulcer, kidney troubles, or if the individual cannot run or walk 100 meters or climb a staircase – he or she is classified as having physical health problems. The variable is dichotomous and takes the value 1 for individuals who are considered as having poor physical health.

Health status in 1991 and the development of health between 1991 and 2000 are both used as measures of health in the analyses. The latter indicator was calculated as health status in 2000 minus health status in 1991. Consequently, a positive score indicates a decline in health between 1991 and 2000.

Lundberg (1990, 1991A, 1991B) has used these indicators of mental well-being and physical health (with minor divergences) in studies of health-related social mobility and health inequalities on data from the Swedish Level of Living Surveys in 1968, 1974 and 1981.

The measure of labour market exit is a dichotomous variable, taking the value 1 for individuals employed in 1991, but not employed in

---

[3] The answers were coded 0 for *"No"*, 1 for *"Yes, minor"* and 3 for *"Yes, severe"*.

[4] An additive index based on three questions concerning aches: *"aches in shoulders"*, *"aches in the back/hips"* and *"aches in hands, elbows, legs or knees"*. The answer *"No"* is coded 0, *"Yes, minor"* is coded 1 and *"Yes, severe"* is coded 3.

[5] An additive index based on four questions concerning stomach problems: *"stomach pain"*, *"sickness"*, *"vomiting"* and *"diarrhea"*. The answer *"No"* is coded 0, *"Yes, minor"* is coded 1 and *"Yes, severe"* is coded 3.

[6] An additive index based on four questions concerning circulatory problems: *"chest pain"*, *"heart weakness"*, *"high blood pressure"* and *"dizziness"*. The answer *"No"* is coded 0, *"Yes, minor"* is coded 1 and *"Yes, severe"* is coded 3.

2000[7]. The indicator for change of industry is a dichotomous variable, coded 1 if the employee is working in 2000, but has changed industry in comparison with 1991.

Furthermore, a dichotomised variable was constructed, indicating the position of class, taking the value 1 for white-collar workers and 0 for blue-collar workers. In addition, age, sex, years of education and skill requirements of the job are included as control variables, since these are of significance for health-related mobility. The method used for the multivariate analyses is logistic regression.

B. Results from Panel Analyses

The descriptive statistics show that workers in private service with reduced mental well-being and in poor physical health in 1991 changed industry more often compared to individuals with health problems in 1991 employed in other industries (cf. table 1). Moreover, employees in private service with reduced mental well-being and in poor physical health 1991 have left the labour market by 2000 to a greater extent than employees with poor mental and physical health in manufacturing and public service, though the difference between industries regarding poor physical health and labour market exits is small in general.

Table 1: The share of employees in poor health in 1991 that have changed industry or left the labour market in 2000, by industry (%)

Industry	Employees with reduced mental well-being in 1991		Employees with poor physical health in 1991	
	Change of industry 2000	Labour market exit 2000	Change of industry 2000	Labour market exit 2000
Manufacturing 1991	30.0	32.6	27.2	22.7
Private service 1991	48.3	34.7	29.9	23.4
Public service 1991	18.1	26.5	13.2	21.5

Note: 9.0% of all employees (227 individuals) are categorised as having reduced mental well-being in 1991, and 36.1% of all workers (908) are classified as having poor physical health in 1991. The total sample size is 2517 individuals.

---

[7]   I.e. unemployed, pensioners, students, housekeepers or individuals who responded "other things". The analyses have been conducted both with and without including self-employed people in the category "exits from the labour market", and though this affected the estimates to some extent, it did not have any implications for the significance or direction of the interaction terms (health*industry).

C. Mobility between Industries

In table 2 the influence of mental well-being and physical health status on sectoral mobility is analysed.

Table 2: Mobility between industries.
Logistic regression, odds ratios. Standard errors in brackets

	Mental well-being				Physical health			
	Model 1a	Model 1b	Model 1c	Model 1d	Model 2a	Model 2b	Model 2c	Model 2d
Male	0.852 (0.105)	0.845 (0.105)	0.836 (0.103)	0.849 (0.105)	0.832 (0.102)	0.835 (0.103)	0.831 (0.102)	0.830 (0.102)
Age	0.973*** (0.006)	0.972*** (0.006)	0.973*** (0.006)	0.974*** (0.006)	0.973*** (0.006)	0.973*** (0.006)	0.973*** (0.006)	0.973*** (0.006)
Years of education	1.052* (0.024)	1.051* (0.024)	1.050* (0.024)	1.050* (0.024)	1.050* (0.024)	1.051* (0.024)	1.049* (0.024)	1.050* (0.024)
White-collar worker	1.211 (0.165)	1.206 (0.164)	1.209 (0.165)	1.215 (0.165)	1.218 (0.166)	1.213 (0.165)	1.216 (0.165)	1.207 (0.164)
Skill requirements of the job	0.800 (0.109)	0.796 (0.109)	0.801 (0.109)	0.803 (0.110)	0.802 (0.109)	0.797 (0.109)	0.802 (0.109)	0.804 (0.109)
Manufacturing	3.343*** (0.541)	3.498*** (0.591)	3.319*** (0.536)	3.275*** (0.534)	3.314*** (0.535)	3.696*** (0.714)	3.313*** (0.535)	3.254*** (0.528)
Private service	3.559*** (0.522)	3.523*** (0.542)	3.504*** (0.513)	3.342*** (0.498)	3.495*** (0.511)	3.859*** (0.685)	3.494*** (0.511)	3.418*** (0.502)
Poor health in 1991	1.572* (0.333)	1.698 (0.524)			1.027 (0.126)	1.267 (0.275)		
Health decline 1991-2000			1.008 (0.153)	0.765 (0.199)			1.012 (0.099)	0.834 (0.152)
Poor health in 1991 * manufacturing		0.535 (0.287)				0.724 (0.224)		
Poor health in 1991 * private service		1.309 (0.649)				0.750 (0.219)		
Health decline 1991-2000 * manufacturing				1.210 (0.454)				1.257 (0.321)
Health decline 1991-2000 * private service				1.897 (0.697)				1.353 (0.320)
Pseudo-R2	0.07	0.07	0.07	0.07	0.07	0.07	0.07	0.07
Observations	1,947 (2,517)	1,947 (2,517)	1,938 (2,517)	1,938 (2,517)	1,949 (2,517)	1,949 (2,517)	1,949 (2,517)	1,949 (2,517)

Reference categories are: female, blue-collar worker, jobs without skill requirements other than compulsory school, public service and employees without symptoms related to mental well-being or physical health problems in 1991.
Significance levels: ***p≤0.001, **p≤0.01, *p≤0.05.

The results show that mobility between industries is more common for employees in manufacturing and in private service compared with workers in public service. Furthermore, individuals with reduced mental well-being in 1991 are more likely to change industry (cf. table 2, model 1a).

However, sectoral mobility is not related to physical health (cf. table 2, model 2a). Besides, employees with a negative development regarding mental well-being or physical health during the 1990s are not more likely than other workers to change industry (cf. table 2, model 1c and 2c). Most importantly, there is no greater risk for individuals with reduced mental well-being or in poor physical health employed in manufacturing to change industry compared with such workers in other industries (cf. table 2, model 1b and 2b). Neither is there an increase of sectoral mobility for manufacturing workers who have experienced a health decline during the 1990s compared with employees who have a similar health development in other industries (cf. table 2, model 1d and 2d).

Furthermore, the results in table 2 suggest that higher age lowers the odds of changing industry, while a long education gives the opposite effect.

D. Labour Market Exits

A possible impact of mental well-being and physical health status on labour market exits is analysed in table 3. There is an increased risk for employees with reduced mental well-being or in poor physical health in 1991 to leave the labour market (cf. table 2, model 1a and 2a). Nonetheless, the interaction terms between industry and health are not significant (table 3, model 1b and model 2b). This indicates that there is no great risk for workers within manufacturing who have poor health to leave employment, compared with the risk of exits among individuals in other industries with symptoms related to mental well-being or physical health problems. Neither has a manufacturing worker who experienced a declining situation regarding mental well-being or physical health during the 1990s a greater risk of labour market exit compared with a worker in another industry who has a similar development regarding health (cf. table 3, model 1d and 2d).

The estimates of the variables controlled for in table 3 indicate that higher age and being female increases the risk of labour market exits, while long education, white-collar work and having a job with high skill requirements reduces this risk.

Table 3: Labour market exits. Logistic regression, odds ratios. Standard errors in brackets

	Mental well-being				Physical health			
	Model 1a	Model 1b	Model 1c	Model 1d	Model 2a	Model 2b	Model 2c	Model 2d
Male	0.725* (0.097)	0.728* (0.098)	0.705** (0.094)	0.703** (0.094)	0.715* (0.096)	0.716* (0.096)	0.692** (0.092)	0.687** (0.092)
Age	1.057*** (0.007)	1.057*** (0.007)	1.057*** (0.007)	1.057*** (0.007)	1.056*** (0.007)	1.056*** (0.007)	1.057*** (0.007)	1.057*** (0.007)
Years of education	0.935** (0.023)	0.935** (0.023)	0.931** (0.023)	0.931** (0.023)	0.941* (0.023)	0.942* (0.023)	0.932** (0.023)	0.932** (0.023)
White-collar worker	0.688** (0.099)	0.691** (0.100)	0.706* (0.101)	0.705** (0.101)	0.732* (0.105)	0.730* (0.105)	0.700* (0.100)	0.698* (0.092)
Skill requirements of the job	0.680** (0.097)	0.679** (0.097)	0.684** (0.097)	0.683** (0.097)	0.678** (0.097)	0.677** (0.096)	0.677** (0.096)	0.679** (0.096)
Manufacturing	1.044 (0.181)	0.996 (0.185)	1.015 (0.175)	1.012 (0.178)	1.035 (0.180)	1.070 (0.247)	1.027 (0.177)	1.015 (0.176)
Private service	1.290 (0.194)	1.246 (0.200)	1.225 (0.183)	1.235 (0.188)	1.234 (0.186)	1.319 (0.270)	1.238 (0.185)	1.193 (0.181)
Poor health in 1991	2.603*** (0.458)	2.285** (0.572)			2.033*** (0.251)	2.162*** (0.408)		
Health decline, 1991–2000			1.236 (0.186)	1.254 (0.270)			1.014 (0.108)	0.887 (0.144)
Poor health, 1991 * manufacturing		1.351 (0.599)				0.934 (0.293)		
Poor health, 1991 * private service		1.257 (0.526)				0.873 (0.248)		
Health decline, 1991–2000 * manufacturing				1.040 (0.386)				1.088 (0.296)
Health decline, 1991–2000 * private service				0.915 (0.329)				1.404 (0.345)
Pseudo-R2	0.09	0.09	0.08	0.08	0.09	0.09	0.08	0.08
Observations	2,270 (2,517)	2,270 (2,517)	2,262 (2,517)	2,262 (2,517)	2,272 (2,517)	2,272 (2,517)	2,272 (2,517)	2,272 (2,517)

*Reference categories are: female, blue-collar worker, jobs without skill requirements other than compulsory school, public service and employees without symptoms related to mental well-being or physical health problems in 1991. Significance levels: ***p≤=0.001, **p≤=0.01, *p≤=0.05.*

E. Conclusion Concerning a Healthy Worker Effect

The analyses on Swedish panel data for 1991 to 2000 do not indicate any increased risk for individuals employed in manufacturing with symptoms of reduced mental well-being or in poor physical health in 1991 to change industry or to experience labour market exits compared with employees in poor health in other industries. Neither are employees in manufacturing who have experienced a decline in mental well-being or physical health during the 1990s in a more vulnerable position than workers in other industries who have experienced a similar deterioration in health. However, the results show that an employee with reduced mental well-being in 1991 is more likely to change industry. Moreover, individuals with a decline in mental well-being or in poor physical health in 1991 have a much higher risk of labour market exits compared with other employees. Nevertheless, this could not be linked to any specific industry. Hence, the results suggest no apparent support for a healthy worker effect, i.e. there are no tendencies for health-related selection as regards mobility between industries or labour market exits that can be connected to a particular industry. Similar analyses have been carried out on employees in the panel of the Swedish Level of Living Survey (LNU) in 1981 and 1991 with the same results, i.e. the analyses do not support a health-related mobility that could be linked to manufacturing industry (results not presented).

Obviously, conclusions about a healthy worker effect must be drawn with care since the results only refer to the Swedish labour market, and possibly important events taking place between the two interviews are not considered. Nonetheless, the results on this specific case are very clear. In the absence of evidence to the contrary from other cases they indicate that the bias emanating from a healthy worker effect with regard to mobility differences across industries is small.

Health Inequalities in a Combined Framework of Work, Gender and Social Class

Lucía ARTAZCOZ, Joan BENACH,
Carme BORRELL & Imma CORTÉS

Introduction

A large number of studies have examined men's and women's health from different social perspectives. Research on men's health has been dominated by a structural framework focusing on occupational class differentials in morbidity and mortality, whereas women's health has been studied primarily using a role framework, emphasising women's roles as housewives and mothers, with paid employment seen as an additional role (Sorensen & Verbrugge 1987). The dominance of the role framework in studying women's ill health contrasts with the paucity of attention given to family roles and their influence on health in men, as well as to gender inequalities in health emanating from the unequal distribution of family demands (Hall 1992, Hunt & Annandale 1993). On the other hand, studies on women's health have neglected the role of social class as a social category.

These different approaches are consistent with the traditional sexual division of society that assigns men a primary role in the public and labour spheres, whereas women occupy a primary role in family life. The division of labour dictates that men of working age are expected to devote themselves primarily to their professional life, whereas women, especially married women and/or mothers, are expected to devote themselves primarily to unpaid domestic responsibilities. Being born as a male or as a female implies living in a cultural context that determines different values, beliefs and attitudes, as well as different resources and opportunities, for men and women. This sexual division of labour permeates all levels and spheres of society (even research).

The class position interacts with gender by modifying the traditional allocation of men to paid work and women to domestic work. For example, women with high qualifications are more likely to enter the labour market, and they have a higher attachment to paid jobs than women in a lower socio-economic position do. According to Eurostat (Eurostat 2004), in 2003 the employment rate was 50.7% among EU-15 females aged 35-39 with pre-primary or lower-secondary education levels, whereas the corresponding percentages among those with upper-secondary and post-secondary non-tertiary education levels, and those with tertiary education levels, were 73.8% and 82.9% respectively.

As a consequence, different employment status categories (i.e. employees, unemployed people, full-time homemakers etc.) could have a different meaning for women, depending on their social class; therefore, the impact of employment status on health may differ. For example, losing a high-qualified job could be more detrimental to women than losing a less qualified one (Moss 2002). On the other hand, not only gender differences in the impact of combining job and family life may exist, but also social class differences among women, where those of lower social positions, with less resources, face more difficulties and probably experience a greater negative impact on their health.

Nowadays, in a context of transition from the traditional gender roles to more equal positions of men and women in society, employment has become more and more important in women's lives, while family roles are expected to become more and more important for men. However, the meaning of being a parent, being married or not, and being in paid employment or not, is still likely to be different between men and women, and likely to appear differently depending on social class. Therefore, for western industrial countries we propose an analysis framework of social determinants of health, in which these three social axes: gender, social class and work (paid and domestic work) interact in a complex way. These interactions determine effects on health both through exposure to different structural positions and conditions, and by the different experiences and reactions of men and women to the same structural positions. In the next sections we first analyse the interactions between these three social dimensions, and secondly their influence on health.

Given the paucity of studies that analyse the interactions between these dimensions in determining health status, we illustrate the need for using a combined framework of gender and social class by focusing on some studies carried out in Catalonia (Spain) that systematically analyse the interaction between gender, employment status, family roles and social class (Artazcoz *et al.* 2001a, Artazcoz *et al.* 2004a, Artazcoz *et al.* 2004b, Artazcoz *et al.* 2005). In addition, we compare our results with other studies of social inequalities in health.

1. Social Inequalities in the Labour Market

A. *Labour Force Participation*

Throughout Europe, women's labour participation is significantly lower than men's (table 1). Moreover, whereas in all the EU-15 countries parenthood significantly reduces women's employment, men's employment either does not significantly change or even increases (table 2). In general, qualified women are better integrated into the labour market than the less qualified ones. Furthermore, educational level plays an even bigger role when women have children and other family responsibilities. In all the EU-15 countries, the participation of mothers in full-time work increases in accordance with their level of qualifications (Ballarin *et al.* 2004).

There is a horizontal division of the labour market, with the female working population densely concentrated in certain sectors of activity and in certain professions. It is precisely in these sectors that the levels of remuneration are the lowest. Vertical segregation of the labour market, i.e. the concentration of women in the lower categories of the professional hierarchy, reinforces the effects of horizontal segregation and also accounts for women's low wages. In the EU-15, men's wages are 15% higher than women's, with significant differences between countries (table 3).

Table 1: Labour force participation in the EU-15 by gender (2003)

	Men	Women	Gender Difference
European Union	**65.8**	**48.1**	**17.7**
Belgium	60.5	43.6	16.9
Denmark	71.4	59.8	11.6
Germany	65.4	49.7	15.7
Greece	60.4	37.9	22.5
Spain	66.5	42.8	23.7
France	62.8	49.7	13.1
Ireland	71	49.7	21.3
Italy	62.2	37.1	25.1
Luxembourg	65.4	44.7	20.7
Netherlands	73.1	56.4	16.7
Austria	70.2	54.7	15.5
Portugal	66.2	58.4	7.8
Finland	70.6	54.9	15.7
Sweden	65.8	48.1	17.7
United Kingdom	60.5	43.6	16.9

Source: Eurostat.

**Table 2: Employment rate in EU-15 countries by number
of children 0-14 and gender, among people 25-49 years old (2003)**

	Men				Women			
	0	1	2	>2	0	1	2	>2
European Union	**83.8**	**92.2**	**93.2**	**88.1**	**74.4**	**67.7**	**60.9**	**45.4**
Belgium	85.7	79.6	89.1	-	70.2	76.8	72.9	-
Germany	87.9	-	-	-	78.5	-	-	-
Greece	81.6	89.7	91.6	85.1	80.3	70.8	60.9	41.5
Spain	86.0	96.3	96.8	94.9	61.9	56.3	54.1	45.4
France	81.9	92.6	93.8	90.8	64.8	55.0	48.4	41.1
Ireland	83.6	92.5	92.6	88.9	77.9	77.1	67.8	46.2
Italy	87.8	-	-	-	67.2	-	-	-
Luxembourg	82.1	94.0	94.4	91.4	61.9	54.7	47.3	35.9
Netherlands	89.3	96.6	96.9	95.0	77.4	67.7	54.4	41.0
Austria	89.4	93.1	94.9	92.0	82.2	74.3	71.8	59.9
Portugal	83.7	94.9	94.0	92.8	75.3	78.9	77.2	63.1
United Kingdom	84.4	-	-	-	79.0	-	-	-

Source: Eurostat.

Table 3: Gender salary difference in the EU-15 in percentages (2003)

	Salary gap
European Union	**16**
Belgium	-
Denmark	18
Germany	23
Greece	11
Spain	18
France	12
Ireland	14
Italy	-
Luxembourg	15
Netherlands	18
Austria	17
Portugal	9
Finland	-
Sweden	16
United Kingdom	22

Source: Eurostat.

B. Unemployment

Although unemployment rates vary widely from country to country, women's unemployment rate is higher than men's in 10 of the EU-15 countries (table 4). Consistent with data about labour force participation, the highest unemployment rates among women and the biggest gender gap can be found in countries with a strong male breadwinner model, such as Spain, Greece and Italy. Moreover, less qualified workers are more likely to be unemployed and the gender gap in employment is greater among less privileged workers (table 5).

Societies with a strong version of the male breadwinner model of the gender contract are likely to consider the absence of certain categories of women, i.e. wives and mothers with young children, from the labour market as legitimate. Thus, women in these categories may well be without a job, but they will not be considered, and will probably not consider themselves, to be unemployed to the same extent as men in similar circumstances. Moreover, in countries where the male breadwinner model persists more strongly, unemployment benefits are usually only awarded to those with a continuous type of employment pattern and/or to those who have previously worked for the minimum number of hours per week required to qualify for benefits. Thus, women who have had a career break or who were previously working part-time may not fulfil the conditions needed to receive unemployment benefits (Ballarin *et al.* 2004).

Table 4: Unemployment rates in the EU-15 by gender (2003)

	Men	Women	Gender difference
European Union	**7.4**	**8.9**	**-1.5**
Belgium	7.4	8	-0.6
Denmark	5.1	5.7	-0.6
Germany	10.2	9.3	0.9
Greece	6	14.3	-8.3
Spain	7.9	15.8	-7.9
France	7.5	9.5	-2
Ireland	4.8	4	0.8
Italy	6.9	11.9	-5
Luxembourg	3	4.6	-1.6
Netherlands	3.5	3.8	-0.3
Austria	3.9	4.3	-0.4
Portugal	5.2	7.2	-2
Finland	11	9.9	1.1
Sweden	6.1	5	1.1
United Kingdom	5.4	4	1.4

Source: Eurostat.

**Table 5: Percentages of unemployment by level of education
and gender in EU-15 (2003)**

	Men	Women	Gender difference
Pre-primary, primary and lower-secondary education	10.1	13.4	-3.3
Upper-secondary and post-secondary non-tertiary education	7.4	8.6	-1.2
Tertiary education	4.4	5.6	-1.2

Source: Eurostat.

C. Temporary Work

In recent years employers and policy makers have considered labour market flexibility as a means of improving workers' performance and adaptability to technical change and increasing globalization (OECD 1998). Alongside these changes within production, employment conditions have become less stable. Temporary employment is significantly higher among women, with differences among EU-15 countries (table 6). Interestingly there is no gradient by educational level, and the higher gender differences are found among workers with higher education (table 7).

Temporary work makes it possible to fit the size of the employed workforce and paid working time as closely as possible to the volume of goods and services immediately required. However, it has been pointed out that this job flexibility can legitimise human resource management methods which push workers to their physical and mental breaking points, implying selection of workers, and abdication from responsibility for the consequences of these management methods, both in terms of the human and financial cost of unemployment, and in terms of meeting the health and economic costs of occupationally disabled workers excluded from the labour market (Thébaud-Mony 2001).

2. Social Inequalities in Domestic Labour

The distribution of domestic labour is fundamental in the analysis of women's work. The differences in rates and kinds of employment for men and women are explained to a large extent by the exclusive attribution of the domestic sphere to women. Still, many women in the EU-15 work as full-time homemakers, but important differences between countries exist. In 2003, whereas only half of all women aged 20 to 49 were employed in countries such as Spain or Italy with a predominant male breadwinner model the percentage in Denmark or Finland was about 80% (Eurostat 2005).

Even when they have a paid job, the task of 'domestic management' is undertaken by women of all social classes, also by the most privileged women who earn enough in paid work to delegate some of the domestic tasks that society has assigned to them, to persons outside the home, usually to other women cleaners and childminders (Kempeneers & Leliëvre 1991, Lundberg *et al.* 1994). Although, as has been mentioned before, women are paid less than their male counterparts, they are more likely to use their own salary to remunerate the people hired to carry out domestic tasks or to look after children, than to expect their spouse to make a financial contribution to these costs (Ballarin *et al.* 2004). This unequal distribution of expenditure linked to the smooth running of the household reveals the extent to which women are considered, and may sometimes consider themselves, as being solely responsible for domestic work and childcare. Paid work may also be experienced as something which prevents them from carrying out their domestic work correctly, i.e. according to the standards set by society (De Konink *et al.* 2001). Women often seek to limit the consequences of their employment for their families, either by eroding their free time when they have to do this work themselves (Nickols & Abdel-Ghany 1983, Hochschild 1989, Thrane 2000), or by taking responsibility for the financial cost of finding a substitute worker to cover for their absence (Artazcoz *et al.* 2001a, Artazcoz *et al.* 2001b).

**Table 6: Percentage of temporary employees
in the EU-15 by gender (2003)**

	Men	Women	Gender difference
European Union	8.3	10.6	-2.3
Belgium	4.2	9.1	-4.9
Denmark	5	8.6	-3.6
Germany	6.3	6.8	-0.5
Greece	8.5	11.9	-3.4
Spain	24.1	29.2	-5.1
France	7.2	10.8	-3.6
Ireland	2.1	3.6	-1.5
Italy	6.4	10.4	-4
Luxembourg	1.5	3.5	-2
Netherlands	8	11.8	-3.8
Austria	2.1	3.3	-1.2
Portugal	15.5	18.7	-3.2
Finland	9	16.4	-7.4
Sweden	9.2	12.6	-3.4
United Kingdom	4.1	5.8	-1.7

Note: Temporary employees are defined as salaried workers with fixed-term or non-fixed-term temporary contracts.
Source: Eurostat.

**Table 7: Percentage of temporary employees in the EU-15
by gender and level of education (2003)**

	Men	Women	Gender difference
Pre-primary, primary and lower-secondary education	14.1	16.7	-2.6
Upper-secondary and post-secondary non-tertiary education	6.4	8.7	-2.3
Tertiary education	9.4	13.8	-4.4

Note: Temporary employees are defined as salaried workers with fixed-term or on-fixed-term temporary contracts.
Source: Eurostat.

3. Analysis of the Interaction between Gender, Social Class and Work in Determining Health

The influence of multiple roles – as an employee, a spouse and a mother – on women's health has been examined, but the results are not consistent. The contradictory findings may be due to the insufficient characterisation of each role. In some studies, having multiple roles implies having more than one principal role (thus number of roles is the focus); in others, it means combining job and family responsibilities (i.e. a focus on type of roles) (Sorensen & Verbrugge 1987). However, the relation between multiple roles and health not only depends on the number or the type of roles occupied, but also on the nature of the particular roles. In other words, the exposures related to the job differ by occupational status, or those associated with marital or parental status depend to a great extent on the family demands associated with these roles. Moreover, the effect of family demands on health may be different depending on different employment status – Is being responsible for three children the same for a full-time homemaker as for an employed woman? – and even for the same employment status, there may be differences depending on occupational social class. Women of more privileged classes can finance domestic work provided by other women, thus relieving them of part of this burden.

The limited number of outcomes analysed in most studies is another shortcoming of the research on health inequalities. Many studies merely analyse one outcome, i.e. self-perceived health status, long-standing limiting illness, chronic conditions or mental health. However, determinants of different health conditions may differ, and it is necessary to analyse different health indicators in order to obtain a global picture of the social determinants of health (Macintyre *et al.* 1996).

A systematic analysis of the influence of family, social class and paid work, as well as the multiple interactions among them, should be carried out in both sexes. Given that gender and class determine different values and beliefs as well as resources and opportunities in social life, this approach should combine both a structural perspective that focuses on the objective social positions and conditions of men and women, and a psychological perspective that emphasises the actual experiences and reactions in each of the different social domains.

The epidemiological analysis of such complex interactions among gender, class, paid work and family roles (parental and marital status) is not easy. Many researchers argue that using interaction terms in statistical analysis serves the same purpose as using disaggregated models and has the advantage of preserving parsimony. Even though this position can be defended on statistical grounds, some of the theoretical richness and intuitive interpretability of disaggregated models is lost. Moreover, several significant interaction terms of three or four variables could be found, making it difficult to interpret these relationships (Kunkel & Atchely 1996). In order to understand this complexity, we propose to analyse different pieces of reality by restricting the study populations according to some variables; to fit statistical models separated for the social variables of interest; and to give full theoretical voice to the complexity of the socially constructed meaning of the combined impact of gender, social class and work. For a more intuitive understanding of our proposal we try to answer questions such as, for example, whether having family responsibilities has the same impact on men's and women's health status, whether it is the same for employed or unemployed people and, finally, whether the relationship depends on social class.

Specifically, among people aged 25-64 years (people with active productive and reproductive roles) we will analyse: 1) the role of family demands in shaping women's health by employment status (employed and full-time homemakers) and social class; 2) the impact on health of combining job and family roles by gender and social class; 3) the influence of unemployment status on mental health by gender, family roles, and social class and 4) the impact of temporary work on different psychosocial health domains. Although it can be interesting to analyse other possible combinations of social roles – e.g. previously married people – and additional employment status categories or social situations – such as those of lone parents – these combinations are less frequent and their limited number in health surveys (the main data source used in the studies presented in the next sections) makes them difficult to study.

We illustrate the use of this combined framework of work, gender and social class in explaining health, by focusing primarily on four studies that have systematically analysed the interactions between gender, social class and work (paid jobs and domestic work) carried out in Catalonia, a region in the north-east of Spain which has about 6 million inhabitants (Artazcoz *et al.* 2001a, Artazcoz *et al.* 2004a; Artazcoz *et al.* 2004b). In addition we compare our results with other studies of social inequalities in health.

In three studies the data were taken from the 1994 Catalonian Health Survey (CHS), a cross-sectional survey based on a representative sample of the non-institutionalised population of Catalonia. The survey included self-reported information on morbidity, health status, health-related behaviours and use of health care services as well as socio-demographic data. Fifteen thousand subjects were randomly selected using a multiple stage random sampling strategy. For each of the 8 health regions of Catalonia, the first sampling stage consisted of selecting municipalities (or municipal districts in the case of the Barcelona city health region) according to their population size (8 strata). In each of these strata, cluster random sampling was employed to select individuals by using proportional probabilities according to the weight of the municipality (or district). Trained interviewers administered the questionnaires at home in a face-to-face interview from January to December 1994 to avoid a potential seasonal bias. Only 5.4% of subjects were substituted due to refusal or absence of those initially selected. Half of those in the total sample were aged 25-64 years.

The population selected for the study that compared employed women and full-time homemakers comprised 1,191 female workers and 1,675 housewives aged 25 to 64 years, who were married or cohabiting, (Artazcoz *et al.* 2001). The sample for analysing gender differences in the health impact of combining job and family responsibilities included 2,148 men and 1,191 women aged 25 to 64 years, who were employed, married or cohabiting, (Artazcoz *et al.* 2004a). Finally, the analysis of the effect of unemployment on mental health was based on a sample of 2,422 men and 1,459 women who were employed, and 371 men and 267 women who were unemployed, all aged 25-64 years (Artazcoz *et al.* 2004b). To avoid a possible reverse causation effect, those individuals reporting a limiting long-standing illness (LLI) during the 12 months prior to the survey, and those unemployed who were not actively looking for work, were excluded from the analysis. Among the employed, 8% of men and 12% of women reported LLI in the last 12 months, whereas the prevalences of LLI among the unemployed were 10% and 17% respectively.

In the study about flexible employment and psychosocial health (Artazcoz *et al*. 2005), the data were derived from the 2002 Catalonian Health Survey (CHS), a cross-sectional study based on a representative sample of 8400 persons. For the purposes of this study we selected a subsample of all salaried workers aged 16-64 with no LLI (1474 men and 998 women).

A. Differences in Health Status between Employed and Full-time Homemaker Females

It is generally assumed that women engaged in paid work have better health than full-time homemakers (Nathanson 1980, Verbrugge 1983, Nathanson 1995, Waldron & Jacobs 1998, Annandale & Hunt 2000). It has been reported that family-role occupancy benefits the well-being of employed women in two ways: partnered women report higher well-being than single women, and the quality and experience in each role makes an independent contribution to subjective well-being (Barnett & Marschall 1991). Moreover, some studies have confirmed that the better health of employed women does not simply reflect a 'healthy worker' effect (Passannante & Nathanson 1985, Arber 1997, Waldron & Jacobs 1998). The job environment can offer opportunities to build self-esteem and confidence in one's decision-making, social support for otherwise isolated individuals, and experiences that enhance life satisfaction (Sorensen & Verbrugge 1987). Additionally, income provides women with financial independence and increases their power in the household unit. These findings support the role enhancement hypothesis.

However, other studies support the role-overload or role-conflict hypotheses. It has been reported that employment has beneficial effects on the health of unmarried women, but has little or no effect for married women (Waldron *et al*. 1998). Also, that the health benefits for mothers with a job are restricted to those working part-time (Bartley *et al*. 1992, Walters *et al*. 1996, Bartley *et al*. 1999). The provision of support and care may be emotionally satisfying and may also provide some social status for the woman. Yet, for women in paid work, taking care of their family and the associated domestic work can be very draining and impair their health. Therefore, it seems that when the total workload is high, combining job and family demands can be detrimental to health.

Significant interactions between employment status and structural disadvantage, measured through marital status and housing tenure, have been reported in the analysis of social determinants of women's health status (Arber 1991). A study carried out in Spain concluded that among married females aged 25-64, employed women showed an overall better health status than full-time homemakers, regardless of social class, although the employed had more unfavourable health-related behaviours (Artazcoz *et al.* 2001a). Moreover, health advantages depended on the health indicator analysed and were more consistent for workers who had a low socio-economic position (figure 1).

Figure 1: Different health indicators among female full-time homemakers with low education as compared to employed women with low education

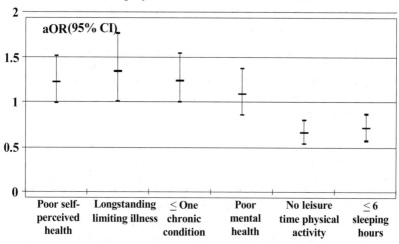

Source: Artazcoz L., Borrell C., Benach J., Cortès I., Rohlfs I., "Women, family demands and health: The importance of employment status and socio-economic position". Soc Sci Med 2004; 59: 263-74.

Additionally, living with children under 15 was not related to health among employed women but it had a positive effect on mental health among more privileged full-time homemakers (Artazcoz *et al.* 2004a). Research on the impact of parenthood on health overall shows that, among women, having children at home either decreases psychological well-being or has no impact at all (Ross *et al.* 1990). In favourable circumstances children could improve the well-being of women (Ross & Mirowsky 1988). Whereas for women of low educational level the financial strain and the domestic work associated with having children can be important sources of stress, for more privileged women who enjoy high household material standards, children mainly mean a source of satisfaction.

Although many studies about health differences between employed women and full-time homemakers have focused on mental health, recent studies have found more differences in terms of physical health (Khlat *et al.* 2000). However, in Spain, a higher consumption of sleeping pills or tranquillisers has been reported among housewives in both low and high socio-economic positions as compared with employed women, after adjusting for age and family demands (Artazcoz *et al.* 2004a). The consumption of these drugs could mask an excess of poor mental health among housewives, and thus explain why differences by employment status were not found. These findings illustrate the importance of examining different health indicators when analysing social determinants of health.

It is interesting to note the reported poorer health status of full-time homemakers although their health behaviours (sleeping time and physical exercise during leisure time) are more favourable, and that this paradox is independent of social class (Artazcoz *et al.* 2004a). Both short sleeping time and insufficient physical exercise during leisure time are to a great extent related to lack of time. In the long run one might suspect that without increased gender equality in family responsibilities, a paid job could have negative health effects for female workers.

B. Social Inequalities in Health Related to the Combination of Job and Family Demands

Despite the dramatic increase of women in the labour market in recent decades, there has often been no significant change in the distribution of domestic work, even when both partners are working (Bartley *et al.* 1992). The sexual division of labour remains unchanged; when women have a paid job outside the home, they will still typically have the main responsibility for childcare and housework. Women do not yet have the power to force men to undertake an equal share of domestic labour and childcare, no matter how high the status of their employment is (Bartley 1999). These inequalities in private life may be a cause of gender inequalities in health.

Moreover, social class can be an important element in shaping the association between family demands and health among people exposed to the double burden of paid and domestic work. Lennon and Rosenfield (Lennon & Rosenfield 1992) reported that the degree of control at work (higher among more qualified workers) moderates the effects of demands in the family setting. On the other hand, more privileged female workers have more resources for facing domestic work. Cleary (Cleary & Mechanic 1983) found a positive relationship between the number of children in the household and depression in women with paid employment, but this relationship was non-significant after controlling for family income. A high income makes it possible to hire paid help with domestic tasks and childcare, thus relieving working women of some of the overload.

In a study carried out in Catalonia (Spain) (Artazcoz *et al.* 2001a), among workers who were 25-64 years old, family demands were not associated with different health indicators either among men or among women of high socio-economic position. However, family demands were consistently related to different forms of ill health as well as with sleeping less than 6 hours a day and being sedentary during leisure time (figure 2). It has been reported that a working mother's ability to work and to sustain time spent in childcare is 'financed' by reductions in her personal care time (including sleep) and in passive leisure such as watching television (Hill & Stafford 1980). A lack of time is the most commonly cited barrier for participation in physical activity (Pate *et al.*1995); caring for children means not only work overload, but also constraints on autonomy and consequent difficulties for leisure-time physical activities, to an even greater extent for married women with a low educational level.

In a study based on a health survey carried out in Barcelona (Spain) (Artazcoz *et al.* 2001b), hiring a person to do domestic tasks was associated with good self-perceived health status among married female workers after adjusting for age and social class. No such association was found among married male workers. Interestingly, female domestic workers in Catalonia have been shown to have poorer health indicators after adjusting for age and occupational social class (Artazcoz *et al.* 2003).

It is interesting to note that in Spain, a protective effect of living with people older than 65 was found among employed married females with a low education. Nowadays, people older than 65 years of age have few limitations in their daily activities as compared with some years ago (Ruigómez *et al.* 1991). It seems likely that the negative association between living with older adults may be mediated by the emotional and/or instrumental support they provide (for example, the fact that they can look after the children at home). Given that the population of elderly people is growing rapidly, it is important to examine this topic in depth.

According to a report of the European Commission Unit for Equal Opportunities, although the provision of formal services is increasing, in most countries the non-formal network continues to be the main resource for childcare among employed mothers. The only exception is the Nordic countries, where publicly financed formal services are used all the more (Deven *et al.* 1998). In a study carried out in Madrid (Spain), 37% of families with children under 13, where both parents were in paid employment, reported receiving frequently or very frequently, the assistance of a female parent in caring for children, and 13% received such assistance from a male parent (Meil 1999).

Figure 2: Association between household size and different health indicators among manual female workers aged 25-64 years who are married or cohabiting (Reference: 2 members)

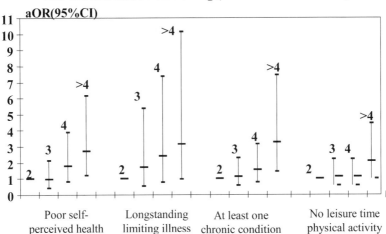

Source: Artazcoz L., Borrell C., Benach J., "Gender inequalities in health among workers: the relation with family demands". J Epidemiol Community Health *2001; 55: 639-47.*

C. Unemployment and Mental Health

One of the most studied health effects of unemployment is that of psychological distress among the unemployed (Bartley 1994, Dooley *et al.* 1996, Janlert 1997). However, despite the high prevalence of unemployment and mental health disorders among women, the different position of men and women in the labour market, and the gender differences in the social determinants of mental health (Piccinelli & Wilkinson 2000, Qin *et al.* 2000, Doyal 2001), the potential gender differences in health effects of unemployment have rarely been addressed. Indeed, many studies on unemployment have included only men (Bartley & Owen 1996, Leino-Arjas *et al.* 1999).

In a study concerning the impact of unemployment on mental health that systematically examined the potential interaction between gender, family roles (marital and parental status) and social class (manual and non-manual workers), three main findings were reported: 1) the beneficial effects of unemployment compensations are not equally distributed across different categories of gender, family roles, and social class, 2) the higher impact of unemployment on men's mental health is accounted for by workers with family responsibilities: marriage increases the risk of poor mental health for manual men, whereas for women, being married and, primarily, living with children, acts as a buffer; and 3) the mediating effect of social class in the impact of unemployment on mental health differs by gender and family roles (Artazcoz *et al.* 2004b).

In that study, carried out in Catalonia (Spain) (Artazcoz *et al.* 2004b) among people who were married or cohabiting, the negative effect of being unemployed without benefits was higher among male manual workers with family responsibilities (figure 3). The higher risk of poor mental health status in this group, much higher than that for single workers of the same social class, suggests that besides stigmatisation, financial problems may act as an additional source of poor mental health status. It could be that many manual workers live in households with a low income, but higher than that required for receiving social benefits. Therefore, being married can be a source of serious financial strain for unemployed men from lower social classes, primarily when they are the main breadwinners, as may well be the case for most of these workers. Moreover, due to their traditional low involvement in nurturant roles, for males, family responsibilities cannot successfully replace a job as an alternative source of goal and meaning in life.

Conversely, marriage and primarily motherhood, was seen to have a protective effect for women. Even when they are unemployed and not receiving benefits, most married women have their basic financial needs guaranteed by their husbands' income, just as parents guarantee those of most single unemployed females (in Spain almost all of them living with their parents). But for women, who still have a principal role in the family in developed countries (Bartley *et al.* 1992), nurturant roles could replace the rewards that were once provided by the job, as their reason to go on through the day and from one day to the next. This is consistent with the role enhancement hypothesis (Sorensen & Verbrugge 1987) that states that when troubles arise in one role – as is the case of unemployment – the others – caring for children for example – may be an alternative reward. Moreover, single unemployed women with no unemployment benefits receive financial support from their parents, for nothing in exchange, and this can have a stigmatising effect. Conversely, looking after the children can be the exchange for the financial support that married women receive from their husbands. Therefore, contrary to what some authors have suggested (Jahoda 1982, Lahelma 1992), it seems that it is the higher involvement of women in family responsibilities, rather than their lower attachment to the job, that explains the lower impact of unemployment on female workers' mental health.

D. *Job Flexibility and Psychosocial Health*

Although increasing job flexibility is one of the main features of current labour market policies, in comparison with literature about unemployment, very little research has been done to analyse the impact of flexible employment on individuals' health and living conditions. Such knowledge is likely to complement the arguments of those who advocate greater flexibility in the labour market for reasons of productivity. Recently a handful of studies have explicitly analysed the association between different forms of unstable contractual employment arrangements and mortality (Kivimäki *et al.* 2003) or other health outcomes (Benavides *et al.* 2000, Virtanen *et al.* 2002, Rodríguez 2002, Bardasi & Francesconi 2004, Benach *et al.* 2004), but their findings are inconsistent.

One of the shortcomings of studies about job flexibility is their lack of consideration of the potential interaction between gender and social class. Moreover, the impact of unstable contractual employment could reasonably be suspected to have negative effects on e.g. partnership formation or the decision to become a parent, but such associations have not been analysed.

A study carried out in Catalonia (Spain) (Artazcoz *et al.* 2005) showed that the effect of flexible contractual arrangements, other than fixed-term temporary contracts, on mental health was higher among less privileged groups (women and manual male workers), and that the impact of flexible employment, either fixed-term or non-fixed-term contracts, in family formation was more pronounced among men. In most countries, holding a job is an important predictor for cohabitation, marriage and parenthood among men. Moreover, in countries with a strong male breadwinner model, long-term and full-time employment for men is considered necessary in order to consolidate the financial basis considered as necessary for these transitions (Baizán *et al.* 2002).

Figure 3: Impact of unemployment with no financial compensations on the mental health of workers who are married or cohabiting, by gender and social class (Reference: employed people of the same sex and social class)

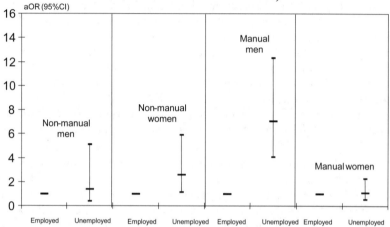

Source: Artazcoz L., Benach J., Borrell C., Cortés I., "Unemployment and mental health: Understanding the interactions among gender, family roles, and social class". Am J Public Health 2004; 94: 82-8.

4. Implications for Policies and Research

It has been pointed out that particular attention needs to be paid to the dialectical relationship between what happens to men and women in the employment sphere and their behaviour in the family, the production-reproduction interface. According to Battagliola (Battagliola 1984), the sexual differentiation of jobs and career paths is based on the different positions of men and women in the domestic sphere of reproduction, but is not a direct result of it. Personnel management policies, along with a number of informal rules and strategies of individuals, also play an important role in producing and reproducing the sexual division of labour, with regard to both paid and unpaid work. Moreover, welfare systems can also work either in favour of or against women entering the labour market, as well as positively or negatively affecting their chances of keeping their jobs when they are responsible for dependent children or adults.

It has been shown that the mechanisms of this dialectical relationship play a key role in the development of atypical employment patterns for women, particularly regarding part-time work. According to Kergoat's (Kergoat 1984) analysis of women's part-time work in France, it is often the case that women from households which are reasonably well-off, and whose efforts to gain promotion never meet with success, choose to take extended unpaid parental leave or to work part-time in an effort to distance themselves from unrewarding and monotonous jobs. Therefore it appears that in many cases the family situation of these women cannot explain their subordinate positions in the labour market, rather it serves as a relief from their limited professional career prospects. In much the same way, expectations about the breadwinner role of men serve to justify their promotion opportunities (Battagliola 1984).

Employment practices will thus tend to reflect the gender system or gender contract of society as a whole. If this contract is based on the idea that women's priorities remain in the home, employers will favour members of the gender group who are considered most likely to respond to their expectations. By operating a gender-differentiated system of staff management, employers contribute in turn to the reinforcement of gender norms. Women who have been socialised into these norms, and who experience objective discrimination in the labour market, will tend to transfer their personal aspirations to the one domain that is likely to satisfy them: the family. By adopting employment patterns that help them to cope with the domestic burden, i.e. career breaks, part-time work, etc., they will soon find themselves dependent on the professional success of their spouse. In order for the spouse to maximise his promotion prospects, the woman is likely to take on an even greater share of the domestic tasks and family responsibilities which they shared, more or less equally, when she was working full-time (Ballarin *et al.* 2004).

Women's informal caring for children, the elderly and the sick can have severe consequences for their health, employment, financial status and citizenship rights, primarily among less privileged women. Mothers and childminders supplement or substitute for the shortages of welfare-state services for children at a minimum cost to the welfare state that depends on an informal infrastructure of services usually provided by women. Any labour necessary for the maintenance of life which the state refuses to undertake, and which cannot be paid for through privatisation, is usually taken on by unpaid women, thus reducing their ability to participate in the paid labour market.

Social policies in different areas such as labour, health or gender-equal opportunities should take into account the combined impact of job and family on women's and men's health, as well as the dialectical relationship between the two domains. They should also take into account the modifying effect of gender and social class by analysing both spheres, their impact on health and the greater needs of less privileged persons.

Our results also have implications for future research. They point out the importance of using a combined framework of work, gender and social class in analysing the social determinants of health. This framework needs to analyse the interaction between gender, social class and work (paid and domestic work), combining a structural approach that emphasises different positions and conditions of men and women in society, with a psychological approach that considers the different gender experiences and reactions to the same structural conditions. Moreover, more attention should be paid to the role of family as an important determinant for the health and well-being of both men and women.

Ackowledgements

Funding: This study was partially funded by the Red de Investigación Temática de Salud y Género (exp. G03/042) and the Red de Centros de Investigación de Epidemiología y de Salud Pública (exp. c03/09).

References

ANNANDALE E., HUNT K. 2000. "Gender inequalities in health: Research at the crossroads". In ANNANDALE E., HUNT K., *Gender inequalities in health*. Buckingham: Open University Press: 1-35.

ARBER S. 1991. "Class, paid employment and family roles: Making sense of structural disadvantage, gender and health status". *Soc Sci Med* 32: 425-36.

ARBER S. 1997. "Comparing inequalities in women's and men's health in Britain in the 1990s". *Soc Sci Med* 44: 773-88.

ARTAZCOZ L., BENACH J., BORRELL C., CORTÉS I. 2005. "Social inequalities in the impact of flexible employment on different domains of psychosocial health". *J Epidemiol Community Health* 59: 761-7.

ARTAZCOZ L., BENACH J., BORRELL C., CORTÉS I. 2004b. "Unemployment and mental health: Understanding the interactions among gender, family roles, and social class". *Am J Public Health* 94: 82-8.

ARTAZCOZ L., BORRELL C., BENACH J., CORTÉS I., ROHLFS I. 2004a. "Women, family demands and health: The importance of employment status and socioeconomic position". *Soc Sci Med* 59: 263-74.

ARTAZCOZ L., BORRELL C., BENACH J. 2001a. "Gender inequalities in health among workers: the relation with family demands". *J Epidemiol Community Health* 55: 639-47.

ARTAZCOZ L., BORRELL C., ROHLFS I., BENI C., MONCADA A., BENACH J. 2001b. "Trabajo doméstico, género y salud en población ocupada (Housework, gender and health in the working population)". *Gac Sanit* 15: 150-3.

ARTAZCOZ L., CORTÉS I., BENACH J., BENAVIDES FG. 2003. "Les desigualtats en salut laboral a Catalunya (Occupational health inequalities in Catalonia)". In BORRELL C., BENACH J., *Les desigualtats en la salut a Catalunya* (Inequalities in health in Catalonia). Barcelona, Mediterrània: 251-82.

BAIZAN P., BILLARI F., MICHIELIN F. 2002. "Political Economy and Lifecourse Patterns: the Heterogeneity of Occupational, Family and Household Trajectories of Young Spaniards". *Demographic Research* 6: 189-240.

BALLARIN P., EULER C., LE FEUVRE N., RAEVAARA E., "Women in the European Union". [page visited: 02 09 04]. Accesible in: http://www.helsinki.fi/science/xantippa/wee/wee1.html.

BARDASI E., FRANCESCONI M. 2004. "The impact of atypical employment on individual wellbeing: evidence from a panel of British workers". *Soc Sci Med* 58: 1671-88.

BARNETT R., MARSCHALL N. 1991. "The Relationship Between Women's Work and Family Roles and their Subjective Well-being and Psychological distress". In FRANKENHEAUSER M., LUNDBERG U., CHESNEY M., *Women, Work and Health. Stress and Opportunities*. New York: Plenum Press: 111-36.

BARTLEY M., OWEN C. 1996. "Relation between socio-economic status, employment and health during economic change, 1973-93". *BMJ* 13: 445-9.

BARTLEY M., POPAY J., PLEWIS I. 1992. "Domestic conditions, paid employment and women's experience of ill-health". *Sociology of Health and Illness* 14: 313-43.

BARTLEY M., SACKER A., FIRTH D., FITZPATRICK R. 1999. "Social position, social roles and women's health in England: changing relationships 1984-1993". *Soc Sci Med* 48: 99-115.

BARTLEY M. 1999. "Measuring women's social position: the importance of theory". *J Epidemiol Community Health* 53: 601-2.

BARTLEY M. 1994. "Unemployment and ill health: understanding the relationship". *J Epidemiol Community Health* 48: 333-7.

BATTAGLIOLA F. 1984. "Employés et employées. Trajectoires familiales et professionnelles". In *Le sexe du travail: structures familiales et système productif*. Grenoble: 57-70.

BENACH J., GIMENO D., BENAVIDES FG., MARTINEZ JM., TORNE M., DEL M. 2004. "Types of employment and health in the European Union. Changes from 1995 to 2000". *Eur J Public Health* 14: 314–21.

BENAVIDES FG., BENACH J., DIEZ-ROUX AV., ROMAN C. 2000. "How do types of employment relate to health-indicators? Findings from the Second European Survey on Working Conditions". *J Epidemiol Community Health* 54: 495-501.

CLEARY PD., MECHANIC D. 1983. "Sex differences in psychological distress among married people". *J Health Soc Behav* 24: 111-21.

DE KONINK M., MALENFANT R., TARDIF J., POULIN V. 2001. *Maternité et précarisation de l'emploi*. Québec : Haute-Ville-Des-Rivierès : *CLSC-CHSLD*, 70 p.

DEVEN F., INGLIS S., MOSS P., PETRIE P., "Revisión de les investigaciones realizadas en Europa sobre conciliación de la vida laboral y familiar por hombres y mujeres y calidad de los servicios de atención. Informe final para la Unidad de Igualdad de Oportunidades de la Comisión Europea". Madrid: *Ministerio de Trabajo y Asuntos Sociales*: 1998.

DOOLEY D., FIELDING J., LEVI L. 1996. "Health and unemployment". *Annu Rev Public Health* 17: 449-65.

DOYAL L. 2001. "Sex, gender, and health: the need for a new approach". *BMJ* 323: 1061-3.

EUROSTAT. "Population and social conditions". [page visited: 02-09-04]. Accessible in: http://europa.eu.int/comm/eurostat/.

EUROSTAT. 2005. *News Release, Reconciling work and family life in the EU-25 in 2003*: 3.

HALL EM. 1992. "Double exposure: The combined impact of the home and work environments on psychosomatic strain in Swedish men and women". *Int J Health Serv* 22: 239-60.

HILL CR., STAFFORD FP. 1980. "Parental care of children: time diary estimates of quantity, predictability and variety". *Journal of Human Resources* 15: 202-39.

HOCHSCHILD A. 1989. *The second shift: working parents and the revolution at home*. New York: Viking Press, 309 p.

HUNT K., ANNANDALE E. 1993. "Just the job? Is the relationship between health and domestic and paid work gender specific?". *Sociology of Health and Illness* 15: 632-64.

JAHODA M. 1982. *Employment and unemployment: A Social Psychological Analysis*. New York: Cambridge University Press.

JANLERT U. 1997. "Unemployment as a disease and diseases of the unemployed". *Scand J Work Environ Health* 23 : suppl 3: 79-83.

KEMPENEERS., M. LELIËVRE., E. 1991. "*Famille et emploi dans l'Europe des Douze. Eurobaromëtre 34 (Family and employment in the Europpe 12. Eurobarometer 34)*". Brussels: European Communities Commission, 187 p.

KERGOAT D. 1984. *Les femmes et le travail à temps partiel*. Paris : La Documentation Française, 227 p.

KHLAT M., SERMET C., LE PAPE A. 2000. "Women's health in relation with their family and work roles: France in the early 1990s". *Soc Sci Med* 50: 1807-25.

KIVIMÄKI M., VAHTERA J., VIRTANEN M., ELOVAINIO M., PENTTI J., FERRIE JE. 2003. "Temporary employment and risk of overall and cause-specific mortality". *Am J Epidemiol* 158: 663-8.

KUNKEL SR., ATCHELY RC. 1996. "Why gender matters: Being female is not the same as not being male". *Am J Prev Med* 12: 294-6.

LAHELMA E. 1992. "Unemployment and mental well-being: elaboration of the relationship". *Int J Health Serv* 22: 261-74.

LEINO-ARJAS P., LIIRA J., MUTANEN P., MALMIVAARA A., MARTIKAINEN E. 1999. "Predictors and consequences of unemployment among construction workers: prospective cohort study". *BMJ* 319: 600-5.

LENNON MC., ROSENFIELD S. 1992. "Women and mental health. The interaction of job and family conditions". *J Health Soc Behav* 33: 316-27.

LUNDBERG U., MARDBERG B., FRANKENHAEUSER M. 1994. "The total workload of male and female white collar workers as related to age, occupational level, and number of children". *Scand J Psychol* 35(4): 315-27.

MACINTYRE S., HUNT K., SWEETING H. 1996. "Gender differences in health. Are things really as simple as they seem?". *Soc Sci Med* 42: 617-24.

MEIL G. 1999. "Cambio familiar y política de conciliación de vida laboral y familiar en España" (Family change and policies of reconciling job and family life in Spain). *Revista del Ministerio de Trabajo y Asuntos Sociales* 1: 11-40.

MOSS NE. 2002. "Gender equity and socioeconomic inequality: a framework for the patterning of women's health". *Soc Sci Med* 54: 649-61.

NATHANSON CA. 1995. "Illness and the feminine role: a theoretical review". *Soc Sci Med* 9,57-62.

NATHANSON CA. 1980. "Social roles and health status among women: The significance of employment". *Soc Sci Med* 14: 463-71.

NICKOLS, S.Y., & ABDEL-GHANY M. 1983. "Leisure time of husbands and wives". *Home Economics Research Journal* 12: 189-98.

OECD. 1998. *Organization of Economic Cooperation and Development. Economic Outlook.* Paris.

PASSANNANTE MR., NATHANSON CA. 1985. "Female labour force participation and mortality in Wisconsin, 1974-1978". *Soc Sci Med* 21,655-65.

PATE RR., PRATT M., BLAIR SN., HASKELL WL., MACERA CA., BOUCHARD C., BUCHNER D., ETTINGER W., HEATH GW., KING AC. 1995. "Physical activity and Public Health. A recommendation from the Centers for Disease Control and Prevention and the American College of Sports Medicine". *JAMA* 273: 402-7.

PICCINELLI M., WILKINSON G. 2000. "Gender differences in depression". *Br J Psychiatry* 177: 486-92.

QIN P., AGERBO E., WESTERGÅRD-NIELSEN N., ERIKSSON T., MORTENSEN PB. 2000. "Gender differences in risk factors for suicide in Denmark". *Br J Psychiatry* 177: 546-50.

RODRÍGUEZ E. 2002. "Marginal employment and health in Britain and Germany: does unstable employment predict health?". *Soc Sci Med* 55: 963-79.

ROSS CE., MIROWSKY J., GOLDSTEEN K. 1990. "The impact of the family on health. The decade in review". *Journal of Marriage and the Family* 52: 1059-78.

ROSS CE., MIROWSKY J. 1988. "Child care and emotional adjustment to wives' employment". *J Health Soc Behav* 29: 127-38.

RUIGÓMEZ A., ALONSO J., ANTÓ JM. 1991. "Salud percibida y capacidad funcional de la población anciana no institucionalizada de Barcelona (Perceived health and functional capacity of a non-institutionalised elderly population in Barcelona)". *Gac Sanit* 24: 117-24.

SORENSEN G., VERBRUGGE LM. 1987. "Women, work, and health". *Annu Rev Public Health* 8: 235-51.

THÉBAUD-MONY A. 2001. "Casualisation and flexibility: Impact on Worker's Health". In: "What knowledge and research is needed for healthy work in the New Century?". *TUTB newsletter* 15: 16-22.

THRANE C. 2000. "Men, women, and leisure time: Scandinavian evidence of gender inequality". *Leisure Sciences* 22,109-122.

VERBRUGGE LM. 1983. "Multiple roles and physical health of women and men". *J Health Soc Behav* 24: 16-30.

VIRTANEN P., VAHTERA J., KIVIMAKI M., PENTTI J., FERRIE J. 2002. "Employment security and health". *J Epidemiol Community Health* 56: 569-74.

WALDRON I., JACOBS JA. 1998. "Effects of labour free participation on women's health: New evidence from a longitudinal study". *J Occup Med* 30: 977-83.

WALDRON I., WEISS CC., HUGHES ME. 1998. "Interacting effects of multiple roles on women's health". *J Health Soc Behav* 39: 216-36.

WALTERS V., DENTON R., FRENCH S., EYLES J., MAYR J., NEWBOLD B. 1996. "Paid work, unpaid work and social support: a study of the health of male and female nurses". *Soc Sci Med* 43: 1627-36.

PART III

SUMMARY AND CONCLUSIONS

Does Work Promote or Reduce Inequalities in Health?

Ingvar LUNDBERG, Tomas HEMMINGSSON
& Christer HOGSTEDT

This chapter is an extended summary of the chapters in the book. It will discuss our findings regarding the social class distribution of unfavourable working conditions, and the extent to which working conditions may explain social class differences in health. We will conclude by discussing the implications of recent changes in the labour market and in working life, for the magnitude of social class differences in Europe in the near future.

1. The Relationship between Working Conditions and Ill Health

It is obvious that most working conditions that are detrimental to health accumulate in lower social classes. This is particularly true for chemical hazards and muscular load, and is demonstrated in data from all countries. It is also true for job control, usually measured as a combination of skill discretion, i.e. the opportunity to learn new things at work, and decision authority. In any hierarchical system, job control will be distributed in this way, since higher positions must entail greater decision authority, at least in the long run. However, this is not true for job demands, i.e. how hard you have to work, how fast, and how difficult your tasks are to carry out. Although high job demands, as they are usually measured, are generally related to poorer self-rated health (SRH) (see for example (Rahkonen *et al.* 2006) (Laaksonen *et al.* 2006)) and to psychological distress (see for example (Stansfeld *et al.* 1995) (Niedhammer *et al.* 1998)), they are more common in higher social classes.

Unfavourable working conditions may explain social class differences in ill health if they are risk factors for ill health and occur more commonly in lower than in higher social classes. To what extent are working conditions risk factors for ill health? A number of chemicals in the workplace are established carcinogens or may cause other diseases. The International Agency for Research on Cancer has published a large number of monographs evaluating the carcinogenicity of various chemicals (www.iarc.fr). A large number of studies, although few with a longitudinal design, have shown that there is a relationship between high job demands and low social support at work, i.e. components of the demand-control-support model (JDCS), and depressive symptoms. Most of these studies use questionnaires to measure the outcome but a few studies have used a diagnosis of depression, obtained through a psychiatric interview (Stansfeld *et al*. 1995) (Niedhammer *et al*. 1998) (Wang 2004). The results for job control are more ambiguous. At present it is reasonable to conclude that at least high job demands and insufficient social support at work are risk factors for depression. A number of studies have also shown an association between serious life events at work and post-traumatic stress disorder (Cothereau *et al*. 2004) (Farmer *et al*. 1992).

A vast number of studies have investigated the effects of the components of the job demand-control model (JDC) and JDCS on other outcomes, primarily the relationship with cardiovascular disease. A recent review concludes that out of 17 well-performed longitudinal studies on the JDC model, eight showed significant results and three non-significant results in line with the hypothesis. Six out of nine case-control studies supported the hypothesis. Most of the studies, and those which provided the best evidence, were performed among men. The authors concluded that "job strain is a major CVD risk factor" (Belkic *et al*. 2004). However, some authors argue that the association between job control and CVD may be due to other, unmeasured, true risk factors, appearing particularly during earlier periods of the life course (Davey Smith *et al*. 2002).

The extent to which muscular load and psychosocial conditions at work may actually cause musculoskeletal disorders is somewhat controversial. However, a major report from the US National Research Council and Institute of Medicine recently concluded that "the weight of the evidence justifies the identification of certain work-related factors for the occurrence of musculoskeletal disorders of the low and upper extremities" and that "modification of those physical and psychosocial factors could reduce substantially the risk of symptoms for low back and upper extremity disorders" and that "the weight of the evidence justifies the introduction of appropriate and selected interventions… to reduce physical as well as psychosocial stressors. (through) the development of integrated programs that address equipment design, work procedures, and organisational characteristics". Among risk factors for low back pain are listed manual materials handling, frequent bending or twisting, heavy physical load, static work postures and whole-body vibrations, as well as high job demands, monotonous work, low social support, and low job satisfaction. Risk factors listed for upper extremity disorders included repetitive work, force, vibration, high job demands, low decision latitude, low social support and few rest break opportunities (Punnett and Wegman 2004). In another review similar findings emerged (Ariens *et al.* 2001).

In conclusion there seems to be evidence that certain working conditions are associated with certain health outcomes.

2. Unfavourable Working Conditions in Social Classes, Development over Time

Information on the occurrence of working conditions in repeated surveys over time in social classes was available only from Sweden, where work environment surveys on random samples of working people have been conducted every second year since 1989. The summary of the data on working conditions in social classes will be based on the Swedish data, with comments on the findings from other countries in relation to the Swedish findings.

A. Swedish Data

In Sweden, comparisons were made between social classes regarding a number of self-reported working conditions in 1991, 1995 and 2001: years when the same questions on the relevant exposures were used in the surveys.

The higher the social class, the more common were high job demands in both sexes. The only exception was a lack of difference between unskilled and skilled manual workers among men. There seemed to be no difference in the prevalence of high job demands between men and women. Over time there was a continuous increase in the prevalence of high demands among skilled and unskilled manual workers among men, and in all classes except higher non-manual employees among women.

The lower the social class, the more common was low decision authority among men. Among women there seemed to be no prevalence difference between skilled and unskilled manual workers, or between lower and intermediate non-manual employees, but otherwise the distribution of low decision authority followed the expected gradient. Low decision authority seemed almost twice as common among women as among men.

Among men the prevalence of low decision authority increased over time, particularly among skilled manual workers but also among unskilled manual workers. Among non-manual employees there seemed to be no such increase between 1991 and 2001. There was a marked increase in the prevalence of low decision authority (from around 35 to almost 50%) among female manual workers, a smaller increase among female intermediate non-manual employees, and no increase among female higher non-manual employees.

The prevalence of low social support was rather similar in the social classes, although the highest prevalence of low support was found among higher non-manual employees at all time points and in both sexes. There were no obvious differences over time in any social class in either gender. In all social classes the prevalence of low social support was markedly higher among men than women.

The proportions reporting musculoskeletal load were much higher among manual than non-manual employees of both genders. Over time the proportion that stated musculoskeletal load in each class did not seem to change.

Physical and chemical exposure was markedly more common among manual than non-manual employees, and more common among men than women in the manual classes. The proportion stating chemical exposure did not seem to change over time in any social class or gender, except for a possible small increase over time among female skilled workers.

B. *Working Conditions in Social Classes in Countries other than Sweden*

Data from other countries regarding time trends in the social class distribution of working conditions was scarce. However, from most countries there were data on the social class distribution of working conditions at one time point. The findings from a national survey in Spain in 1999 were similar to the Swedish findings regarding the social distribution of physical and chemical risks and musculoskeletal load, as well as decision authority and skill discretion, psychological demands and social support at work.

The findings from Denmark were also similar concerning musculoskeletal load, physical and chemical exposures in 1995, and psychological demands, low decision authority, low social support and low skill discretion in 1990. Job insecurity was also more common in lower than in higher social classes.

An index of self-reported physical working conditions (based on questions about noise, dirty work, smell, danger and physically heavy work) in the Netherlands in 2000 followed a gradient where such conditions were much more common among labourers than among self-employed people, lower employees, intermediate employees and those in higher jobs (in that order), among men as well as women.

In France in 1994 the social distribution of an indicator of physical risk (including exposure to noise, heat and cold) as well as an indicator of ergonomic problems (including repetitive movements, vibrations, standing more than half of the work time, manual handling of materials) followed the expected social group distribution in that such exposures were more common among blue-collar workers than among clerks and service workers, associate professionals and managers. National surveys of self-reported psychosocial working conditions (e.g. questions related to job demands and job control) were carried out in 1991 and 1998. In 1998 questions related to autonomy at work showed that autonomy was always less common among blue-collar workers than among clerks and service workers, associate professionals and managers, in that order.

The findings of an investigation within the GAZEL cohort, i.e. of a specific company, in 1997 were similar to those in Sweden regarding the social distribution of physical demands, decision latitude, psychological demands and social support, although male managers seemed to have a more favourable situation than other men.

There is a lack of national studies of working conditions in Germany. However, from a number of studies, it seems that the prevalence of effort-reward imbalance increases with lower social class.

A national survey study in England in 1995 showed that high pace of work was more common, the higher the social class, while low control at work showed the opposite distribution. Low variety in work was also more common, the lower the social class. The results were similar among men and women. Similar results have been obtained in a number of papers from the Whitehall II project.

The Norwegian Surveys of Level of Living in 1980-1983 and 1991-1995 were used to investigate the distribution of unfavourable working conditions in social classes. Physical and chemical exposures as well as inappropriate muscular load were much more common the lower the social class in both time periods and in both sexes. There was no evident change over time in any class.

Questions related to work control were distributed in the expected way by social class among men. Among women, however, there were smaller social class differences, and in the last time period the most favourable situation concerning opportunity to decide on working speed and plan one's own work schedule was obtained from unskilled workers and higher salaried employees. Very large class differences in the expected direction were obtained in the question on varied work. There were small social class differences concerning hectic work situation.

C. Time Trends in Working Conditions
   in Countries other than Sweden

Concerning time trends in working conditions, questions related to job demands and job control in national surveys from 1991 and 1998 in France, showed a generally negative development among French wage earners. This trend seemed rather independent of social class. In Norway self-reported hectic work situations seemed to increase in all social classes among men between 1980-1983 and 1991-1995. However, the increase was smaller in the two highest than in the other social classes, and in the last time period there was no longer any difference between social classes regarding hectic work situations.

In order to support our findings we have also analysed data from the second and third surveys of working conditions in Europe, performed in 1995 and 2000 (Paoli *et al.* 2000). We have used data from Belgium, Denmark, Germany, Greece, Italy, Spain, France, Ireland, Luxemburg, the Netherlands, Portugal, the United Kingdom, Finland, Sweden and Austria. From each country 1,500 individuals were interviewed each year. Analyses have been performed for job decision authority, skill discretion and job demands. The interview question to measure decision authority was: "Are you able to choose or change: 1) the order of your tasks, 2) your methods of work, 3) your speed or rate of work", with the response alternatives "yes" or "no". The question on skill discretion was: "Generally, does your main paid job involve, or not, learning new things", with the response alternatives "yes" or "no". The questions on work demands were: "Does your job involve: 1) working at a very high speed, 2) working to tight deadlines". In both cases the response alternatives were a seven-grade scale from 1 ("all the time") to 7 ("never").

The results are shown for the occupational groups used in the surveys. There were small differences in job demands, as measured, between the groups among both men and women. The results were also much the same between the two years.

The results for decision authority are shown in table 1 and 2 for women and men respectively. The tables show the well-established differences in decision authority between men and women, although the gender differences in decision authority, as measured, seem greater for higher non-manual than for lower non-manual and manual occupational groups. Between 1995 and 2000 a decreased proportion reported high decision authority among, particularly, service and sales workers in both sexes and elementary occupations among men.

Table 1: High job decision authority in occupational groups among European women in 1995 and 2000

	1995	2000
Legislators, senior officials and managers	75	75
Professionals	61	62
Technicians, associate professionals	54	60
Clerks	53	51
Service workers and shop and market sales workers	57	42
Crafts and related trade workers	44	46
Plant and machine operators and assemblers	28	22
Elementary occupations	46	47

Table 2: High job decision autority in occupational groups among European men in 1995 and 2000

	1995	2000
Legislators, senior officials and managers	81	78
Professionals	71	71
Technicians and associate professionals	67	62
Clerks	52	50
Service workers and shop and market sales workers	56	50
Crafts and related trade workers	50	47
Plant and machine operators and assemblers	31	30
Elementary occupations	44	35

Regarding skill discretion, the differences between occupational groups were as expected in both genders (tables 3 and 4). Men and women in non-manual jobs showed skill discretion to the same extent but in non-manual jobs men more often showed skill discretion. Between 1995 and 2000 there were pronounced reductions in skill discretion among women in elementary occupations and among male service and sales workers, although these occupational categories also showed reduced skill discretion in the opposite sex.

Table 3: Skill discretion in occupational groups among European women in 1995 and 2000

	1995	2000
Legislators, senior officials and managers	71	65
Professionals	92	92
Technicians, associate professionals	88	86
Clerks	78	76
Service workers and shop and market sales workers	70	64
Crafts and related trade workers	67	61
Plant and machine operators and assemblers	54	55
Elementary occupations	45	33

**Table 4: Skill discretion in occupational groups
among European men in 1995 and 2000**

	1995	2000
Legislators, senior officials and managers	81	76
Professionals	93	90
Technicians and associate professionals	89	85
Clerks	73	73
Service workers and shop and market sales workers	75	62
Crafts and related trade workers	74	73
Plant and machine operators and assemblers	60	58
Elementary occupations	56	51

D. Summary of Information on Working Conditions in Social Classes

To summarise, chemical and physical hazards as well as inappropriate ergonomic conditions are distributed in the expected way in all countries, i.e. the lower the social class, the more common are the exposures. Low job control is distributed in a similar way in all countries, while social support at work most often seems unrelated to social class and high job demands are usually more common, the higher the social class.

In Sweden as well as in France and Norway there are indications of deteriorating psychosocial working conditions during the 1990s. There were no data provided from other countries that could show whether the development there was similar. However, this may be likely, since there was an increase in unemployment in most countries during these years, combined with pressure for increased productivity in all sectors. Norway was one of the countries least seriously hit by the crisis.

Among social classes, deterioration of working conditions seems to have been most pronounced among manual workers. This was confirmed by our analyses of measures of decision authority and skill discretion in the European surveys of working conditions in 1995 and 2000. Over time, manual workers showed deterioration in decision authority and skill discretion that was not present among higher non-manual workers. It also seems likely that this development is based on the higher levels of unemployment and increased competition for work in lower social classes. However, at least in Sweden, it is known that the deterioration was most pronounced among women working in the fields of care and education, mostly in the public sector, and that these problems seem to have affected all social classes in these sectors, although manual employees somewhat more than non-manual employees.

Thus it seems that decision authority may have decreased conspicuously among manual workers in both sexes during the 1990s, while there was no correspondent decrease among higher non-manual employees in either of the sexes. Simultaneously, job demands have increased continuously during the 1990s in the manual classes, although this was not reflected by our measure in the European surveys. The data from Sweden and Norway indicate that these findings may vary by gender and that women have experienced a more unfavourable development than men with regard to psychosocial working conditions.

3. How much do Work Environment Conditions Contribute to Social Class Differences in Health?

This question was analysed differently in different countries. Different outcomes were used, the social classes were defined differently and the exposures studied as explanations were different. Almost all analyses were cross-sectional, which is associated with certain problems discussed below. Depending on access to data, different data sets were used. National surveys were used in most countries (Sweden, Norway, Netherlands, Germany, Denmark) but analyses were also based on regional data (Spain) or specific companies or workplaces (France, UK, Germany).

A. *Self-Reported Health (SRH)*

Analyses of the importance of working conditions for social class differences in self-rated health were performed in France, the UK, Holland, Spain and Sweden. Denmark provided data on self-reported health in social classes but no further analyses. Self-rated health is based on the question: "How do you regard your state of health?" or something similar. The response alternatives are usually: "very good", "good", "fair", "poor" and "very poor". Self-rated health was dichotomised so that those with less than good self-rated health were regarded as having poor SRH.

Social Class Differences in SRH

In all countries with data, poor SRH was reported more often in lower than in higher classes. In Sweden and Spain the five classes of unskilled and skilled manual workers and lower, intermediate and higher non-manual employees were used, and among participants in surveys in 1996/97 in Sweden and Spain (2000) there was an increase in the prevalence of self-reported health with each step down in the hierarchy in both sexes. In Denmark (2000) the same finding emerged in both sexes combined. In the UK data from the Whitehall study in 1993 and

1998 were used. With three classes (top, middle and low grades) the prevalence of poor SRH followed the same pattern.

In Holland (2000) and France (1997-1998) classes were defined differently and class differences seemed smaller. In France, however, craftsmen among men and clerks among women seemed to have worse SRH than other groups. In Holland there were no differences in SRH among women between the social groups studied. Among men higher workers showed better self-reported health than three intermediate classes with similar SRH (one of them self-employed). Labourers stated poor SRH more often than any of the other classes.

Working Conditions as Explanations of Social Class Differences in SRH

In cross-sectional analyses, working conditions explained a substantial part of the social class differences in SRH in all countries. In Spain physical working conditions (musculoskeletal load, chemical exposure etc.) explained 20-40% (dependent on class) of the social class differences among men. Among women, only about 10% of social class differences were explained by such factors. Psychosocial working conditions (job control, demands and social support) explained around 10% of social class differences among both men and women. The combined effects of physical and psychosocial working conditions on social class differences were 25-45% among men or 10% or less among women. In Sweden similar working conditions were studied. Among men, physical working conditions explained 10-30% of the class differences in SRH. When psychosocial working conditions were included in the analysis, 20-40% of the differences between social classes were explained. Among women, about 50% of the, originally smaller, social class differences were explained by physical working conditions alone or by the combination of physical and psychosocial working conditions. A problem in these analyses was that job demands were used as an explanatory factor in the analyses. Since job demands show a social distribution with the highest levels in the higher strata, job demands cannot explain social class differences but rather increase them, depending on how strong a risk factor the demands are.

In the UK only psychosocial working conditions were analysed and both genders were combined in the analyses. Decision authority explained about 50% of the excess risk of poor SRH in middle or low grades. Including psychological work demands in the analysis either did not change or reduced somewhat the explanatory power of psychosocial working conditions.

In Holland there were no initial differences among women between the social groups studied, and accordingly no social class differences that could be explained by working conditions. Among men, skill discretion (learning new things at work) explained around 30% of the SRH difference between higher workers and labourers, and less of the difference between higher workers and other social groups.

As mentioned above, the initial social group differences were rather small in France, with the exception of the difference between managers and engineers, and craftsmen among men and clerks among women. However, a major part of the differences was explained by a combination of decision latitude (the combination of skill discretion and decision authority) and physical demands. For male craftsmen and female clerks, around 50% of the differences were explained, compared with percentage for managers and engineers.

In a prospective analysis of new cases of poor SRH over one year, the social group differences were rather similar to those in the cross-sectional analyses, but for unclear reasons very little of the explanation for these differences was found in working conditions.

B. Long-Standing Illness (LSI)

Long-standing illness (LSI), or long-standing medical condition, as a questionnaire response, was studied in the UK (Whitehall data from 1993 and 1998), in Sweden (nationally representative data from 1996/1997) and in Norway (nationally representative data from 1980-1995).

In the UK there were no initial grade differences in LSI.

In Norway three indicators of working conditions were used: an index of harmful environment (chemical hazards), an index of ergonomic strain (musculoskeletal load) and decision latitude. Among women there were no initial social class differences. Among men there were initial expected differences in LSI between the five social classes although the differences were not very large. However, among men all social class differences were explained by the combination of the indices of working conditions.

In Sweden, male higher non-manual employees reported less LSI than other classes but there were no other differences between classes. Among women the expected gradient over the classes was found, except that the highest prevalence of LSI was found among skilled workers. Among men, about 50% of the difference between higher non-manual employees and unskilled workers was explained by working conditions, among which physical conditions were most important. Among women a similar proportion of the differences between these classes were explained by working conditions.

C. Other Health Measures

In Germany self-reported symptoms (an index of symptoms: musculoskeletal, gastrointestinal, fatigue, sleeping problems, common cold, nausea, vertigo) were used as the outcome in a study of public transport employees; the two sexes were combined in the analysis. Three classes were identified: unskilled and skilled manual workers and non-manual employees. Initially there was a large difference in symptom levels between the classes which was markedly reduced by adjustment for an index of physical and chemical hazards or for effort-reward imbalance. If both indices were simultaneously adjusted for, the differences between the classes disappeared completely.

A study of a nationally representative sample of people employed in 1998 was also performed in Germany. The outcome was self-reported musculoskeletal symptoms. There were large differences in musculoskeletal symptoms between the social classes, with the expected gradient. After adjustment for effort and resources the differences increased somewhat. However, after adjustment for physical and chemical hazards the difference in musculoskeletal symptoms between unskilled workers and professionals was reduced by almost 70% among women as well as men.

In the Netherlands, analyses were performed with a dichotomised index of psychosomatic complaints as the outcome. Among men such complaints were most common among lower non-manual employees, while higher workers and self-employed people stated such complaints most seldom. Among women, those who were self-employed stated more complaints than the other social groups. Among men, skill discretion explained a large part of the difference between labourers and higher workers but very little regarding other differences between social groups. Among women, working conditions did not contribute to explain social group differences.

D. Summary and Conclusions

The results presented in this section indicate that in cross-sectional analyses, unfavourable working conditions, muscular load as well as physical and chemical exposures and psychosocial working conditions, may explain a substantial part of social class differences in different forms of self-reported health. This is particularly true if, of the psychosocial conditions, only job control and not job demands are included in the analyses.

However, cross-sectional analyses cannot determine causality. Social class differences are likely to be underestimated because of differential selection of ill people from lower social classes out of the labour market. Neither could conclusions be drawn regarding whether working conditions are caused by ill health, or if working conditions cause ill health or are incompatible with ill health. Moreover, what appear to be effects of working conditions could be the effects of risk factors appearing earlier in the life course and forming pathways to lower social class. This possible bias has not been adjusted for in any previous study on working conditions and social class differences in health. However, apart from this bias our cross-sectional analyses are in accordance with the results of previous longitudinal studies reviewed in the introductory chapter.

4. Further Observations on Work and Labour Market Related Inequalities in Health and Predictions for the Future

A number of themes related to changes in the occurrence of labour market and working conditions and their importance for social inequalities in health were brought up in the chapters of this book. In this section we will comment on some of these themes.

A. The 'Healthy Worker' Effect

One particular problem in our studies is the continuous exchange between the working part of the population and those who are unemployed or outside the labour market. This is the basis for the so-called 'healthy worker' effect. The higher the proportion of employed in the population, the more unhealthy people will be employed; and the lower the proportion of employed people, the healthier those working will be. Hence it is likely that the lower the proportion of employed people, the smaller the social class differences in health will be in cross-sectional analysis.

The proportion of the male population that is employed seems to have diminished slowly but continuously in most countries during recent decades. The opposite has occurred among women. However, the proportion of women in employment has still not reached the proportion among men in any country. Moreover, a large fraction of the employed women work part-time. Although few men still work part-time, there seems to be an increasing trend of part-time work among men in most countries. The employment rates between countries are hard to compare due to varying definitions and variations in the constructions of the social insurance systems. However, among men there seem to be no major differences, although the rates are lower in Spain. Thus, when comparing the countries studied, pure employment differences can hardly be a reason for different effects of working conditions on social class differences in health among men.

The trends for part-time work obviously vary from country to country. In the Netherlands the increase in female employment between 1980 and 2000 has almost only concerned part-time employment, which increased from 12 to 32%, while full-time employment did not change (18% in 2000). In Germany and in France part-time employment among women increased similarly. In all cases this was due to a shrinking number of housewives. In Sweden, part-time employment actually decreased among women during the period 1980-2000 (from 47 to 34%) due to an increased number of full-time workers. Hence, among women, employment rates are clearly different between countries, and may partly explain the small social class differences in self-reported health among women in Holland. The different definitions of social classes used from country to country may certainly also contribute to different magnitudes of social class differences between countries.

B. High Levels of Unemployment

Since the 1980s, or in some cases the early 1990s, unemployment levels have been higher than previously during the post World War II era in most countries in Western Europe. Several researchers claim that the high unemployment is not only due to business cycles but might also have structural causes. A higher rate of growth than previously may now be needed to attain higher employment levels (Magnusson and Ottosson 2002). The increase in unemployment has occurred simultaneously with an increase in different forms of temporary employment and part-time employment in almost all countries. The number of self-employed people has also increased in some countries but has also diminished in other countries, so this tendency is not universal and the discrepancies are probably related to differences in the welfare systems, taxation legislation etc. between different countries.

According to many neoclassical economists, the labour market in Western Europe is characterised by the fact that wage and salary differences are too small, and that unemployment benefits are too high to make people sufficiently active on the labour market. Other problems according to these economists include taxes on labour, particularly in low-wage sectors, to increase the demand for labour in these sectors (Boeri *et al.* 2001). The growing black labour market in such sectors in several countries is taken as an indication of this.

C. Increased Educational Requirements for Employment

The educational requirements for employment seem to have increased in all countries, particularly in the last 10-15 years. A vast number of jobs have disappeared in manufacturing and been partly replaced by jobs requiring a higher level of education, with more varied and wider responsibilities, and requiring an ability to adapt to change by acquiring new competencc. As we have seen, within a short period of time these developments have increased the age at which people become established in the labour market by several years, i.e. the number of years spent in education is increasing, allowing a smaller number of years for employment unless the age of retirement is raised. Simultaneously there are indications of over-education, where an increasing number of people have to take jobs below their actual level of qualifications. Probably these changes will also lead to a decrease in the employment of low educated individuals in jobs requiring less education, since the average employer tends to employ applicants with the highest education.

During the last few decades, however, there has also been a continuous decrease in the average age of leaving the labour market. In most countries, however, changes in the pension systems are being discussed, or have already been introduced to make it financially beneficial to retire from the labour market at a later age.

D. Organisations in the Labour Market and their Impact on Social Inequalities in Health

The labour market is the hub of social activity. Both welfare and health in a society are dependent on human production, and production is dependent on the activities in the labour market. This is where powerful interests, primarily the employers and their organisations, are competing to increase their share of the wealth created through production. It is the employers who decide what should be produced, as well as how, when and where; they also decide who should be employed or not, and about wages and salaries etc. Hence, they also decide about working conditions. However, it is not likely that employers' organisations will take a primary interest in diminishing social class differences in health unless these differences threaten efficiency and productivity. States, or supranational structures, have in many cases provided legislation to ensure that working conditions do not fall short of minimum standards, and that people who are not fit to work according to current requirements in the labour market are provided with necessary allowances. In general, states do not consider that large health inequalities between social classes are justified, and ways to combat such inequalities have been considered in several states such as the UK and Sweden (Acheson 1999) (Health 2005). In Sweden, improvement of work environments is one of eleven goals specified in the public health policy (Health 2005). Finally, the trade unions were established to support workers in wage bargaining, as well as to fight for increased democracy and participation of the workers in enterprises. According to the inquiries presented in this book it seems that, so far, unions in most countries have taken rather little interest in health issues overall, and we have found no unions that have specifically mentioned social inequalities in health as an area of interest. However, in the Norwegian country paper there is an interesting discussion on 'decommodification' of labour, which has been a cornerstone of Norwegian labour market policies. Espen Dahl and Jon Ivar Elstad argue that Norwegian trade unions may have contributed to lowering social class differences in health by a dedication to economic growth simultaneously with an emphasis on collective bargaining systems covering large parts of the labour market.

E. Increased Income Differences and Globalisation

While income differences between social classes diminished during the era of the homogenous industrial society until the 1960s, such differences seem to have increased during the last few decades in most countries. They seem to increase also in countries where trade unions are relatively strong but have been more pronounced in the USA, Australia, the UK and Canada than in other countries in Western Europe (Magnusson 2000). The relative strength of the trade unions in some countries has probably contributed to this development. In all countries those at the top of the income distribution seem to rapidly increase their income in comparison with other groups. However, in the USA the widening of income differences seems to occur over the entire gradient of incomes (Subramanian and Kawachi 2004). One of the reasons for widening income differences is that, compared with the era of the homogenous industrial society, an increasing part of the salaries for an increasing part of the workforce are related to skills and abilities specific to the person employed. This also means that the costs involved in finding replacements for those who are employed has increased.

It is also important to remember that income from work is only part of the total income and that capital gains also contribute to the increasing differences between social classes (for example see the chapter on the situation in Sweden). Capital has become increasingly mobile across borders since the 1970s, resulting in the increase of profits in comparison with wages since the 1970s. Through this process, international competition for work has increased; to begin with it has mainly affected manual employees in industrialised societies but it will probably start to affect also non-manual employees. If, or when, this happens, wage differences are likely to start to decrease again. However, for the time being, wage differences and thus social class differences in health are likely to continue to increase.

It is common to consider globalisation to be an important cause of increased wage inequalities and rising unemployment in developed countries (Deardorff 2003) (Deardorff and Stern 2002). However, research also shows that globalisation defined in economic terms has not affected employment stability or job mobility in Sweden, and has not led to an increased risk of unemployment among individuals with low education, compared with other groups (Korpi and Tåhlin 2006a) (Korpi and Stern 2006b). In a paper in this volume Halldén has examined whether economic globalisation may lead to increased work intensificaty which in turn might imply health inequalities between social classes. The paper defines globalisation as growing international flows of trade, capital and labour. Using data on increased total trade as a share of GDP in 1990-2000, EU-countries are described in terms of globalisation rate. Data from the European Survey on Working Conditions (Paoli and Merllié) were used to assess increase in work intensity between 1995 and 2000, as well as a potential connection between increased economic globalisation, raised work intensity and an increase in psychological distress. The analysis was based on the assumption that if globalisation had a major effect on work intensification (largely equivalent to quantitative work demands) leading to psychological distress, this would mainly affect manual workers in the manufacturing industry, since these workers would be those primarily affected by increased international competition. Moreover, workers in unskilled work in such industries would be at higher risk. It was found that work demands increased in all sectors but no more in the manufacturing industry than in other sectors. Nor had work demands increased more for manual workers in the manufacturing industry than for manual workers in other sectors. Finally, there was an increase in psychological distress in all sectors which was no greater in manufacturing than in the other sectors. Hence, there was no increase in social class differences in indicators of psychological distress, mediated by work intensity. An investigation was also performed to elucidate whether the findings could be related to health-related selection out of the manufacturing industry in Sweden but this was not the case. The main interpretation is that economic globalisation *per se* is not the cause of the increasing work demands and the increase in psychological distress seen in the last decade. Another interpretation is that trade between developed and developing countries is still a minor part of the total trade in developed countries. A final possibility may be that computer technology has increased the demands for skills in firms in developed countries. If so this, rather than globalisation, could explain the low demand for unskilled labour together with increasing wage inequalities (Adams 1997) (Acemoglu 2003).

F. Conclusions Regarding the Development of Work and Labour Market Related Social Inequalities in Health

In the near future it is likely that most of the tendencies observed regarding the development of working and labour market conditions will result in increasing social class differences in health. This is due to the widening income disparities between classes, to the higher unemployment rates compared with the more recent past, the decreasing demand for low educated labour and the increased educational requirements for employment. The fact that the strength of the trade unions has diminished, although to very different extents in different countries, may also contribute to this development.

In the longer run developments are difficult to predict since an abundance of conditions may contribute.

G. The Need for a Combined Social Class – Gender Framework in the Analysis of Work and Labour Market Related Inequalities in Health

In their chapter in this book Artacoz *et al.* point to the fact that gender may fundamentally modify the effects of work and labour market conditions on social class differences in health. They give abundant examples of the necessity to use such a framework in the analysis. The fact that women in all countries in Europe have, and take on, considerably more family responsibilities than men, and work in sectors where salaries are lower, implies that work often occurs in different contexts for men and women. In most countries, women typically also belong to lower social classes than men.

5. Suggestions for Research and Development

The importance of labour market and working conditions for social class differences has only been studied to a limited extent and we believe that there are several areas where more, or new, research and development efforts are needed.

A. Lack of Exposure Data

Regular surveys of working and labour-market conditions are lacking in most countries. Such data are necessary in order to understand, in particular, the importance of working conditions for social class differences in health over time. This needs to be improved. There are no external assessments of psychosocial working conditions whatsoever, and this hampers comparisons over time. The situation concerning muscular load may be somewhat better but some external assessment would be beneficial also in this case. Surveys should preferably also include data on other living conditions and contain data on education and income.

B. Studies on More Outcomes

Studies on labour-market and working conditions as a cause of social class differences in health have so far been concentrated to a few outcomes: self-reported health and self-reported long-standing illness, psychological distress, and coronary heart disease. Studies of other outcomes are needed, in particular of musculoskeletal disorders and lung cancer, as well as accidents and all-cause mortality.

C. Recruitment to Social Classes

The initial recruitment to social classes may be associated with risk indicators, as we have shown in the introductory chapter. There is a need to investigate whether this applies to countries other than Sweden and Finland, and whether it applies to women as well as men. There are very few studies that explore the effects of risk factors from before labour market entry together with working conditions, and these studies have only examined the time period until the participants have reached their mid-1930s (Power *et al.* 1998) (Matthews *et al.* 2001) (Matthews and Power 2002). There will be a need to bring social, life course, epidemiology and occupational health epidemiology together, in the context of social class differences in health.

D. Does Politics Matter?

Comparisons of general characteristics of politics between countries and how this affects working conditions and social class differences in health are needed. A few such efforts have been made in other areas, for example regarding social consequences of illness (Burstrom *et al.* 2000) (Burstrom *et al.* 2003), regarding the health situation among lone mothers (Whitehead *et al.* 2000) and regarding the different welfare policies of countries with different dominating political currents (Navarro 2002).

E. Gender and Class

Although there is abundant literature on gender and health issues, there is very little on labour market and working conditions, social class and health. As pointed out by Artazcoz *et al.* in this volume, research on working conditions by gender and class needs to analyse the combined impact of job and family on women's and men's health, as well as the interdependence between these two domains.

F. Other Issues

Today there is limited public interest in social class differences in health. Are there social forces, trade unions, political organisations or other groups, who are likely to engage themselves in diminishing social class differences in health? Do social class differences in health provoke more action to improve health in lower social strata than everyday occupational health efforts to improve health among workers, or vice versa? Are social class differences more or less unacceptable to the general public than income differences or differences in other areas of life?

References

ACEMOGLU D. 2003. *Technology and Inequality*. Cambridge: National Bureau of Economic Research.

ACHESON D. 1999. *Independent inquiry into inequalities in health report*. London.

ADAMS J. 1997. *Technology, trade and wages*. Cambridge: Working Paper 5940.

ARIENS G. A., VAN MECHELEN W., BONGERS P. M., BOUTER L. M. and VAN DER WAL G. 2001. "Psychosocial risk factors for neck pain: a systematic review". *Am J Ind Med* 39: 180-93.

BELKIC K. L., LANDSBERGIS P. A., SCHNALL P. L. and BAKER D. 2004. "Is job strain a major source of cardiovascular disease risk?" *Scand J Work Environ Health* 30: 85-128.

BOERI T., BRUGIAVINI A. and CALMFORS L. 2001. *The role of unions in the twenty-first century: a report for the Fondazione Rodolfo Debenedetti*. Oxford: Oxford University Press.

BURSTROM B., WHITEHEAD M., LINDHOLM C. and DIDERICHSEN F. 2000. "Inequality in the social consequences of illness: how well do people with long-term illness fare in the British and Swedish labor markets?" *Int J Health Serv* 30: 435-51.

BURSTROM B., HOLLAND P., DIDERICHSEN F. and WHITEHEAD M. 2003. "Winners and losers in flexible labor markets: the fate of women with chronic illness in contrasting policy environments – Sweden and Britain". *Int J Health Serv* 33: 199-217.

COTHEREAU C., DE BEAUREPAIRE C., PAYAN C., CAMBOU J. P., ROUILLON F. and CONSO F. 2004. "Professional and medical outcomes for French train drivers after 'person under train' accidents: three year follow up study". *Occup Environ Med* 61: 488-94.

DAVEY SMITH G., BEN SHLOMO Y. and LYNCH J. 2002. "Life course approaches to inequalities in coronary heart disease risk". In M. S. Stansfeld and M. MARMOT [eds.]. *Stress and the heart. Psychosocial pathways to coronary heart disease*. London: BMJ Books: 20-49.

DEARDORFF A. 2003. "What might globalization's critics believe? ". *The World Economy* 26: 639-658.

DEARDORFF A. and STERN R., "What you should know about globalization and the world trade organization". *Review of International Economics* 10: 404-423.

FARMER R., TRANAH T., O'DONNELL I. and CATALAN J. 1992. "Railway suicide: the psychological effects on drivers". *Psychol Med* 22: 407-14.

HEALTH, S. N. I. o. P. 2005. *The 2005 Public Health Policy Report – Summary*, Stockholm.

KORPI T. and TÅHLIN M. 2006a. "The impact of globalization on men's labour market mobility in Sweden". In H. BLOSSFELD, M. MILLS and F. BERNARDI (eds.). *Globalization, Uncertainty and men's careers: An International Comparison*. Edward Elgar: UK: Cheltenham and USA: Northampton MA.

KORPI T. and STERN, C. 2006b. "Globalization, Deindustrialization and the Labour Market Experiences of Swedish Women 1950 to 2000". In H. BLOSSFELD and H. HOFMEISTER (eds.). *Globalization, Uncertainty, and Women's Careers: An International Comparison*. Edward Elgar: UK: Cheltenham and USA: Northampton, MA.

LAAKSONEN M., RAHKONEN O., MARTIKAINEN P. and LAHELMA E. 2006. "Associations of psychosocial working conditions with self-rated general health and mental health among municipal employees". *Int Arch Occup Environ Health* 79: 205-12.

MAGNUSSON L. 2000. "Den tredje industriella revolutionen (The third industrial revolution) ". In SWEDISH. Stockholm: Arbetslivsinstitutet.

MAGNUSSON L. and OTTOSSON J. 2002. "Introduction: 11-19". In L. MAGNUSSON and J. OTTOSSON (eds.), *Europe – One Labour Market.*, Brussels P.I.E.-Peter Lang.

MATTHEWS S. and POWER C. 2002. "Socio-economic gradients in psychological distress: a focus on women, social roles and work-home characteristics". *Soc Sci Med* 54: 799-810.

MATTHEWS S., POWER C. and STANSFELD S. A. 2001. "Psychological distress and work and home roles: a focus on socio-economic differences in distress". *Psychol Med* 31: 725-36.

NAVARRO V. 2002. "The World Health Report 2000: can health care systems be compared using a single measure of performance? ". *Am J Public Health* 92: 31, 33-4.

NIEDHAMMER I., GOLDBERG M., LECLERC A., BUGEL I. and DAVID S. 1998. "Psychosocial factors at work and subsequent depressive symptoms in the Gazel cohort". *Scand J Work Environ Health* 24: 197-205.

PAOLI P. and MERLLIÉ D., *Third European Survey on Working Conditions 2000*. European Foundation for the Improvement of Working and Living Conditions 2000. www.Eurofound.eu.int.

POWER C., MATTHEWS S. and MANOR O. 1998. "Inequalities in self-rated health: explanations from different stages of life". Lancet 351: 1009-14.

PUNNETT L. and WEGMAN D. H. 2004. "Work-related musculoskeletal disorders: the epidemiologic evidence and the debate". *J Electromyogr Kinesiol* 14: 13-23.

RAHKONEN O., LAAKSONEN M., MARTIKAINEN P., ROOS E. and LAHELMA E., "Job control, job demands, or social class? The impact of working conditions on the relation between social class and health". *J Epidemiol Community Health* 60: 50-4. 2006,

STANSFELD S., FEENEY A., HEAD J., CANNER R., NORTH F. and MARMOT M. 1995. "Sickness absence for psychiatric illness: the Whitehall II Study". *Soc Sci Med* 40: 189-97.

SUBRAMANIAN S. V. and KAWACHI I. 2004. "Income inequality and health: what have we learned so far? *Epidemiol Rev* 26: 78-91.

WANG J. 2004. "Perceived work stress and major depressive episodes in a population of employed Canadians over 18 years old". *J Nerv Ment Dis* 192: 160-3.

WHITEHEAD M., BURSTROM B. and DIDERICHSEN F. 2000. "Social policies and the pathways to inequalities in health: a comparative analysis of lone mothers in Britain and Sweden". *Soc Sci Med* 50: 255-70.

Appendix

The main questions to be addressed in the conclusion of each country's chapter were:

1. How much of the relationship between social class and health among men and women may be explained by working conditions in the country? Development over time.

2. How do these relationships relate to the labour market policies and social insurance policies of the country? The findings could be interpreted in the light of:

- the economic benefits of early retirement, unemployment, or sick leave,
- whether there is commitment to full employment (among both men and women) and to what age,
- how sickness insurance is constructed and the levels of compensation,
- requirements for early retirement,
- policies to facilitate geographical or occupational mobility to areas or occupations (retraining) where there is a demand for work,
- policies to increase the participation of older workers in the workforce,
- publicly financed incentives for employers to make work environments healthier,
- the organisation of work-related rehabilitation, e.g. regulations that demand rehabilitation after some period of sick leave, and public incentives for employers to organise rehabilitation,
- the extent to which occupational health services are available.

  In other words, no formal data collection is needed on labour market, social insurance and work environment policies, but the above points for data collection should instead be used as a checklist when discussing the relationships between working conditions and social class differences in health.

3. How is the relationship between work-related conditions, social class and health likely to develop during the next 10-20 years? (1-3 pages).

In order to reach these conclusions, information is needed on the following points:

1. The size of socio-economic groups among men and women in the country. By socio-economic groups we mean something close to the five classes: higher, intermediate and lower non-manual employees, and skilled and non-skilled manual workers. In addition, information on farmers and self-employed people would be beneficial. The social classes used should be defined in the text. If socio-economic group/occupational class is not available, information should be given on the proportions of inhabitants with different levels of education (something on the lines of: up to and including 9 years of education, 10-14 years, and 15+ years, which would roughly correspond to elementary school, intermediate education and university education in most countries). Some information on income levels by social class or educational group is beneficial. The number of immigrant workers by social class (or education should be given). Development since 1980. (around 2 pages).

2. What is known about the labour market in the country, i.e. the proportions of people who are long-term and short-term employed, self-employed, early retired, homemakers (women and men), studying, on long-term sick leave, unemployed (i.e. trying to find work); the proportion of women and men in precarious work (workers on short-term contracts or in temporary employment); the sizes of different branches of industry? Development since 1980. (2-4 pages)

3. What is known about the relation between social class and health among men and women? Social class should be measured by socio-economic group (or by education if socio-economic group is not available). Health should be measured by overall mortality and mortality in cardiovascular disease (ICD10 chapter IX or I0-99). Long-standing illness or self-reported health should be additional health measures and available from survey studies in most countries. The development of the number of fatal occupational accidents (divided into those occurring at work and on the way to and from work) since 1980. (around 5 pages).

4. What is known about the development of working conditions in the country? The conditions should if possible include measures of muscular load, of psychosocial conditions (information on job demands, job control and job social support should be given if available) and some information on chemical and physical hazards. Development over time. Finally, the proportion of men and women in the population who are working at ages 25, 45 and 60 (or in similar age groups) in different social classes should be used as an indicator of the extent to which work environment conditions, labour market and social policies allow full

employment. Information on this point would in all countries come from population samples. (around 5 pages).

5. The degree of unionisation. How powerful are the trade unions in relation to work-life factors that may affect health? Are there trade union policies on social class differences in health? (1 page).

6. A short summary of ongoing research on social class and health in the country, with particular emphasis on research concerning social class, working conditions, labour market policies and health. (1 page).

7. A summary of potential existing national goals and strategies to reduce inequities in health, including work-related health, and an evaluation of the resources, implementation and effects of the strategy (policy research). (1 page).

A short description of any data sets that would be suitable for international and comparative analyses of work-related inequity in health (1 page).

Presentation of the Contributors

Marcelo Amable

Degree in Sociology, Master in Prevention of Occupational Health Risks and PhD in Public Health. He has a large experience in teaching occupational epidemiology and health policies in the University of Lanus, Institute Lazarte of Rosario and the University of Buenos Aires (Argentina). Assistant professor at University Pompeu Fabra where he teaches Occupational Health. His professional experience includes the development of health promotion programs and training on occupational health in the Ministry of Health in Argentina. His main research fields include flexible and precarious employment and health and occupational health inequalities where he has published a number of papers, book chapters, and his PhD dissertation: "Precarious employment and its impact on health" (2006).

Lucía Artazcoz

Lucía Artazcoz heads the Institute of Community Services in the Public Health Agency of Barcelona. She has been working for a number of years in the field of Occupational health viewed in a public health perspective. Her current research is focused on work-related health inequalities. Her research also deals with the psychosocial work environment and mental health.

Mona Backhans

Mona Backhans has a MSc in Sociology and is a research officer at the Swedish National Institute of Public Health (SNIPH). Within the Institute's remit she has worked with issues related to questionnaire construction, labour market policy, working conditions and sickness absence. She is a PhD student at Karolinska Institutet, Department of Public Health Sciences. Her dissertation deals with welfare state policies and their impact on social inequalities in health in a comparative perspective.

Joan Benach

Degree in Medicine, Master in Public Health, Specialist in Preventive Medicine and Public Health and PhD in Public Health. Senior researcher and associate professor at Pompeu Fabra University (Barcelona, Spain) where he is member of the Occupational Health Research Unit. His main research fields of interest include topics such as health inequalities, precarious employment, small area geographical analysis, and health policy priorities, where he has published over a hundred articles, reports and books. Among his publications we can mention the "Spanish Black Report on Health Inequalities", the Atlases of small-areas mortality in Spain and Catalonia, several reports on employment conditions and health, the causes of occupational injuries, or his book "Learning to look at health. How social inequalities damage our health".

Fernando G. Benavides

Graduated with a Degree in Medicine, Doctor in Medicine and Surgery and Specialist in Preventive Medicine and Public Health. Associate professor at Pompeu Fabra University and member of the Occupational Health Research Unit. Author of over a hundred articles published in Medline-indexed scientific journals and several books and chapters, among which we highlight the Occupational Health Manual. Drafted the Report on Occupational Hazards Prevention (Durán Report) and co-edited the Report on Occupational Health. Director of Archivos de Prevención de Riesgos Laborales, the only journal in Spanish on occupational health with peer review. Director of the Mutual Cyclops-UPF chair in Labour Medicine and of the Occupational Health Observatory (UPF-ISTAS-UM).

Carme Borrell

Carme Borrell heads the Health Observatory of Barcelona in the Public Health Agency of Barcelona. She has been working for years in health information systems. Her field of research is the study of social class inequalities in health and use of health care services, having many articles and projects related with this. She has coordinated two reports on Health Inequalities in Catalonia and the Report of the Spanish Society of Public Health of 2004 on Public Health in Spain from the gender and social class perspective. She is also an associate professor of the Pompeu Fabra University and participates in the coordination of the Master of Public Health.

Imma Cortès

Imma Cortès is the responsible for the Occupational health unit of Barcelona, a department of the Public Health Agency of Barcelona who provides support to primary health care centres in issues related to occupational health. Her current research is focused in work-related health inequalities, the psychosocial work environment and mental health.

Espen Dahl

Espen Dahl is a professor at Oslo University College where he heads the research programme Care, health and Welfare. His main research interests are health inequalities, social exclusion and labour market participation among disadvantaged groups, and social and health policies in a comparative perspective.

Jon Ivar Elstad

Jon Ivar Elstad has a PhD in sociology. He is Senior Researcher at Norwegian Social Research, Oslo, and currently also Adjunct Professor at the Institute of Sociology and Human Geography, University of Oslo. His main research interest is social inequalities in health, and he has published a number of articles and book chapters on that topic.

Marije Evers

Marije Evers is an industrial and organisational psychologist who started her career in 2003 as a researcher at TNO Work and Employment. Her main field of interest is occupational health services for people with chronic illnesses. She has contributed to the evaluation of an intervention for hospital workers with heavy work and has been involved in the European Stress Impact project (5th Framework programme of the EC). Currently she examines the effectiveness of an occupational health intervention for people who on sick-leave due to low back pain.

Peeter Fredlund

Peeter Fredlund, BSc, MPH., works as a statistician and computer programmer at the Centre for Epidemiology, Swedish National Board for Health and Welfare, Sweden. He has a special interest in health problems related to the psychosocial aspects of the labour market and the work environment.

Karin Halldén

Karin Halldén is a PhD student at the Swedish Institute for Social Research (SOFI), Stockholm University. Her dissertation deals with working life and labour market careers in a cross country comparative perspective. One forthcoming publication is "Agency and Capabilities to Create a Worklife Balance in Diverse and Changing Institutional Contexts" (with Hobson, B. and Duvander, A.-Z.), in J. Lewis (ed.), Children, Family Policies and Welfare State Change, London: Edward Elgar. She presented the paper "Testing the Gender Differential in Overeducation: Local Labour Markets and Productivity Dominance. Analyses on Swedish Partner Data" at the EqualSoc Conference in Torino, January 2006. During 2005, she completed a three month internship at the International Labour Organization (ILO) in Geneva, Switzerland.

Eva Støttrup Hansen

Eva Støttrup Hansen is an associate professor at the Institute of Public Health, University of Copenhagen, Denmark. She is an epidemiologist and works within the field of Occupational and Environmental Health. To this field she has contributed on theoretical and ethical as well as on empirical issues. She also teaches occupational health to medical students.

Tomas Hemmingsson

Tomas Hemmingsson, BA, has a PhD in Public Health Sciences from the Karolinska Institute where he was appointed Associated Professor in 2006. He is currently at the division of Social Medicine, Department of Public Health Sciences, at the Karolinska Institutet. Tomas Hemmingssons' research interests concern the socioeconomic distribution of mortality and morbidity and its explanations. The main interest is in life course epidemiology.

Christer Hogstedt

MD in 1971, PhD in 1980 and Associate Professor at the University of Linköping the same year. From 1982 to 2000 Professor in Occupational Medicine at the National Institute for Working Life and the Karolinska Institutet, Sweden. From 2001 Head of the Research Department at the Swedish National Institute of Public Health, Stockholm.

His main research activities used to be occupational epidemiology with applications mainly in cancer, cardiovascular, musculoskeletal and neuropsychological epidemiology.

Since 2001 he has also researched evidence-based public health interventions, social epidemiology, policy analysis and the effects of globalization with health equity and the wider determinants of health as primary foci.

He is the Swedish research counterpart for two major, long-term R&D programmes on Work and Health in Central America and southern Africa..

Irene Houtman

Irene Houtman works at TNO Work and Employment, the Netherlands, since 1990. Before 1990 she worked at the Free University of Amsterdam where she obtained her PhD (thesis: 'Stress and Coping in Student Teachers'). Since 1995 she is a senior researcher at TNO Work & Employment, and in 2002 she was awarded a senior research fellowship by TNO. She is involved in a large number of projects within the area of 'work, stress and health'. The projects range from small to quite large scale national as well as international projects. In international projects she is acting as the national correspondent for the Netherlands (e.g. in the EWCO, for the European Foundation for the Improvement of Living and Working Conditions), as a partner representing the Netherlands in the JACE (Biomed-1), as well as in the Stress Impact project (5th Framework programme of the EC). Irene has also been active in the Topic Centres for Practice and Research, in the ESF-Scientific Programme on Social Variations in Health Expectancy, and is acting as a WHO consultant on mental health and work.

Martin Hyde

Martin Hyde is a research fellow at University College London. His main research areas are in psychosocial work environment factors, globalisation and new patterns of labour market exit. He has been involved in the development of both the English Longitudinal Study of Ageing (ELSA), the Survey of Health, Ageing and Retirement in Europe (SHARE) and the Swedish Longitudinal Occupations and Health Survey (SLOSH). He is currently writing his Phd on the relationships between globalisation and later life.

Annette Leclerc

Annette Leclerc is a senior researcher in epidemiology at the National Institute for Health and Medical Research (INSERM) in France. In cooperation with specialists in occupational health and ergonomists she is responsible for research projects on work-related musculoskeletal disorders. The specific aims include: to assess the occurrence and the consequences of these disorders in the general population, the long-term effects of occupational exposure, and the contribution of biomechanical stressors at work to health inequalities. A part of her activity focuses on social inequalities in mortality, including changes over time in the magnitude of inequalities. She was the first author of "Les inégalités sociales de santé" (La Découverte 2000), a book on various aspects of health inequalities in France, with more than 50 contributors.

Ingvar Lundberg

MD in 1976, Specialist in Occupational and Environmental Medicine in 1993. PhD in 1986 (Doctoral thesis: "Health effects of organic solvent exposure in the paint industry"), Associate Professor of Occupational Medicine at the Karolinska Institutet since 1993. From 2002 to 2007 Professor of Occupational Epidemiology at the National Institute for Working Life. Since 2007 Professor at Uppsala University.

Previous research has mainly concerned epidemiological studies of health effects of organic solvents. Current research is based on epidemiological methods and concerns occupational causes of psychiatric disorders, health related selection to social classes and occupations, work as a determinant of social inequalities in health, and pesticide health effects.

María Menéndez

Degree in Medicine, Master in Epidemiology and Technical Specialist in the Prevention of Occupational Health Risks of Higia-CONC (Girona, Spain). María Menéndez has worked in many public health research, health care activities and gender projects in Nicaragua and Cuba. She has been former director in several Primary Care Health Centers in Nicaragua and Sub-director of the Regional Direction of Hygiene and Epidemiology, in Matagalpa and Jinotega. Nicaragua. She has participated and coordinated many projects on occupational health psychosocial risk factors, occupational health inequalities and various gender issues. Her main areas of research include the analysis of psychosocial work environment, occupational health inequalities by gender, and the impact of Safety Reps activities on occupational health.

Carles Muntaner

Degree in Medicine, PhD is Research Chair at the Social Equity and Health Section, Center for Addictions and Mental Health, and Professor at the University of Toronto. He has conducted research in deprived communities in the Americas, the EU, and Africa and has been working with the Bolivarian government to reduce health inequalities in Venezuela. He has conducted pioneering work in social class measurement, effects of work organisation on psychiatric disorders, contextual effects, the conceptualisation of race, and the critique of "social capital" and "psychosocial factors". Recognised internationally as a scientist with more than 130 publications and recipient of the 2004 Wade Hampton frost Award of the Epidemiology Section of the APHA.

Isabelle Niedhammer

Isabelle Niedhammer is a senior researcher at the National Institute for Health and Medical Research (INSERM) in France. As an epidemiologist specialised in occupational health, her main research fields have been psychosocial work factors and shift work. She has developed and validated the French versions of several instruments measuring psychosocial work factors, and constructed job exposure matrices. Her current research also focuses on workplace bullying and the contribution of work to social inequalities in health.

Richard Peter

Richard Peter is a professor of Medical Sociology and head of the Working Group Medical Sociology at the University of Ulm, Germany. His background as sociologist determined his interest in social inequality in health and in the impact of psychosocial work-related factors on health. Since about 10 years Richard Peter investigates the association between social status and premature morbidity and mortality in Germany. Since nearly 20 years he has contributed to the development and empirical testing of one of the effort-reward imbalance stress model. His work is published in leading scientific journals. For more information please go to http://www.uni-ulm.de/epidemiologie/.

Kimberley Rauscher

Kimberly Rauscher is currently working for the Massachusetts Department of Public Health's Occupational Health Surveillance Program. She recently completed her Doctorate in Work Environment Policy at the University of Massachusetts Lowell. Her research focus is on young workers in the US, particularly with respect to health and safety, work quality and the class dimensions of youth employment. (krauscher26@comcast.net)

David H. Wegman

Dean of the School of Health and Environment at the University of Massachusetts Lowell, USA, David Wegman has published over 150 articles in the scientific literature on epidemiologic studies of occupational respiratory disease, musculoskeletal disorders, and cancer and on public health and policy issues related to worker health and safety. He has served as a member of several US National Academy of Science committees and has chaired the Academy's committees on Youth Workers and on Older Workers; currently he chairs the Academy's Framework Committee for Review of the National Institute for Occupational Safety and Health Research. He chaired the 2006 International Evaluation Group (IEA) assisting in the evaluation of Swedish occupational health research and has also been active in a number of national and international professional societies including as a member of the Executive Council and Treasurer of the International Epidemiologic Association. Dr. Wegman is co-editor of one of the standard textbooks in the field of occupational health, "Occupational and Environmental Health: Recognizing and Preventing Disease and Injury", published by Lippincott, Williams and Wilkins in 2006.

John Wooding

John Wooding is currently the Provost at the University of Massachusetts, Lowell. He is the former Chair of the Department of Regional Economic and Social Development at Lowell and a political scientist. He has written widely on issue of work environment policy, occupational health and safety regulation and on the theory of the capitalist state.

"Work & Society"

The series "Work & Society" analyses the development of employment and social policies, as well as the strategies of the different social actors, both at national and European levels. It puts forward a multi-disciplinary approach – political, sociological, economic, legal and historical – in a bid for dialogue and complementarity.

The series is not confined to the social field *stricto sensu*, but also aims to illustrate the indirect social impacts of economic and monetary policies. It endeavours to clarify social developments, from a comparative and a historical perspective, thus portraying the process of convergence and divergence in the diverse national societal contexts. The manner in which European integration impacts on employment and social policies constitutes the backbone of the analyses.

Series Editor: Philippe POCHET, Director of the Observatoire
Social Européen (Brussels) and Digest Editor
of the Journal of European Social Policy

Recent Titles

No.59 – *Changing Liaisons. The Dynamics of Social Partnership in 20th Century West-European Democracies*, Karel DAVIDS, Greta DEVOS & Patrick PASTURE (eds.), 2007, 268 p., ISBN 978-90-5201-365-7.

No.58 – *Work and Social Inequalities in Health in Europe*, Ingvar LUNDBERG, Tomas HEMMINGSSON & Christer HOGSTEDT (eds.), SALTSA, 2007, 538 p., ISBN 978-90-5201-372-5.

No.57 – *European Solidarities. Tensions and Contentions of a Concept*, Lars MAGNUSSON & Bo STRÅTH (eds.), SALTSA, 2007, 355 p., ISBN 978-90-5201-363-3.

No.56 – *Industrial Relations in Small Companies. A Comparison: France, Sweden and Germany*, Christian DUFOUR, Adelheid HEGE, Sofia MURHEM, Wolfgang RUDOLPH & Wolfram WASSERMANN (eds.), SALTSA, 2007, 229 p., ISBN 978-90-5201-360-2.

No.55 – *The European Sectoral Social Dialogue. Actors, Developments and Challenges*, Anne DUFRESNE, Christophe DEGRYSE & Philippe POCHET (eds.), SALTSA/Observatoire social européen, 2006, 342 p., ISBN 978-90-5201-052-6.

No.54 – *Reshaping Welfare States and Activation Regimes in Europe*, Amparo SERRANO PASCUAL & Lars MAGNUSSON (eds.), SALTSA, 2007, 319 p., ISBN 978-90-5201-048-9.

No.53 – *Shaping Pay in Europe. A Stakeholder Approach*, Conny Herbert ANTONI, Xavier BAETEN, Ben J.M. EMANS & Mari KIRA (eds.), SALTSA, 2006, 287 p., ISBN 978-90-5201-037-3.

No.52 – *Les relations sociales dans les petites entreprises. Une comparaison France, Suède, Allemagne*, Christian DUFOUR, Adelheid HEGE, Sofia MURHEM, Wolfgang RUDOLPH & Wolfram WASSERMANN, 2006, 243 p., ISBN 978-90-5201-323-7.

No.51 – *Politiques sociales. Enjeux méthodologiques et épistémologiques des comparaisons internationales / Social Policies. Epistemological and Methodological Issues in Cross-National Comparison*, Jean-Claude BARBIER & Marie-Thérèse LETABLIER (eds.), 2005, 2nd printing 2006, 295 p., ISBN 978-90-5201-294-0.

No.50 – *The Ethics of Workplace Privacy*, Sven Ove HANSSON & Elin PALM (eds.), SALTSA, 2005, 186 p., ISBN 978-90-5201-293-3.

No.49 – *The Open Method of Co-ordination in Action. The European Employment and Social Inclusion Strategies*, Jonathan ZEITLIN & Philippe POCHET (eds.), with Lars MAGNUSSON, SALTSA/Observatoire social européen, 2005, 2nd printing 2005, 511 p., ISBN 978-90-5201-280-3.

N° 48 – *Le Moment Delors. Les syndicats au cœur de l'Europe sociale*, Claude DIDRY & Arnaud MIAS, 2005, 2nd printing 2005, 349 p., ISBN 978-90-5201-274-2.

No.47 – *A European Social Citizenship? Preconditions for Future Policies from a Historical Perspective*, Lars MAGNUSSON & Bo STRÅTH (eds.), SALTSA, 2004, 361 p., ISBN 978-90-5201-269-8.

No.46 – *Restructuring Representation. The Merger Process and Trade Union Structural Development in Ten Countries*, Jeremy WADDINGTON (ed.), 2004, 414 p., ISBN 978-90-5201-253-7.

No.45 – *Labour and Employment Regulation in Europe*, Jens LIND, Herman KNUDSEN & Henning JØRGENSEN (eds.), SALTSA, 2004, 408 p., ISBN 978-90-5201-246-9.

N° 44 – *L'État social actif. Vers un changement de paradigme ?*, Pascale VIELLE, Philippe POCHET & Isabelle CASSIERS (dir.), 2005, 2e tirage 2006, ISBN 978-90-5201-227-8.

Peter Lang—The website

Discover the general website of the Peter Lang publishing group:

www.peterlang.com

C. Dufour, A. Hege, S. Murhem, W. Rudolph & W. Wassermann

Industrial Relations in Small Companies
A Comparison: France, Sweden and Germany

Reference is often made to small companies, but little is known about them, especially regarding industrial relations. How can small companies be defined? Is their small size a sufficient feature for them to be considered the same? If they are different from each other, what makes them so? Is the distinction between them and other companies – big ones – relevant? In what way is life organised in such units, where employer and employees are in very close contact with each other? In order to answer these questions, the authors of this innovative book carried out surveys together in France, Sweden and Germany. They met employers, employees, union members and industrial relations specialists. Comparisons of these three national cases show that small companies do have common features that transcend frontiers. They do, however, also have national characteristics. They, therefore, warrant being analysed and understood in something other than merely negative terms. It thus appears that small companies are not so far off resembling big ones...

Christian Dufour, sociologist, is deputy director of IRES (Institute for Economic and Social Research, France) and a specialist in French and international industrial relations.

Adelheid Hege, sociologist, is a researcher at IRES (France) and specialises in international comparative industrial relations.

Sofia Murhem, economist and historian, was a researcher at the National Institute for Working Life (Arbetslivsinstitutet, Uppsala, Sweden)

Wolfgang Rudolph is a researcher at the Office for Social Research (Büro für Sozialforschung, Kassel, Germany). His main areas of research concern the development of works councils, employee representation in small companies and regional development.

Wolfram Wassermann, sociologist, is a researcher at the Office for Social Research (Büro für Sozialforschung, Kassel, Germany). His research concerns codetermination, the sociology of small companies and the trade unions.

Brussels, P.I.E. Peter Lang, 978-90-5201-360-2, 2007

SFR 47.00 / €* 32.00 / €** 32.90 / € 29,90 / £ 20.90 / US-$ 35.95
* includes VAT - only valid for Germany
** includes VAT - only valid for Austria

Amparo SERRANO PASCUAL & Lars MAGNUSSON (eds.)

Reshaping Welfare States and Activation Regimes in Europe

The activation-based intervention paradigm is being adopted by several European countries resulting in major reforms to the social welfare system. The spread of the activation paradigm has had major repercussions, not only for welfare interventions aimed at combating unemployment, but also for the political regulation of the social question and citizenship. Citizenship is being redefined in contractual terms and greater emphasis is being placed on its economic aspects. Nevertheless, a wide range of policies are labelled with recourse to this interpretative framework and a pluralistic approach to implementation could serve just as well to empower as to weaken workers'/citizens' position in society.

This book analyses the extent of these changes from a cross-cultural perspective. Institutional settings as well as prevailing work values and social representation of social exclusion (activation regimes) have a key role in defining the instruments to be used in national activation strategies to regulate the behaviour of job seekers. In this book, a discussion about the range of social welfare model reforms throughout Europe and a typology of activation regimes is proposed.

Amparo Serrano Pascual is Lecturer and Researcher at the Complutense University in Madrid (Faculty of Political Sciences and Sociology). She has published and edited several books and articles on the concept of activation and employability, comparative labour market policies, the European Employment Strategy, the European social model, the regulatory nature of the EU institution and gender mainstreaming.

Lars Magnusson is Vice-rector of Uppsala University and Professor and Chair in Economic History at the same university. He is the Chairman of SALTSA and has published a number of works dealing with the political economy of Europe, the social dimension of Europe and the European Employment Strategy. He is a regular visitor at the European University Institute in Florence.

Brussels, P.I.E. Peter Lang, 978-90-5201-048-9, 2007

SFR 51.00 / € * 35.20 / €** 36.20 / € 32.90 / £ 23.00 / US-$ 38.95
* includes VAT - only valid for Germany
** includes VAT - only valid for Austria

C. H. ANTONI, X. BAETEN, B. J.M. EMANS & M. KIRA (eds.)

Shaping Pay in Europe
A Stakeholder Approach

"Shaping Pay in Europe: A Stakeholder Approach" focuses on pay systems applied in the European Un-ion. Giving due attention to the institutional setting of the European pay systems, the book discusses how European companies may approach pay as an integral part of their operational and strategic framework. Pay is an important topic for several stakeholders on the labour market. The book discusses the perspec-tives of various stakeholders – employees, employers, trade unions, and employer associations – on the issue of pay. Secondary analysis of earlier statistical studies and new empirical material on European pay systems is also presented in the book.

The book also aims at contributing to a better understanding of pay systems. If one wants to understand the various pay systems of a company, which pay elements and pay characteristics should one focus on? Which are the essential pay characteristics shaping an individual's pay and how could these characteristics be studied or audited? The book provides answers to both questions by presenting a practical, yet sophisti-cated model of essential pay characteristics.

Conny Herbert Antoni is the professor for Work and Organizational Psychology at the University of Trier. His research interests include reward and performance management, socio-technical system design and organ-izational development.

Xavier Baeten is a manager at Vlerick Leuven Gent Management School, and responsible for the school's activities on reward management.

Ben J.M. Emans is an associate professor in HRM and Organizational Behaviour at the faculty of Man-agement and Organization of the University of Groningen. His research interests and publications are all in the field of organizational behaviour.

Mari Kira has worked as a European Commission Marie Curie Fellow at University of Kassel, Germany. Her research interests include sustain-ability in work organizations and reward system development.

Brussels, P.I.E. Peter Lang, 978-90-5201-037-3, 2007

SFR 46.00 / €* 31.60 / €** 32.50 / € 29.50 / £ 20.70 / US-$ 34.95
* includes VAT - only valid for Germany
** includes VAT - only valid for Austria